REIMAGINING THE HUMAN SERVICE RELATIONSHIP

Reimagining the Human Service Relationship

Jaber F. Gubrium
Tone Alm Andreassen
Per Koren Solvang

EDITORS

COLUMBIA UNIVERSITY PRESS NEW YORK

COLUMBIA UNIVERSITY PRESS
Publishers Since 1893
New York   Chichester, West Sussex

cup.columbia.edu

Library of Congress Cataloging-in-Publication Data

Names: Gubrium, Jaber F., editor. | Andreassen, Tone Alm, editor. | Solvang, Per, editor.
Title: Reimagining the human service relationship / edited by Jaber F. Gubrium, Tone Alm Andreassen, and Per Koren Solvang.
Description: 1 Edition. | New York, NY : Columbia University Press, 2016. | Includes bibliographical references and index.
Identifiers: LCCN 2015040350 | ISBN 9780231171526 (cloth : alk. paper)
Subjects: LCSH: Human services. | Physician and patient. | Interpersonal relations.
Classification: LCC HV40 .R364 2016 | DDC 362—dc23
LC record available at http://lccn.loc.gov/2015040350

Columbia University Press books are printed on permanent and durable acid-free paper.
Printed in the United States of America

Cover design: Lisa Hamm
Cover image: Carrie House, HOUSEdesign llc

Everything you can imagine is real.

—PABLO PICASSO

CONTENTS

PREFACE

THIS BOOK TURNS OUR ATTENTION to two important developments in human service provision. One is the changing relationship between professionals and service users. The traditional lines of demarcation between service providers such as social workers, counselors, nurses, and therapists on the one side and service users on the other side have been shifting. Old dichotomies are disintegrating, replaced by roles with overlapping goals and responsibilities. Professionals increasingly apply, and some resist applying, user-oriented sensibilities and understandings. They also work together with other professionals within managed service organizations to incorporate the voices of service users into their missions and into the way they function. Conversely, having access to and developing competence in evidence-based knowledge, service users increasingly are taking on the semblances of professional expertise, and some have become adamantly antiprofessional in the process.

The other development is the widespread feeling that human service provision has lost its way, that it is more concerned with systems of accountability, with rules and regulations, than it is with service and care. The moral terrain and working environment of both service providers and service users have been overshadowed by administrative imperatives. In the scramble to develop and implement models of optimal functioning, the seminal unit of service provision—the human service relationship—has become a nexus of cardboard figures designed through management rationalities. In this environment, the experiences of those in need as well as those of professionals in the know are turned into lifeless ghosts of what they are on their own. The strategic quality of social interaction, the inexorable interpretations and negotiations, the shifting allegiances, and the diffuse groundings of trust and collaboration are nowhere to be found.

The chapters in this book seek to reimagine that relationship by bringing its everyday moral bearings into view, restoring its diverse meanings and complex agency. The chapters are informed by the premise that the relationship should be seen as taking shape and developing in the interactive space between those who ostensibly provide human services and those who ostensibly receive them, not by way of experience-distant images of that. The tentativeness is meant to underscore the relationship's working contours—the roles, institutional divisions, means, and aims of which are neither fixed nor clear-cut. These cannot be gauged as if set in stone or as always in tow, but rather must be comprehended as developing in the very process of providing and receiving services. This foregrounds fluid and morally variegated terrain and cultural contradiction, whose essential qualities are rendered invisible, if not otherwise deemed irrational, in experience-distant perspective.

The service relations considered in the book range from child welfare, addiction treatment, social enterprises, and mental health to physical disability, doctoring, dementia, and palliative care. Bringing into focus everyday life, the chapters show in compelling detail how the workings of service provision can be at considerable odds with what is presumed in model-inspired welfare policies. An experience-near approach speaks loudly to the working, not the prescribed, significance of structures and interests. At the same time, the chapters are not blind to the difficulties that an experience-near approach reveals. If anything, they recommend an enduring openness to, and critical reflection on, the competing rationalities of the service relationship.

The approach of this book does not stand comfortably in the rush to rationalize the service relationship, the aim of which is to turn human troubles into discrete, assessable, and treatable problems. It is instead an approach that is centered in the grounded practices of living and relating to one another in service and care. Some refer to it as an everyday-life perspective. Characteristically, others resist reifying it with a label and simply take the view that nothing in life is inherently normal, troubling, or problematic, but rather derives its meaning and is rendered actionable in the course of living. It is an approach that features service providers and service users as collaborative agents of their affairs, not privileging one over the other in the search for understanding and effectiveness. The approach upholds the primacy and lasting value of the service relationship, affirming the productive role it plays in the work and lives of providers and users.

The chapters are supported by research dealing with human relations at the organizational crossroads of service intervention. While most of them analyze specific bodies of empirical material, others are rooted in longstanding programs of empirical work. All draw inspiration from experience-near studies of subjective understanding and the interactions of providers and users. None focuses exclusively on political debates or formal policy agendas, yet each is critically attuned to issues of practice stemming from them. None takes social problems for granted, but instead—in the breathing room that practice provides—they turn our attention to the reflexive linkages between the troubles and problems that enduringly traipse through the service terrain.

The book is organized into four parts. The introductory chapter in Part I begins from the perspective that feelings persuade us as much as reason. Titled "From the Iron Cage to Everyday Life," it presents in deliberate textual detail what it refers to as a "lurking" image of organized service relations. Drawing from Max Weber and Franz Kafka, who wrote in the early twentieth century and were key makers of the image, the chapter traces how its administrative imperatives have resonated through the sentiments of related concerns in the decades that followed. The imperatives still ring loudly in debates about how to conceptualize the service relationship. The chapters of Part II take up the views and actions of service provision from the standpoint of users. Their distinct attitudes and stakes in intervention are front and center. The chapters of Part III deal with everyday facets of professional work, from arts-based interventions to what the authors of Chapter 11 call "civil disobedience." Professionals are presented as regularly crossing the ostensible divides of service provision, from shifting the employment of service providers to client control, to methods for sustaining relational citizenship in dementia care. The concluding chapters, which make up Part IV, present illustrations of reimagined service relationships, from the border crossings of mental health self-healing groups to the ineluctable identity shifts and border work of all service venues.

Taken together, the chapters reimagine the service relationship by making visible the working relevancies of service delivery. Whatever the concern—be it the day-to-day interpretation of policy, dealing with organizational efficiency, managing diverse understandings, or applying professional ethics—their standpoint is that there is a basis in everyday life for viewing these as matters of practice. Everyday life's diverse rationalities cannot be subject to systems of accountability that erase difference, ambiguity, and ambivalence. They demand a form of accountability whose point of reference is the ordinary equity and novel sensibility that undergird all sides of the relationship. This is not to say that reimagination can be free of contradiction, but rather that it must resist approaches that elide it.

ACKNOWLEDGMENTS

GERALDINE FOLEY AND VIRPI TIMONEN ARE GRATEFUL to the Health Research Board of Ireland for funding the study reported on in Chapter 6, and they sincerely thank all participants in the study.

Karen-Lee Miller and Pia Kontos owe sincere thanks to all participants in the study reported on in Chapter 8, and to the families and private sitters for facilitating residents' involvement. They also warmly thank Romeo Colobong for insightful research contributions and flawless study coordination, Gilles Gagnon for sensitive and professional videography services, and Jessica Babineau for library assistance. Clown scholars and teachers such as Lee-Fay Low, Peter Spitzer, and Bernie Warren were sage sources for both grant development and the clown intervention, and the authors deeply appreciate their assistance.

Tarja Pösö wishes to thank the Academy of Finland for funding the project Child Welfare Care Orders as Interventions—A Process View from the Inside, which made Chapter 9 of this book possible.

Amanda Grenier and Cristi Flood are grateful to the individuals and organizations that participated in their research reported on in Chapter 10. They thank Rachel Weldrick and Brian Budd for their assistance in the preparation of this chapter. Research discussed in this chapter was funded by the Social Sciences and Humanities Research Council (SSHRC) of Canada.

Signe Mie Jensen and Kaspar Villadsen wish to thank the elderly care center in the municipality of Tønder for generously granting them access to observe their meetings reported on in Chapter 11. They also would like to thank FOA (the trade union for social workers and health care workers in Denmark) for inviting them to evaluate the leadership development project sponsored by the union.

Tom Shakespeare and Rachael Collins thank the Great Britain Sasakawa Foundation for funding the UEA mental health self-knowledge workshop reported on in Chapter 12. They also thank Kohji Ishihara, Geoffrey Reed, Helen Simpson, Alice Whieldon, and Jon Wilson for their support with this chapter.

Erik Eriksson and Katarina Jacobsson thank Anna Meeuwisse, Malin Åkerström, and the editors for their helpful comments on previous versions of Chapter 13. Thanks are also given to the Swedish Foundation for Humanities and Social Sciences for partial funding.

REIMAGINING THE HUMAN SERVICE RELATIONSHIP

PART | I

The Human Service Relationship

WHAT IS THE HUMAN SERVICE RELATIONSHIP? Chapter 1 presents its interactional terrain as a distinctive social form. The chapter starts by describing how contemporaries Max Weber and Franz Kafka in the 1920s imagined the divisions, roles, and regulations that were to become the organizational nexus of professional service provision. Weber worried that the bureaucratic mediation of human service was eclipsing its moral bearings. Kafka offered a frightening portrait of the segregation of outsiders. With the images of Weber and Kafka lurking in the background, the chapter goes on to discuss the service relationship as it expanded rapidly in the decades following World War II, when human service provision became highly specialized, credentialed, and proprietary. Centered on issues of knowledge, skill, and autonomy, debate over the position and scope of professionalism was heated. Moving beyond formal organization and turning to the everyday logics of troubles and problems, Chapter 1 features the contrasting practice of the service relationship, contending that what Weber and Kafka imagined nearly a century ago and still lingers in thinking about service organization can be reimagined and realized in alternative terms.

1

From the Iron Cage to Everyday Life

▸ *JABER F. GUBRIUM*

ERVING GOFFMAN (1983) ARGUED FORCEFULLY that human relations transpire in a domain of their own, with diverse subjectivities, sentiments, and strategies for action. The domain is influenced by personality and social structure, but it is not determined by them. Positioned at the public margins of inner life, personality presents itself, in Goffman's (1959) view, as a function of judgments strategically communicated in sites of interaction. Situated outside of inner life, structures such as governments and institutions are in continuous need of local articulation in what Dorothy Smith terms the experience-near "relations of ruling" (Smith 1987). Influential images and ideas of what these structures are and intend play out in the contingencies of practice. Uneasy with experience-distant perspectives, Goffman (1983) called the domain the "interaction order," which is the relational context central to the concerns of this book.

In an era of hyperindividualism, it is easily forgotten that we experience life in relationships. From the relations of family living and schooling to the relations of work and retirement and the relations of sickness and care, relationships deploy ways of being and prompt directions for action. Relationships are ever present in life, mediating identities as much in the flow of interaction as in the personal monitoring of thought and feeling. Relational worlds and relational sequences—first parental, then educational, and later occupational—provide life with substance and patterning, giving shape to experience through time and space. While some would claim that individual identity is a fundamental presence in life, in practice, who and what we are are socially constructed, with manifold identities being formed in the process (Mead 1934).

Increasingly prevalent today is the organized service relationship. It is the kind of relationship that leads the way in turning troubles into problems and discerning pathways for intervention and recovery (Gubrium and Järvinen 2014). The service relationship is professionally mixed and institutionally diverse. It varies from the relations of doctoring, nursing, and physical therapy to the relations of counseling, social service, and personal assistance. The relationship is as wide-ranging in context as the differences between solo practice and corporate management. More and more, it is a relationship that is mixed in its values, as the logic of administrative accountability and efficiency operates alongside the logics of service and care (Gill 2012; and see Jensen and Villadsen, Chapter 11, this volume).[1] As Everett Hughes pointed out decades ago, contemporary experience, especially its troubles, is being drawn through and rendered actionable by a sundry world of "going concerns" (Hughes 1984 [1957]).

This book deals with that relationship as it functions in the interaction between service providers and service users. It is concerned with state and institutional policies as far as they bear on the ordinary practice of that relationship. It does not feature a specific sector such as doctoring, nursing, or social work but rather approaches the service relationship as a social form in its own right, opening its borders, actors, and logics to critical scrutiny and reconsideration. While individual chapters have points of departure in particular national contexts and organizational venues, all proceed with an eye toward recognizing the fluid complexity of the service relationship and, on that basis, what it can mean to provide and receive just and humane service and care for all concerned across the board.

IMAGE OF THE IRON CAGE

Forever lurking around the service relationship is a troubling image of organizations, official insiders, and their connection with outsiders that Max Weber nearly a century ago likened to an iron cage.[2] The image persists to this day and is quietly ominous in the chapters of this book, even while organization theory is now highly variegated in its metaphorical bearings (Alvesson 2012; Gabriel 2000; Gubrium and Holstein 2001;

Hatch 2012; Morgan 1985; Reed and Hughes 1992; Silverman 1970). The image depicts rigid rules of interaction, an unsparing application of official responsibility, and a sharp demarcation of the separateness of outsiders and the transparency of their circumstances. Weber focused on the inner borders of officialdom, while his literary contemporary Franz Kafka portrayed the borders of access for outsiders.[3]

As administrative imperatives increasingly influence the service relationship, it is instructive in this introductory chapter to begin with Weber's and Kafka's portrayals. Noteworthy is the dismal future they foresee for the relationship. This calls on us to imagine something different but invisible in what Weber and Kafka wrote about. In what follows, I deliberately dwell on pertinent texts of theirs as a way of communicating their portrayals' deeply emotional contours—what it feels like on all sides to be caught in the web of the iron cage—which continues to raise hackles, resentment, and calls for action.

Inner Borders

Weber was distressed by the increasing rationalization of contemporary life, the ideal form of which he described as bureaucratically organized. He viewed modernity as rooted in the rationalization process. In his book *The Protestant Ethic and the Spirit of Capitalism* (1985 [1930]), Weber drew linkages between the ascetic ethic of Puritanism, capitalist accumulation, and modern organization. Guided spiritually by tenets designed to achieve maximum efficiency, unbridled accumulation, and ultimately salvation, the actors Weber envisioned fashioned rules of rational production, which informed and bound the very actions that produced them, generating his infamous iron cage. If Weber's prose was characteristically neutral and systematic, the metaphor he applied accompanies enduring anguish over what he sought to understand.

Maximally efficient rationality is concisely described in Weber's principles of bureaucracy. He sharpens the description by contrasting it with what he idealizes as a premodern form of social organization. Modern capitalist organization's ironclad and global inevitability is compared nostalgically with a long-lost form of moral order capable of "throw[ing] aside [such confining encumbrances] at any moment like a light cloak":

> When [Puritan] asceticism was carried out of monastic cells into everyday life, and began to dominate worldly morality, it did its part in building the tremendous cosmos of the modern economic order. This order is now bound to the technical and economic conditions of machine production which to-day determine the lives of all the individuals who are born into this mechanism, not only those directly concerned with economic acquisition, with irresistible force. . . . [Rather than being able to throw this aside at any moment like a light cloak], fate decreed that the cloak should become an iron cage. (Weber 1985:181)

This appears to be the only place in Weber's voluminous writing where he used the iron-cage metaphor. If seeming to be a passing trope, it nonetheless has become standard usage for principles of organization that Weber simultaneously figured to be pernicious.

The principles are presented in a section of his book *Economy and Society* (1968 [1922]) titled "Characteristics of Modern Bureaucracy." The first of Weber's six principles is the "principle of official *jurisdictional areas*" (Weber 1968:956). Fixed rules govern the range of official activities. Weber explains that "the authority to give the commands required for the discharge of [official] duties is distributed in a stable way and is strictly delimited by rules concerning the coercive means, physical, sacerdotal, or otherwise, which may be placed at the disposal of officials" (p. 956).

Weber's second principle is the "principle of *office hierarchy* and of channels of appeal [that] stipulate a clearly established system of super- and subordination in which there is a supervision of the lower offices by the higher ones" (p. 957). This applies to all modern bureaucracies, both private and public. Control and accountability are top-down, not bottom-up, in other words.

The third principle refers to "the management of the modern office, [which] is based upon written documents (the 'files'), which are preserved in their original or draft form, and upon a staff of subaltern officials and scribes of all sorts" (p. 957). The modern office is not governed by random application of rules, nor does it abide discretion, but instead operates in terms of written and stable guidelines.

The fourth principle deals with the education of officials, which "usually presupposes thorough training in a field of specialization" (p. 958). Official posts are not filled helter-skelter from an available labor market but draw from pertinent expertise, again regardless of whether the bureaucracy is private or public.

Fifth is the principle of "*full working capacity*" (p. 958). This refers, in the first instance, to the full on the job separation of the public and private lives of occupants. In the second instance, the principle rests on the understanding that the maximum efficiency of modern bureaucracy stems from work time that is purely engaged with organizational, not personal, goals and commitments.

And, finally, Weber's sixth principle is "the management of the office follows *general rules*, which are more or less stable, more or less exhaustive, and which can be learned" (p. 958). The rules apply regardless of circumstances. Ideally, there is no room for compromise, only straightforward execution.

According to Weber, the principles are exhaustive and are applicable without exception; deviation hampers maximum efficiency. Practice is subject to principle, in other words, not the other way around. The concept of frontline discretion, eloquently described by Michael Lipsky (1980) in his book *Street-Level Bureaucracy*, would be a form of border disruption tantamount to a violation of assigned authority and designated hierarchy. There is no indication that the modern relationship Weber portrays could be otherwise in his idealized scheme of things, such that practice instead is foundational, and principle is applied locally and strategically for everyday purposes.

Oddly enough, the first to express frustration and a desire for something different—a reimagination, if you will—was Weber himself. He lamented principles that turned officials into mere cogs of efficient organization, whirling with disenchantment away from traditional values such as trust, care, collaboration, and gratitude, losing touch with people's basic humanity. Referencing J. P. Mayer (1943), biographer Reinhard Bendix (1960) quotes Weber berating the bureaucrat, a role that the chapters of this book show is more complex in practice than Weber could (or would dare to) imagine (see Barnes, Chapter 15, this volume):

> It is horrible to think that the world could one day be filled with nothing but those little cogs, little men clinging to little jobs and striving towards bigger ones—a state of affairs which is to be seen once more, as in the Egyptian records, playing an ever-increasing part in the spirit of our present

> administrative system, and especially of its offspring, the students. This passion for bureaucracy . . . is enough to drive one to despair. It is as if in politics . . . we were deliberately to become men who need "order" and nothing but order, who become nervous and cowardly if for one moment this order wavers, and helpless if they are torn away from their total incorporation in it. (Bendix 1960:464)

Borders of Access

Franz Kafka's novels *The Trial* (1925) and *The Castle* (2009 [1926]) are stark portrayals of the borders of access to the iron cage. While Kafka did not use the metaphor, he featured outsiders trapped by its consequences. Unlike Weber's formal prose, which reflects his bureaucratic principles, Kafka's own writing—like his outsider—meanders with resignation from one off-putting circumstance to another. I will use *The Castle* to identify parallel, but in Kafka's case implicit, principles of outsidership.

Featured in the novel is the protagonist K, the outsider who has been summoned by castle officials to do a land survey. A key symbol is the Castle Inn, which is frequented by officials, not "rustics" and other villagers. The latter frequent the distant Bridge Inn, which K stumbles on late one night in the dead of winter when he arrives in the village. The portrait is hardened by villagers who have little sense of what officials do, or the reason for the castle's governance over village affairs. They could care less and are stunningly complicit in sustaining the local order of things. Except for K. He is a stranger to the village and, to a fault, dutifully seeks access to the castle to learn the details of his assignment. Failing with frontline officials and even with those who ostensibly have castle connections, K is determined to contact Klamm, the arbiter of castle affairs. The villagers naturally resent this. As K persists, his relations with villagers sour and his chance engagement with girlfriend Frieda disintegrates.

Exemplary excerpts offer the basis for identifying principles of action on this side of the divide. The first excerpt is taken from the novel's opening pages and hearkens a principle of *exclusion and respect*. Soon after K arrives at the Bridge Inn and falls asleep from exhaustion, he is awakened by the landlord and the son of the castle warden. The following annotated exchange transpires. WS is the warden's son, who bristles at the idea that K is crossing a line, the principle of which, like Weber's rules, is applicable regardless of circumstances.

WS [*To K*] This village belongs to the castle, so anyone who stays or spends the night here is, so to speak, staying or spending the night at the castle. And no one's allowed to do that without a permit from the count. However, you don't have any such permit, or at least you haven't shown one.

K [*Groggily sitting up*] What village have I come to, then? Is there a castle in these parts?

WS There most certainly is. Count Westwest's castle.

K And I need this permit to spend the night here?

WS [*Derisively*] Yes, you need a permit. [Turning to the landlord and other guests] Or am I wrong? Doesn't he need a permit?

K [*Yawning*] Well, I'll have to go and get a permit, then.

WS Oh yes? Who from?

K Why, from the count. I suppose there's nothing else for it.

WS [*Shouting*] What, go and get a permit from the count himself at midnight!?

K [*Unruffled*] Is that impossible? If so, why did you wake me up?

WS [*Beside himself*] The manners of a vagrant! I demand respect for the count's authority! I woke you up to tell you that you must leave the count's land immediately. (Kafka 2009:5–6)

The next excerpt depicts a second principle and is taken from Chapter 9, titled "Opposition to Questioning." The principle is *the ultimate truth of bureaucratic files and records*. The principle designates that what is written in official documents should be taken to be more credible than the events and experiences they describe. In the presence of the Bridge Inn's landlady (L), who is growing increasingly impatient with K's behavior, K asks a castle representative, Mr. Secretary (MS), about the need to complete records in order to get an interview with Klamm.

K However, now, Mr. Secretary, I'll ask you to tell me whether the landlady is right, I mean in saying that the records you want me to help you complete could result in my getting an interview with Klamm. If that is the case, then I'm prepared to answer all your questions at once. Yes, if it comes down to that I'm ready for anything.

MS No, there's no such connection. My business is only to get a precise account of this afternoon's events down on paper for Klamm's village registry. The account is drawn up already, there are just two or three gaps I want you to fill to make sure it's all in order. There was no other purpose, nor can any other purpose be achieved.

L [*to MS*] I've been telling him forever, I tell him today and I always will, that he hasn't the slightest prospect of an interview with Klamm, and if there isn't any prospect of it then he won't get one through your records. Can anything be clearer? (Kafka 2009:101)

A third principle is the *acceptance of miscommunication*. The border of miscommunication is one-way only. Since officials are experts, all communication from them is correct. Mistakes derive from how communication is interpreted on the other side of the border among those who receive it. In the case of human services, this means the users. This is portrayed at the start of Chapter 10 of *The Castle* in an encounter K has with Barnabas (B), a minor official who has been uncommonly understanding of K's circumstances. Barnabas at first seems to be bringing good news, but soon K complains of a miscommunication, which, incidentally, Weber on the other hand idealizes as perfect communication because it comes from experts.

B [*Greeting K*] Yes, indeed I was coming to find you with a letter from Klamm.

K [*Overjoyed*] A letter from Klamm! [Reading the letter] "To the Land Surveyor at the Bridge Inn. I appreciate the surveys you have carried out so far. The work of your assistants is praiseworthy too; you know how to keep them busy. Do not desist from your zealous labors! Bring the work to a happy conclusion. Any interruption would be irksome to me. Furthermore, rest assured that the matter of your remuneration will be decided very soon. I am keeping an eye on you." [K turns to Barnabas] This is a misunderstanding. [Holding the letter in Barnabas's face] See what the gentleman says to me. The gentleman has been misinformed. I have not carried out any surveys, and you can see for yourself what my assistants are worth. I clearly can't interrupt work that I am not doing. I can't even be irksome to the gentleman, so how could I have earned his appreciation. And I feel I can never rest assured of anything.

B I'll go and pass that message on. (Kafka 2009:105–106)

A fourth principle deals with outsiders' responses to what they take to be miscommunication. Curiously enough, outsiders are not simply puppets in the scheme of things. They do have agency, but it is a form of agency set against crossing borders. The underlying principle here is the *freedom to wait*. Desperate, late one evening K attempts to meet the elusive Klamm at the Castle Inn. Earlier in the novel, K had seen what appeared to be Klamm there. But, try as he might, K encounters yet another minor official, who after several exchanges with K just disappears, leaving his sleigh driver behind. Ignoring K, the driver goes about his business, putting away the horse and the sleigh. But K insistently stays put, and Kafka writes:

> It seemed to K as if all contact with him [the driver] had been cut, and he was more of a free agent than ever. He could wait here, in a place usually forbidden to him, as long as he liked, and he also felt as if he had won that freedom with more effort than most people could manage to make, and no one could touch him or drive him away, why, they hardly had a right even to address him. But at the same time—and this feeling was at least as strong—he felt as if there was nothing more meaningless and more desperate than this freedom, this waiting, this invulnerability. (Kafka 2009:95)

The fifth and final principle of outsidership relates to desperation. It offers a happy ending of sorts, one that keeps officials safely ensconced on one side of the divide and villagers and K optimistically anxious on the other side. That principle is *the gift of hope*—hope for understanding, hope for involvement, and hope for resolution. Following an earlier altercation with the Bridge Inn landlady and Mr. Secretary, K admits to being wrong about his view of official due process, for which he apologizes. The following patronizing exchange with the landlady ensues:

K If that's the case, madam, then I must apologize to you, and I've misunderstood you, for I thought, mistakenly as it now turns out, I had gathered from your earlier remarks that there was in fact some kind of hope for me, however small.

L Exactly, just as I was saying. You're twisting my words again, only this time in the opposite direction. [As if explaining to a child] In my view such a hope for you does exist, and it is indeed to be found solely in these records. But it is not the case that you can simply ask Mr. Secretary aggressively, "If I answer your questions, can I see Klamm?" If a child says something like that we laugh at it; if an adult does so, it is an insult to Klamm's office, and the secretary kindly covered up for the insult with the elegance of his reply. However, the hope I mean lies in the fact that through the records you have, or perhaps you may have, a kind of connection with Klamm. Isn't that hope enough? If you were asked what merits you possess to make you worthy of the gift of such hope, could you come up with the slightest thing? To be sure, nothing more precise can be said about that hope. (Kafka 2009:101–102)

TRENDS AT THE BORDERS

Decades later, debate in the late 1960s and 1970s about future trends at the borders of the service relationship dealt with ideas that would come to challenge Weberian and Kafkaesque principles. One trend related to limits on the scope of professional expertise and autonomy that accompany the increasing availability of expert knowledge in society at large. The other trend related to the condition and scope of control on the user side of the service relationship, particularly the degree to which nonprofessional involvement in service provision can be accommodated.

Scope of Professional Expertise and Autonomy

Marie Haug's (1972) skeptical foresight is palpable in debates about the first trend. Haug's recollection of the issues targets what she calls "syrupy ideas about the future" (Haug 1988:49). In the 1960s, social scientists such as Daniel Bell (1968) and Eliot Freidson (1971) had argued that following the postwar growth of scientific knowledge of all kinds and the related expansion of expertise, the future would be dominated and guided by professionals. The claim rested on professionals' long training, expert knowledge, cultivated objectivity, and selfless service. Sounding Weberian without the morbid undertones, the argument perpetuated an avalanche of celebration. It is worth quoting Haug for a description of this felicitous, if not self-serving, perspective:

> We will live, it is said, in a "post-industrial" society. This means, according to Bell (1968, p. 152), that the professional and technical class will be preeminent or, in more general terms, that it will be a "professionalized society" (Freidson 1971, p. 467).... Another related prediction suggests that the service ethos of the professional's style of work is becoming generalized to the total society. In this view, the imputed ideology of the personal service professions—"concern, sympathy and even affection for those who are to be helped by the professional practitioners"—will structure the social order along the ethical lines espoused by the counsellor (Halmos 1970, p. 14). (Haug 1972:195)

Haug recalls a distinct wariness about the celebratory view, expressed as early as 1964 by Harold Wilensky (see Wilensky 1964), but to little effect:

> Wilensky was reacting to claims such as that of Nelson Foote (1953), who argued that even blue-collar workers were becoming professionals. We have forgotten how widespread the enthusiasm was for this idea, which had the golden glow of wiping out status differences.... Not every occupation, [Wilensky] argued, could be successful in struggling to gain ["extraordinary autonomy"].... [Still], seven years after [Wilensky's] paper was published, Eliot Freidson (1971), in the editorial foreword to a special issue of the *American Behavioral Scientist,* forecast a "professionalized society." ... Meanwhile, Paul Halmos (1970) in Britain was predicting that the service ethos of the professions would be generalized to society as a whole. (Haug 1988:48–49)

The celebrants clearly had the human service professions in mind. Against the felicity, and hedging her own prognostication with the word "hypothesis," Haug proposed what she called "an alternate hypothesis for the future" (Haug 1972:195). She hypothesized that in the future we would see the deprofessionalization of the traditional professions. She did not mean that expertise and educated skill would disappear but instead that professionals' work as organizationally unencumbered and exclusive experts would change, drawing nonprofessionals across the borders of expertise. As Glen Randall and Darlene Kindiak echo in recent reflections on social work as a profession, "Marie Haug depicted a process of deprofessionalization in which a profession's monopoly control over a body of specialized knowledge becomes challenged" (Randall and Kindiak 2008:344). This has resulted in "an increasingly educated public demanding greater accountability of professionals" (p. 344). This hypothesis continues to occupy researchers today (see Dent, O'Neill, and Bagley 1999; Freidson 2001; Harrison and Pollitt 1994; Scott et al. 2000).

Haug also pointed to the changing role of the clients of professionals, the outsiders she called the "missing ingredient" in discussions of the professions and professionalization. This missing ingredient, discussed further in the next section of this chapter, is now making itself felt in many ways, from user advocacy groups to policy agendas that consumerize clienthood. Another missing ingredient Haug identified was the impact of technological change, which has made service knowledge databases widely available. And yet another ingredient, one that is now overwhelming in its influence, is that professional practice in many service sectors is taking place within organizations, inserting managerial accountability into the professional autonomy equation. The era of solo practice in medicine, for example, is virtually over, displaced on many fronts by the corporatization of health care. The question now is whether what lies ahead will come full circle and become an all-consuming, "colonized" iron cage, unwittingly drawing its borders around everyone (see Habermas 1984, 1987).

Porous as the borders of expertise have become, there still are legal limits to its application. If expert knowledge is increasingly widespread, not everyone is free to apply its technology. Hanging one's proverbial professional shingle is still shielded by law. Professional jurisdictional disputes notwithstanding (see Abbott 1988), professionals have the privilege of "professing" because they have a legal basis for carrying out activities that others cannot, such as prescribing medication and making welfare service decisions. This line of demarcation has shifted somewhat over the years but remains remarkably tenacious in defining the borders of professionalism and, relatedly, designating who is and who is not expertly professional in service provision.

Human Rights, User Involvement, and User Control

The other trend at the borders of the service relationship deals with the question of who has the mandate to define what is proper conduct or normal in matters such as health and illness, social services, criminality, and disability (Hughes 1958). This is an issue broader than licensure and ultimately deals with human rights. Putting it in Hughes's terms, the question is who has the right to tell society "what is good and right for the individual and for society at large?" (Hughes 1958:79). Now more than ever, it is on this moral and political basis that border crossings are being advocated and undertaken by nonprofessionals, the outsiders whose resources and circumstances Kafka portrayed at their worst.

In contrast to licensure, the good and the right are of general concern, extending to all of society. Taking as a premise that professional knowledge and action have both credentialed *and* moral bearings, Haug (1972) noted that the moral component is accessible to those without formal training, extending to all relationships. Through their long and intimate acquaintance with ailments and caregiving, patients, parents, children, families, friends, and significant others could be just as knowledgeable as the professionals, and as intimately acquainted with what is good and right in matters of service and care.

Experiential knowledge, it has been argued, has moral bearings of its own (Polanyi 1958; Douglas 1970; Borkman 1976; Pollner 1987). It is a categorically distinct form of knowledge, not subordinate to scientific knowledge. Discussed later in relation to troubles and problems, it is a particularizing form of knowledge, inexorably full of ambiguity (see in this volume Järvinen, Chapter 3; Foley and Timonen, Chapter 6), novelty (see in this volume Carr, Chapter 4; Jensen and Villadsen, Chapter 11), and interpretive agency (see Schön 1984; Alm Andreassen, Chapter 2, this volume). Its working sensibilities flow in a different direction than the generalizing acumen of scientific knowledge.

While Haug foresaw the diffusion of expert knowledge and predicted a consequent decline in professionals' status, she did not anticipate the incorporation of experiential knowledge into policymaking and implementation. She certainly did not foresee the growth of a science of everyday life that stood side by side with the conventional sciences of conduct (Pollner 1987; Holstein and Gubrium 2000; Gubrium and Järvinen 2014). What has come to be called "user involvement" keys into this, incorporating knowledge that moves well beyond the formal boundaries of professional expertise (Alm Andreassen 2008; Barnes, Newman, and Sullivan 2007). It extends, for example, to the lay teaching of professionals as ingredients of educational programs and in-house training (see Eriksson and Jacobsson, Chapter 13, this volume), to the involvement of clients and patients in research as co-investigators (Faulkner and Thomas 2002; Trivedi and Wykes 2002; Gubrium and Harper 2013), to expert patients providing peer support in layperson-led educational programs (Edgar 2005; Taylor and Bury 2007; see also Shakespeare and Collins, Chapter 12, this volume), to the professional support of clients' relational citizenship (see Miller and Kontos, Chapter 8, this volume), to client control of personal assistance (see Solvang, Chapter 7, this volume), and to the control and ambivalence of the terminally ill over their remaining life (see Foley and Timonen, Chapter 6, this volume).

This resonates in the persuasive rhetoric of self-help, in demands from laypersons and various user movements for the incorporation of experiential knowledge into service planning and service provision (see Alm

Andreassen, Chapter 2, this volume). It is argued, for example, that only organizations that share the control of service provision with those who have personal experience with disabilities, chronic illness, or mental health problems have a legitimate right to advise and speak on behalf of users (see Solvang, Chapter 7, this volume). Such movements can be stridently opposed to professionals and philanthropic associations that presume to give voice to the experiences and needs of patients and clients, which is taken to be patronizing. The movements combine support to members in nurturing fellowships of equals, and undertake extensive advocacy for equal opportunities in society, for self-determination, political influence, and the right to speak for oneself (McLean 2010; Rose and Lucas 2007; Shakespeare 1993).

For example, Disabled Peoples International, an international umbrella for organizations of disabled individuals, established in 1981, adopted the slogan "Vox Nostra" (our own voice) to underscore this message. Terms for the roles of clients and patients are replaced by the terms "users" or "consumers." The active agency of the user designation and citizenship are emphasized, which is meant to convey that the disabled are not passive and helpless recipients dependent on the expertise of the professionals but instead are interested stakeholders in care and are able to understand their problems and needs. The idea of user participation supports the goal of moving the relations of ruling in a more symmetrical direction (Drake 1992; Beresford and Campbell 1994).

General terms of reference for the receivers of human services are in flux. The meaning of clienthood has rapidly changed (Hall et al. 2003), and existing claims about clientization are being challenged (Gubrium and Järvinen 2014). The concepts of service user and consumer, for example, are not unanimously accepted. Terms such as "consumer" and "customer," for instance, are not accepted by some, because they are applied by neoliberal advocates of human service retrenchment, some of whom aim to dismantle the welfare state. Conversely, the term "user" has been introduced to communicate the altered position of patients and clients vis-à-vis professionals. This designation can imply a rejection of neoliberal concepts such as "customer," which connotes a market relationship. At the same time, the concept of user also is criticized by disability activists for being stigmatizing, because it foregrounds the master status of dependency for those with impairments. The term "citizen" has been suggested as being more egalitarian (see Miller and Kontos, Chapter 8, this volume). Others believe such terms place too much power in the hands of those who are dependent, helpless, or otherwise unable to participate in service intervention. It is claimed that these terms place too much choice in the hands of those incapable of making choices, such as young children (see Pösö, Chapter 9, this volume) and frail elderly (see Grenier and Flood, Chapter 10, this volume).

New professional roles complicate the issue of user involvement and control by bringing different forms of professional alliances into the mix. Dan Goodley (2011) distinguishes two models of professional involvement: professionals allied with professionals and professionals allied with the community. Inspired by disability activist Vic Finkelstein, Goodley views alliances with the community as preferable (see Greener, Chapter 14, this volume). In that model, every professional accepts as a starting point the premise that disabled people can have satisfying lifestyles. Cure and physical rehabilitation are not the default goals. What Goodley calls the "virgin field" of professionals allied with the community "demands professionals to invest less time in pathological views of impairment and more in *challenging the conditions of dis/ablism*" (Goodley 2011:173). A similar perspective is put forth by occupational therapy researcher Karen Hammell, who calls for reforming the field of rehabilitation with inspiration from disability studies. In her view, even if relevant for some people with injuries, professional work in rehabilitation is not about teaching mobility and self-care per se but about "enabling people to get on with their lives" and to "reconstruct their biographies" (Hammell 2006:124).

An important aspect of Goodley's comparison is the models' organizational implications, only one of which—professionals allied with the community—entails significant border crossing. A telling example is drawn from professional interventions for deafness. The World Federation of the Deaf (WFD) is critical of audiologists who orient toward cures with hearing aids. The group believes audiologists want to replace sign language with an incomplete technology, making deaf people second-rate hearing subjects instead of first-class communicators in sign language. One political outcome is that only certain groups of professionals are welcomed at WFD's world congresses. The presentation of papers is largely from the social sciences and linguistic studies, and the majority of participants are the clients (deaf people). The professionals working at the conference are the interpreters, a role drawn from the understanding that, first and foremost, deafness is a culturally significant difference, not a handicap (Solvang and Haualand 2014).

A more radical form of user control is represented by the Independent Living (IL) movement. Informed by a view of the pernicious impact of professionals' interpretation of disability, IL rejects the utility of professional expertise. The key principles of IL are summarized by rehabilitation scholar Gerben deJong in his influential 1979 article (reprinted in 1983 and 2007) in which the IL approach to service production is contrasted with a rehabilitation model. According to deJong, the locus of the problem is not an incapacity but dependence, inadequate support, and barriers in the environment. Hence, the solutions are located not in the professional interventions of a therapist but in peer support, self-help, the removal of barriers, and antidiscrimination efforts. One practical outcome of this approach is making it possible for disabled persons to hire their own personal assistants. This is seen as a "main presupposition for user control and for freeing disabled people from their reliance on welfare professionals and unpaid carers" (Askheim 2003:227). Advocates of this direct payment strategy deemphasize competence in health care and social work as qualifications for hiring assistants.

Whether the view is inclusive but wary of professionals or altogether rejects professional expertise, the impact on the human service relationship can be significant. General policy decisions are increasingly affected by user voices and actions (see in this volume Carr, Chapter 4; Garrow, Chapter 5). The shape of professional and service user encounters is evolving as never before; neither the scope of professionalism nor the purview of user advocacy is likely to dissipate in this landscape. The category of service provider itself is broadening to include the professional input of amazingly diverse perspectives and skills, bringing the humanities and the arts, for example, into the mix as never before (see in this volume Miller and Kontos, Chapter 8; Solvang, Chapter 7).

EVERYDAY LOGICS OF TROUBLES AND PROBLEMS

Trends are historical; they develop through time. In contrast, like everyday life in general, the relational work of service and care cuts across history and forms through practice. Relational work has been present as long as social relations have existed, which returns us to where we began, to the interaction order and specifically to everyday logics of troubles and problems.

Two seminal texts bring into microscopic view the logics' naturally occurring complexity. One is Robert Emerson and Sheldon Messinger's (1977) article "The Micro-Politics of Trouble." The other is Michael Lipsky's (1980) book *Street-Level Bureaucracy: Dilemmas of the Individual in Public Services*. Their purview is everyday life, the discretionary practices of which Weber's idealization of bureaucratic rationality dismisses as extenuating circumstances and Kafka's depiction of outsidership treats as incidental to borders of separation. Emerson and Messinger's angle is interactional and poses *what* and *how* questions: what are everyday troubles, and how do they relate in practice to the construction of serviceable problems? Lipsky's angle is institutional and poses a *where* question: where is social policy and, to use Emerson and Messinger's terms, how does that relate to everyday logics of troubles and problems?

Emerson and Messinger's article is now about four decades old. It endures because it affirms the fruitfulness of distinguishing the logic of troubles from the logic of problems and, most importantly, places them on equal footing in what they call the "micro-politics" of representation. Both troubles and problems operate in the context of everyday life, whether that is the everyday life of professional or nonprofessional practice. While perhaps differentially visible, the logics inexorably and continually work together in practice. This stands in contrast to critics such as Weber a century ago and especially Jürgen Habermas (1984, 1987) today, who would argue that in contemporary life, the logic of problems increasingly "colonizes" the logic of troubles. I will return to this and the issue of differential visibility at the close of the chapter, because it relates directly to the goal of this book.

The Logic of Troubles

Emerson and Messinger begin their article by suggesting that we frequently overlook the fact that whether what ails or otherwise bothers us eventually becomes, say, psychological, medical, or criminal, it was once something less well formulated—a trouble, not a problem. At the time Emerson and Messinger wrote, the highly normative term "deviance" was being used for social problems in sociology, eliding the reflexivity of troubles and problems:

> Our argument assumes that any social setting generates a number of evanescent, ambiguous difficulties that may ultimately be—but are not immediately—identified as "deviant." In many instances what is first recognized is a vague sense of "something wrong"—some "problem" or "trouble." . . . This [article] will explore the processes whereby troubles are identified, defined, responded to, and sometimes transformed into a recognized form of deviance. (Emerson and Messinger 1977:121)

VAGUENESS AND NOTICING

Inspiration for their argument appears immediately in the article. We are introduced to the idea that there are troublesome experiences with an everyday logic that is distinct from, and that does not automatically lead to, the logic of problems. The experiences are only "sometimes transformed" into problems. As the word "evanescent" would have it, matters of concern in the logic of troubles are fleeting, not as settled or as clear-cut as in the logic of problems. This is because troubles are experienced in relation to the particulars of local contingencies such as who in particular is troubled, when the troubles arise, other troubles that are pertinent, time constraints, what besides the troubles is at stake in the matter, and what the troubles' immediate or long-term consequences might be, among endlessly provisional matters. Troubles' key characteristic—*vagueness*—refers to something seemingly wrong or untoward, but it is not clear what that is, how it is so, or what to do about it in the face of its contingencies. It is troubles' everyday "it depends" quality that generates vagueness, a sort of tentativeness with shaky boundaries.

The authors instruct with familiar examples. If the designation of problems begins with formal procedures such as psychological testing, medical diagnosis, or adjudication, the onset of troubles starts with *noticing* that something is wrong. Noticing is the parallel process to the formal procedures by which experiences are identified in the logic of problems. Troubles come in many forms, from the troubles of bodies, behaviors, and minds to troubled relationships and groups. The authors explain:

> The perception of "something wrong" is often vague at the outset: a woman notices that she is gaining weight, or that she is frequently depressed; a hus-

> band realizes that his wife is drinking more than usual, or is beginning to stay out later after work; parents see their daughter getting overly interested in boys, or their son starting to hang out with a tough gang of friends. (Emerson and Messinger 1977:121–122)

Noticings do not necessarily lead to professional consultation or formal assessment.[4] A husband or a wife may notice something wrong with a family member but keep it to himself or herself and do nothing about it since doing something may create more trouble than it is worth (an everyday contingency). Or each may share it with the other and leave it at that (a contingent horizon). They might mention it to the subject of what is noticed. They may or may not bring it to others' attention (other contingent horizons). They might even dismiss and ignore the apparent trouble as being insignificant and nothing to fuss about in the face of other concerns in the larger scheme of things (both contingent contexts). The important difference between the logic of troubles and the logic of problems on this front is that, linked as problems now are to chains of formally organized activation rules, problems lead to relatively predictable outcomes, at least in theory. Troubles, in contrast, are not driven by predesignated activities and formal missions but rather by ongoing interpretations of reality—of "something wrong" and what that might mean in the unfolding scheme of things and immediate skein of contingencies.

It is important to note that neither type of logic is exclusive to either outsiders or insiders, but instead they are different ways of making meaning, of knowing, and of acting that are taken up on all sides of the service divide. The idea that the logic of troubles is the representational bailiwick of service users and that the logic of problems is the representational preserve of professionals is not warranted empirically. While Emerson and Messinger's examples might suggest otherwise, just as the logic of problems can assert itself in the lives of users, the logic of troubles extends to and inserts itself into the professional activities of service providers (see in this volume Barnes, Chapter 15; Grenier and Flood, Chapter 10). Unhindered by demands of formality and expertise, the logic of troubles coexists enduringly and inexorably with the logic of problems across service provision. The principles and sentiments of the freedom to wait and the gift of hope described by Kafka extend in their own fashion to the Castle and its denizens, which Kafka's focus on outsiders fails to recognize. The everyday lives of insiders (and professionals) are as saturated by the vagueness and noticings of troubles, both their own and those of users, as they are beholden to the logic of clearly seeing, and seeing to, the problems over which they have formal oversight.

The Logic of Problems

In contemporary society, it is the ostensible gaze and related application of professional expertise that officially and "logically" transforms troubles into problems. The gaze can be, and often is, adopted by users, but this can be threatening to expertise and largely goes unrecognized or is formally discounted.

CLARITY AND PROBLEMATIZATION

If a key feature of troubles is vagueness, its counterpart in the logic of problems is *clarity*. This is not to say that problems are clear from the start or that they eventually are completely clarified. Clarity is a matter of principle, not practice; it is ultimately a feature of the logic of problems, not concrete problems as such. Problems in society are continually subject to clarification, their historical paths strewn with clarifying claims and counterclaims (see Spector and Kitsuse 1987; Schneider 1985; Best 2012). This is the stock-in-trade of social movements, from political and economic movements to newer identity and self-help movements. As far as clarity is concerned, the goal of social movements is to transform the vagueness of what is troublesome into what is claimed to be clearly problematic—what might be called "problematization." Whether troubles center on the body, behavior, the mind, relationships, or groups, the related mission (if it is taken up) is two-pronged: to concertedly establish the taken-for-grantedness of a problem in what is otherwise vaguely understood and to marshal evidence of that. As John McCarthy and Mayer Zald (1977) instructed years ago, clarification is not just cognitive but entails organization and evidence, without which the clarification process is likely to falter or fail.

The logic of problems extends beyond social movements to what already is established and professionally relevant. Guiding texts, such as various editions of the *Diagnostic and Statistical Manual* (*DSM*) of the American Psychiatric Association and the many versions of the *Big Book* of self-help addictions groups such as Alcoholics Anonymous and Narcotics Anonymous, are well known and widely used for purposes of clarification. They textually inform a huge public and a swath of service providers and organizations of what is presumed to be evidently problematic, not just troublesome, in life. The *DSM* alone details a problematizing system, quantitatively organized in terms of too much or too little, for virtually every conceivable form of experience. It is just one of a panoply of texts whose discursive conventions are well established, indeed professionalized, offering formal guidance for how to problematize troubles by eclipsing vagueness. More and more, problematization is "textually-mediated," as Smith (1987, 1990) would put it. It is organized not only to categorize problems but also to actually write and read them into troubled lives. The textual demands of problematization are now so persuasive and time-consuming as to virtually transform professional practice into being as much a matter of documentation as it is a matter of service and care.[5]

DEPROBLEMATIZATION

Challenges to problem clarity also are the stock-in-trade of social movements. Efforts to *deproblematize* troubles have emerged on many fronts, from the goal of deproblematizing drug use, body weight, and alternative sexualities to the aim of deproblematizing particular groups and relationships. These also are two-pronged. Whether it is being overweight, having a mental illness, being addicted, or courting undesirable peer influences, the mission on one front is to question the assumption that the problems in question are self-evident and on the other front to provide factual proof of that. "Naturalization," "normalization," and "neutralization" are common terms of reference for this process (see Sykes and Matza 1957).

The *Where* Question

As for the *where* question, in his book *Street-Level Bureaucracy*, Lipsky encourages us to explore a space where we might not have considered looking if the borders of the service relationship were as clear-cut as Weber and Kafka made them out to be. Lipsky advises us to open to view the everyday practices of service workers, which "are not reducible to programmed formats." He encourages us to look in order to see and to make visible how policy is realized in the discretionary flux of troubles and problems in the frontline sites of service provision. Arguing that the logic of troubles coexists with the logic of problems in the very practice of providing and receiving services, turning policy into a matter of everyday life, Lipsky collapses the Weberian divide.

If, as Weber would have it, service organizations ideally deploy rules, regulations, and policies that are expert, ironclad, and promote efficiency, Lipsky's description of street-level service provision suggests something strikingly different. The everyday challenges of practice on the front lines, Lipsky argues, move in many directions, inexorably mixing logics and their related rights in the "border work" entailed (see in this volume Carr, Chapter 4; Newman, Chapter 16; Pösö, Chapter 9). Attention to the street-level activities of service provision makes visible the persistent intrusions, shifting alliances, and flux of extenuating circumstances that cross the borders of service intervention. Presenting the central argument of his book and ending with a suggested refocusing on the complex challenges of "client-processing," Lipsky writes:

> The book is grounded in observations of the collective behavior of public service organizations and advances a theory of the work of street-level bureaucracies as individual workers experience it. I argue that the decisions of street-level bureaucrats, the routines they establish, and the devices they invent to cope with uncertainties and work pressures, effectively become the public policies they carry out. I maintain that public policy is not best understood as made in legislatures or top-floor suites of high-ranking administrators. These decision-making arenas are important, of course, but they do not represent the complete picture. To the mix of places where policies are made, one must add the crowded offices and daily encounters of street-level workers. Further, I point out that policy conflict is not only expressed as the contention of interest groups, as we have come to expect. It is also located in the [everyday] struggles between individual workers and citizens who challenge or submit to client-processing. (Lipsky 1980:xiii)

Lipsky points out that, at close range, we can observe that troubles and problems are not distinct entities located in separate places in practice but rather are part and parcel of the service divide itself, reflexively both affecting and constructing it. In practice, providers and users overlap in applications of the logics of troubles and problems. At the street level, some troubles may not be problematized and some problems may be deproblematized, for all practical purposes. Needs and interventions are subject to the ever-present categorical activity, deployed logics, invoked expertise, stakes in the matter, negotiations, and resistances that run through the service relationship (Gubrium and Holstein 2001). Both vagueness and clarification continually wend their way into, out of, and around the alleged problems in question (cf. Gubrium and Buckholdt 1982; Gubrium 1992; Rose 1998; Gubrium and Holstein 2001).[6]

Observed closely and critically, the street level and its discretion are everywhere in the service relationship. If, as Habermas maintains, the "life world" (everyday life?) is increasingly colonized by the logic of problems, the life world's practices on all fronts remain a phenomenon in their own right, uncolonized and ever present within the colonization project (cf. Schön and Rein 1995; and see Newman, Chapter 16, this volume). Ambivalence and ambiguity are unassailable ingredients of the life world (see Järvinen, Chapter 3, this volume), not historically diminished with modernization (Levine 1985). What Habermas calls "system" is strategically used in the life world, as much as the system ostensibly menaces and uses its actors (see Barnes 2000:87–92). New and controversial social policy developments certainly influence, but they do not displace, the everyday practice of engaging what is and what is not a serviceable problem in the encounters between service providers and service users.

If colonization has any concrete meaning in practice, it refers to the process by which only some of what is common to providers and users as everyday members of society is rendered categorically visible. In this regard, the idea of formal organization is as much a mechanism of invisibility as it refers to concerted designs for work and action. Being formal, its articulations systematically make visible the operation and by-products of the logic of problems, while systematically rendering invisible or otherwise tangential the operation and by-products of the logic of troubles. This is what colonization should mean, not the deplacement of everyday life.

• • •

The task of reimagining the human service relationship relates directly to this. It involves rendering visible what has increasingly become invisible in human service provision. Noticing and documenting the differential visibility of troubles and problems is the aim. The contributors' common procedure has been to recognize and trace the everyday sentiments, ambivalences, conceptual tensions, working resilience, strategic agency, and artfulness of the interaction order as it unfolds in concrete sites of human service provision. The iron cage notwithstanding, there is a shared commitment to opening to view the moral complexity and local inventiveness of human service intervention.

As Goffman contended for the interaction order, the chapters of this book argue that the everyday "micro-politics" of troubles and problems is the proper grounding for understanding human service policy. Current experience-distant models of service provision distinguish and describe service actors in terms hardly recognizable in practice. By turning us to everyday life, the chapters problematize such models of service provision. In doing so, they bring our attention and our will to the need for a more realistic and multi-sited vision. The rationalization of everyday life will not disappear. As Weber lamented, its by-products are increasingly apparent in our lives. What he (and Kafka) did not undertake to conceptualize, examine, and document is policy and service in practice, the operating contours of which this book unsettles and reimagines, freeing us from iron-cage necessity.

NOTES

1 While, analytically, it is important to identify the various operating "logics" of action, such as Annemarie Mol (2008) has admirably outlined for care and caring in her book *The Logic of Care*, one might argue that its idealized philosophical horizons can never be realized in everyday life. Everyday life is filled with interactionally contingent and diverse logics, which overlap, confirm, compete with, and resist each other in the flux of practice. Especially important in the following chapters on the human service relationship are the organizational contingencies—the organizational embeddedness—of care (see Gubrium and Holstein 1990, 1997, 2000). The logic of care, in other words, coexists in practice with the logic of service, which would then turn us as much to management and work as to care and caring in reimagining the service relationship (see Alford and O'Flynn 2012). It is the coexisting and increasingly present relational logics of service *and* care that are the focus of this book.

2 American sociologist Talcott Parsons translated *The Protestant Ethic and the Spirit of Capitalism* from the German into English, in which the English "iron cage" was used for Weber's original German "stahlhartes Gehäuse." Peter Baehr suggests that the English "shell as hard as steel" would have been better, given the sense of inescapability present in Weber's depiction (Baehr 2001).

3 There is reason to believe that there was an intellectual line of influence between Weber and Kafka. Max Weber's younger brother, Alfred, was Kafka's professor at

Charles University in Prague, and it is likely that Kafka learned of Max's work from Alfred (see Litowitz 2011).

4 As this volume goes to press nearly forty years after the publication of the micro-politics article, a book-length explication by Emerson of the perspective presented in the article has appeared under the title *Everyday Troubles: The Micro-politics of Interpersonal Conflict* (Emerson 2015). It provides many useful illustrations of the locally contingent character of everyday troubles. But in contrast to the view taken in our book and in the Emerson and Messenger article, the Emerson book frames the development of troubles through time as sequential. According to Emerson's book, the course of troubles progresses from vague beginnings through several stages of social complication until, in the final stage, authorities and/or professionals become involved. The relationship between troubles and problems, in other words, is linear, which stands in contrast to the more reflexive relationship suggested in the micro-politics articles and in part inspires my discussion of the everyday logics of troubles and problems. No matter how clear problems are or become "in theory," all are continually troublesome in practice because they are located in a world of contingencies. The perspective presented in Emerson's book violates a signal ethnomethodological precept, which is not to treat a topic of study (sequentiality) as an explanatory resource (see Heritage 1984). Certainly, empirically, facets of troubles may be patterned through time to eventually become clear and authoritative in practice, but that is something to be conceptually problematized and explained, not something to be taken for granted. As I have shown in a number of monographs empirically centered in "iron cage" human service organizations, the contingent nature of everyday life is always in effect, extending to its temporal organization (Buckholdt and Gubrium 1979; Gubrium and Buckholdt 1982; Gubrium 1992, 1993).

5 See David Buckholdt and Jaber Gubrium's study of a service organization in which the representational burden of problem documentation has overwhelmed its therapeutic activity (Buckholdt and Gubrium 1979). The authors describe ethnographically how an extensive regime of behavioral assessment for children with conduct-control disorders and emotional disturbances is managed in the process of treating the children's problems.

6 That troubles and problems continually wend their way across the landscape of service provision, crossing both informal and formal borders in the process, suggests that they "travel" various sites of articulation (see Clarke et al. 2015). There is no absolute "colonial" power or process that straightforwardly renders the meaning of policy in practice, only the metaphorical semblance of it. As experience-distant policies move between places and organized settings, they prompt varying configurations of understanding about what the policies mean and how providers and users are to apply them. As Clarke and others argue, this requires a process of experience-near "translation." The perspective requires not only a concerted turn to, and documentation of, the local *whats*, *hows*, and *wheres*, but also the *whens*, of the policy process. The chapters in this volume present discussions and examples of located and occasioned "assemblages" of policy articulations and interventions, none of which is reducible to

experience-distant metrics of their components. Assemblages of service provision, instead, must be understood on their own terms sui generis and are grist for reimagining the human service relationship.

REFERENCES

Abbott, A. 1988. *The System of Professions*. Chicago: University of Chicago Press.

Alford, J. and J. O'Flynn. 2012. *Rethinking Public Service Delivery*. Basingbroke, Hampshire: Palgrave Macmillan.

Alm Andreassen, T. 2008. "'Asymmetric Mutuality': User Involvement as a Government–Voluntary Sector Relationship in Norway." *Nonprofit and Voluntary Sector Quarterly* 37(2): 281–299.

Alvesson, M. 2012. *Understanding Organizational Culture*. Thousand Oaks, CA: Sage.

Askheim, O. P. 2003. "Empowerment as Guidance for Professional Social Work: An Act of Balancing on a Slack Rope." *European Journal of Social Work* 6:227–240.

Baehr, P. 2001. "The 'Iron Cage' and the 'Shell as Hard as Steel': Parsons, Weber, and the Stahlhartes Gehäuse Metaphor in *The Protestant Ethic and the Spirit of Capitalism*." *History and Theory* 40:163–169.

Barnes, B. 2000. *Understanding Agency: Social Theory and Responsible Action*. London: Sage.

Barnes, M., J. Newman, and H. Sullivan. 2007. *Power, Participation and Political Renewal: Case Studies in Public Participation*. Bristol: Policy.

Bell, D. 1968. "The Measurement of Knowledge and Technology." In *Indicators of Social Change*, edited by E. B. Sheldon and W. E. Moore, 145–237. New York: Russell Sage Foundation.

Bendix, R. 1960. *Max Weber: An Intellectual Portrait*. New York: Doubleday.

Beresford, P., and J. Campbell. 1994. "Disabled People, Service Users, User Involvement, and Representation." *Disability and Society* 9:315–325.

Best, J. 2012. *Social Problems*. New York: Norton.

Borkman, T. 1976. "Experiential Knowledge: A New Concept for the Analysis of Self Help Groups." *Social Service Review* 50:445–456.

Buckholdt, D. R., and J. F. Gubrium. 1979. *Caretakers: Treating Emotionally Disturbed Children*. Sociological Observations Series. Thousand Oaks, CA: Sage.

Clarke, J., D. Bainton, N. Lendvai, and P. Stubbs. 2015. *Making Policy Move: Towards a Politics of Translation and Assemblage*. Bristol: Policy.

deJong, G. 1979. "Independent Living: From Social Movement to Analytic Paradigm." *Archives of Physical Medicine and Rehabilitation* 60(10): 435–446.

Dent, M., M. O'Neill, and C. Bagley. 1999. *Professions: New Public Management and the European Welfare State.* Stoke-on-Trent: Staffordshire University Press.

Douglas, J. D., ed. 1970. *Understanding Everyday Life.* Chicago: Aldine.

Drake, R. F. 1992. "Consumer Participation: The Voluntary Sector and the Concept of Power." *Disability, Handicap and Society* 7:267–278.

Edgar, A. 2005. "The Expert Patient: Illness as Practice." *Medicine, Health Care and Philosophy* 8:165–171.

Emerson, R. M. 2015. *Everyday Troubles: The Micro-politics of Interpersonal Conflict.* Chicago: University of Chicago Press.

Emerson, R. M., and S. Messinger. 1977. "The Micropolitics of Trouble." *Social Problems* 25:121–134.

Faulkner, A., and P. Thomas. 2002. "User-Led Research and Evidence-Based Medicine." *British Journal of Psychiatry* 180(1): 1–3. doi: 10.1192/bjp.180.1.1.

Foote, N. N. 1953. "The Professionalization of Labor in Detroit." *American Journal of Sociology* 58:371–380.

Freidson, E. 1971. "Editorial Foreword." *American Behavioral Scientist* 14:467–474.

Freidson, E. 2001. *Professionalism: The Third Logic.* London: Polity.

Gabriel, Y. 2000. *Storytelling in Organizations.* Oxford: Oxford University Press.

Gill, M. 2012. "Care and Value at the End of Life." *Poetics* 40:118–132.

Goffman, E. 1959. *The Presentation of Self in Everyday Life.* New York: Doubleday.

Goffman, E. 1983. "The Interaction Order." *American Sociological Review* 48:1–17.

Goodley, D. 2011. *Disability Studies.* Thousand Oaks, CA: Sage.

Gubrium, A., and K. Harper. 2013. *Participatory Visual and Digital Methods.* Walnut Creek, CA: Left Coast.

Gubrium, J. F. 1992. *Out of Control: Family Therapy and Domestic Disorder.* Thousand Oaks, CA: Sage.

Gubrium, J. F. 1993. *Speaking of Life: Horizons of Meaning for Nursing Home Residents.* New York: Aldine de Gruyter.

Gubrium, J. F., and D. R. Buckholdt. 1982. *Describing Care: Image and Practice in Rehabilitation.* Cambridge, MA: Oelgeschlager, Gunn and Hain.

Gubrium, J. F., and J. A. Holstein. 1990. *What Is Family?* Mountain View, CA: Mayfield.

Gubrium, J. F., and J. A. Holstein. 1997. *The New Language of Qualitative Method.* New York: Oxford University Press.

Gubrium, J. F., and J. A. Holstein. 2000. "The Self in a World of Going Concerns." *Symbolic Interaction* 23:95–115.

Gubrium, J. F., and J. A. Holstein, eds. 2001. *Institutional Selves: Troubles Identities in a Postmodern World.* New York: Oxford University Press.

Gubrium, J. F., and M. Järvinen. 2014. *Turning Troubles into Problems: Clientization in Human Service.* London: Routledge.

Habermas, Jürgen. 1984 and 1987. *The Theory of Communicative Action*, vols. 1 and 2. Boston: Beacon.

Hall, C., K. Juhila, N. Parton, and T. Pösö. 2003. *Constructing Clienthood in Social Work and Human Services.* London: Kingsley.

Halmos, P. 1970. *The Personal Service Society.* New York: Schocken.

Hammell, K. W. 2006. *Perspectives on Disability and Rehabilitation.* Philadelphia: Elsevier.

Harrison, S., and C. Pollitt. 1994. *Controlling Health Professionals.* Buckingham: Open University Press.

Hatch, M. J. 2012. *Organization Theory: Modern, Symbolic and Postmodern Perspectives.* Oxford: Oxford University Press.

Haug, M. R. 1972. "Deprofessionalisation: An Alternative Hypothesis for the Future." *Sociological Review Monographs* 20:195–211.

Haug, M. R. 1988. "A Re-examination of the Hypothesis of Physician Deprofessionalization." *Milbank Quarterly* 66:48–56.

Heritage, J. 1984. *Garfinkel and Ethnomethodology.* Cambridge: Polity.

Holstein, J. A., and J. F. Gubrium. 2000. *The Self in a World of Going Concerns.* New York: Oxford University Press.

Hughes, E. C. 1958. "Licence and Mandate." In *Men and Their Work*, edited by E. C. Hughes, 78–87. Westport, CT: Greenwood.

Hughes, E. C. 1984[1957]. "Going Concerns: The Study of American Institutions." In *The Sociological Eye: Selected Papers*, edited by E. C. Hughes, 52–64. New Brunswick, NJ: Transaction.

Kafka, F. 1925. *The Trial.* New York: Trebeca.

Kafka, F. 2009[1926]. *The Castle.* Oxford: Oxford University Press.

Levine, D. N. 1985. *The Flight from Ambiguity.* Chicago: University of Chicago Press.

Lipsky, M. 1980. *Street-Level Bureaucracy: Dilemmas of the Individual in Public Services.* New York: Sage.

Litowitz, D. 2011. "Max Weber and Franz Kafka: A Shared Vision of Modern Law." *Law, Culture and the Humanities* 7:48–65.

Mayer, J. P. 1943. *Max Weber and German Politics*. London: Faber and Faber.
McCarthy, J., and M. Zald. 1977. "Resource Mobilization and Social Movements: A Partial Theory." *American Journal of Sociology* 82:1212–1241.
McLean, A. 2010. "The Mental Health Consumers/Survivors Movement in the United States." In *A Handbook for the Study of Mental Health*, second edition, edited by T. L. Scheid and T. N. Brown, 461–477. Cambridge: Cambridge University Press.
Mead, G. H. 1934. *Mind, Self and Society*. Chicago: University of Chicago Press.
Mol, A. 2008. *The Logic of Care*. London: Routledge.
Morgan, G. 1985. *Images of Organization*. London: Sage.
Polanyi, M. 1958. *Personal Knowledge: Towards a Post-critical Philosophy*. Chicago: University of Chicago Press.
Pollner, M. 1987. *Mundane Reason: Reality in Everyday and Sociological Discourse*. New York: Cambridge University Press.
Randall, G. E., and D. H. Kindiak. 2008. "Deprofessionalization or Postprofessionalization? Reflections on the State of Social Work as a Profession." *Social Work in Health Care* 47:341–354.
Reed, M., and M. Hughes. 1992. *Rethinking Organization: New Directions in Organization Theory and Analysis*. London: Sage.
Rose, D., and J. Lucas. 2007. "The User and Survivor Movement in Europe." In *Mental Health Policy and Practice Across Europe*, edited by M. Knapp, D. McDaid, E. Mossialos, and G. Thornicroft, 336–355. European Observatory on Health Systems and Policies Series. Maidenhead: Open University Press/McGraw-Hill.
Rose, N. 1998. *Inventing Our Selves*. Cambridge: Cambridge University Press.
Schneider, J. W. 1985. "Social Problems Theory: The Constructionist Theory." *Annual Review of Sociology* 11:209–229.
Schön, D. A. 1984. *The Reflective Practitioner: How Professionals Think in Action*. New York: Basic.
Schön, D. A., and M. Rein. 1995. *Frame Reflection: Toward the Resoluton of Intractable Policy Controversies*. New York: Basic.
Scott, W. R., M. Ruef, P. J. Mendell, and C. A. Caronna. 2000. *Institutional Change and Health Care Organizations: From Professional Dominance to Managed Care*. Chicago: University of Chicago Press.
Shakespeare, T. 1993. "Disabled People's Self-Organization: A New Social Movement?" *Disability, Handicap, and Society* 8:249–264.
Silverman, D. 1970. *The Theory of Organizations*. New York: Basic.

Smith, D. 1987. *The Everyday World as Problematic*. Boston: Northeastern University Press.

Smith, D. 1990. *The Conceptual Practices of Power*. Toronto: University of Toronto Press.

Solvang, P. K., and H. Haualand. 2014. "Accessibility and Diversity—Deaf Space in Action." *Scandinavian Journal of Disability Research* 16:1–13.

Spector, M., and J. Kitsuse. 1987. *Constructing Social Problems*. New York: Transaction.

Sykes, G., and D. Matza. 1957. "Techniques of Neutralization." *American Sociological Review* 22:664–670.

Taylor, D., and M. Bury. 2007. "Chronic Illness, Expert Patients and the Care Transition." *Sociology of Health and Illness* 29:27–45.

Trivedi, P., and T. Wykes. 2002. "From Passive Subjects to Equal Partners: Qualitative Review of User Involvement in Research." *British Journal of Psychiatry* 181:468–472.

Weber, Max. 1968[1922]. *Economy and Society*. New York: Bedminster.

Weber, Max. 1985[1930]. *The Protestant Ethic and the Spirit of Capitalism*. Boston: Unwin.

Wilensky, H. 1964. "The Professionalization of Everyone?" *American Journal of Sociology* 70:137–158.

PART II

Service User Perspectives

THE CHAPTERS OF PART II deal with those who use human services, offering windows on their everyday world and the preferences of service provision from their perspective. The chapters reveal their complex sentiments and circumstances, which extend in directions of limited interest to administrative accountability. The latter's formularized and officious metrics erase the existential conditions that both providers and users are up against. This calls for recognition of the contingent character of service provision. The chapters' signal terminology—"ambivalence," "flipping," "negotiation," and the like—tells of a world enormously more vibrant and intricate than Weber and Kafka imagined it. To apply the language introduced in Chapter 1, the chapters of Part II show that the "logic of problems" is intertwined with the "logic of troubles" in users' lives. The everyday agency, as opposed to the organizational docility, of service users is showcased.

2

Professional Intervention from a Service User Perspective

▸ *TONE ALM ANDREASSEN*

IN RECENT DECADES, INCREASED SIGNIFICANCE has been ascribed to the experiential knowledge of clients and patients. The perspectives of clients and patients inform policy-making, planning, and service provision (Alm Andreassen 2008; Barnes, Newman, and Sullivan 2007; Tritter 2009). To affect the practice of professionals, users are involved in the teaching of professionals in educational programs and in-house training, for example (see Eriksson and Jacobsson, Chapter 13, this volume), and in research as co-researchers (Beresford 2002; Faulkner and Thomas 2002; Trivedi and Wykes 2002; McLaughlin 2010; Smith et al. 2009).

Several aspects of service user involvement have been studied, such as opinions about the character, organization, and functioning of user involvement, and the policies required for increased involvement, as well as their different sources, particularly ideas of consumerism and user choice (Aberbach and Christensen 2005; Alm Andreassen 2009; Barnes and Cotterell 2012; Barnes, Newman, and Sullivan 2007; Crawford et al. 2003; Dent 2006b; Martin 2009; Rutter et al. 2004; Veronesi and Keasey 2013; Tritter 2009). Less attention has been paid to the actual experiences of service users conveyed through involvement processes, and to how professional intervention is conceived from the service users' perspective. This is the focus of the research described in this chapter, particularly the opinions of service user spokespersons about the qualities of health care that are important to service users.

The chapter starts with a brief presentation of some key perspectives on professionals and professionalism, with the focus on how the professionals' relationships with patients and clients are perceived. Then, empirical material from service user involvement in a two-year planning process for organizational restructuring within Norwegian health care is described, together with the methodology used for analyzing the statements of the service user spokespersons. Next, a systematized presentation of the messages contained in these statements is outlined. Finally, I discuss the implications of the messages in terms of the common understanding of professionals and professionalism presented at the start, considering especially what this means for reimagining professional intervention from a service user perspective.

PROFESSIONALS AND PROFESSIONALISM

Their Weberian roots palpable, professionals are understood to be highly educated and skilled workers who have learned to apply abstract, esoteric knowledge to specific, individual cases and problems (see Gubrium, Chapter 1, this volume). Professionals treat individual clients, make specific decisions, analyze individual cases, or give specific advice on the basis of learned, abstract insight. Professionals have acquired knowledge, expertise, or a technical base that enables them to know how to treat individual cases. A knowledge base achieved by way of tertiary education, vocational training, and experience is regarded as an essential ingredient of professionalism (Evetts 2013). Expertise is the key aspect of the professions; for some, it is the defining characteristic (Brante 2011). According to Eliot Freidson (2001), professionalism is a logic to be applied when the work is so specialized that it is inaccessible to those lacking the required training and expertise, and where the problems to be contended with lack uniformity and thus create a need for discretion instead of standardized or rationalized work procedures.

Professional work engages with human problems that are amenable to expert service (Abbott 1988). These problems have certain objective qualities, but they are also subjectively defined. Thus, the definition of a problem varies over time and between different kinds of experts, and even laypeople could have an influence on the definition of a problem. The construction of the problem is what connects the problem to the jurisdiction of the expert (see Gubrium, Chapter 1, this volume). Such jurisdictional claims have three parts: claims to classify a problem, to reason about it, and to take action on it—or, in terms that are more formal: to diagnose, to infer, and to treat. Diagnosis and treatment are mediating acts, according to Andrew Abbott. Diagnosis takes information into the professional knowledge system, and treatment brings instructions back from it. Inference is a purely professional act. Professional workers have to make inferences when they treat cases; they must translate between generic knowledge and the specific clients, dossiers, or problems they have before them (Schön 1983).

In the medical context, the client position corresponding to this expert professional is the sick role, as delineated by Talcott Parsons. Patients are in need of expert services because neither they nor their lay associates—families, next of kin—know what is wrong or what to do about it, nor do they have access to the necessary facilities to remedy it (Parsons 2005 [1951]). Thus, according to the norms of the sick role, the sick person is expected to passively perceive the sickness as a problem and thus to seek help—from the professionals. In such descriptions, the professionals act and treat patients, clients, problems, and cases. In this view, the experiential knowledge and strategic agency of patients and clients are invisible.

Occupational Control

Professionalism is a way of organizing work and controlling workers (Evetts 2013). Occupational control of the work by the practitioners themselves is crucial to professionalism (Freidson 2001). Professionalism, in this sense, is a matter of shielding professional practices from external influences. The elements of professionalism are specialized work grounded in theoretical knowledge, exclusive jurisdiction over a field of labor, credentials based on a formal training program, and an ideology that asserts commitment to doing good work rather than for economic gain, and commitment to quality rather than efficiency of work. This ideology requires the professionals to be independent of those they are supposed to serve, to pursue an ideal goal of service and care that reaches beyond the specific goals of those to be served, the employer, or the client (Freidson 2001). According to the logic of professionalism, relationships of trust characterize practitioner–client and practitioner–management interactions since competencies are assumed to be guaranteed by education, training, and licensing (Evetts 2013).

Neglecting the Clients

In the logic of this conceptual environment, research invariably neglects the clients of the professionals. The study of professions and professionalism has centered largely on the professionalization projects of various occupational groups. Their power and privileges, interprofessional relationships and competition, the role of professions in society, the regulation of professionals, the impact of bureaucratic organizations, and the management of professional autonomy have been the major topics of research (Adams 2015).

The actual work of professionals and their relationships with their clients has received less attention. Abbott (1988) has emphasized the need for studies of professionalization to shift the focus from the organizational structure of professions to the content and control of their work. Still, his own analyses mainly have dealt with the relationships between various occupational groups. The exception is that client differentiation is viewed as a source of professional status differentiation.

Service users occasionally enter the descriptions of professionalism in discussions of the related logic of markets (Freidson 2001). This is specifically in terms of issues of consumer control and through perceptions of consumers being competent to choose whom to perform work for them, to determine what tasks they will perform, and to judge the results. Some view the state as disciplining the professionals through patient choice (Dent 2006b, 2006a).

More often than not, service users are portrayed as clients benefitting from and being reliant on professional expertise. Clients are bound to trust the professionals, and professionalism is the guarantee against mistreatment in the asymmetric relationship between knowledgeable experts and unknowing clients. Professionalism requires professionals to be worthy of trust, which means to put clients first, to maintain confidentiality, and not to use their knowledge for fraudulent purposes (Evetts 2013). The actual relationship between the professionals and the service users is rarely a topic of research (Adams 2015; Bourgeault, Hirschkorn, and Sainsaulieu 2011). That patients and clients are being protected by the professionals' code of ethics seems to be taken for granted rather than being something actually researched.

OUTSIDE THE PROFESSIONS DOMAIN

In another body of research—outside the domain of studies of occupations and professions—patients and clients are depicted rather differently, as strategic actors and agents in movements and organized interest groups. Through collective actions, experiences of illness are converted into grievances and requests for governmental policy (Banaszak-Holl, Levitsky, and Zald 2010; Brown et al. 2011). The point of departure is client stakes and interests, with professions and professionalization being an ancillary concern.

In this context, patients also are seen as drivers of medicalization in the widest sense of the term as social movements, interest groups, and consumers strive to turn their troubles into medical problems (Ballard and Elston 2005; Conrad 2005; Gubrium and Järvinen 2014). Patient self-help groups are seen to be among the most determined in demanding medicalization in the form of recognition of their conditions as being caused by objective, even if not yet confirmed, pathological processes. To aspiring patients, medicalization accords some degree of absolution from moral responsibility for their actions or conditions, although such absolution is conditioned on the willingness to accept appropriate advice and treatment from medical professionals. The argumentation is in line with Parsons' description of the sick role (Parsons 2005 [1951]) as a role allowing exemptions from normal responsibilities and obligations, legitimized by the professionals; that the problem cannot be cured by the sick person's acts of will but must be cared for by the professionals.

However, expanded medicalization is by no means an obvious consequence of social movement advocacy. Several analyses of groups struggling with illnesses or disabilities describe how these groups strive to limit professional intrusion in their daily lives and to challenge the mandate of professionals to act politically on behalf of their clients and define what is in their best interests (Barnes 2003; Barnes and Mercer 1996; Haug and Sussman 1969). Among those most prominently advocating human rights, self-determinacy, and a voice of their own are the disability movement and the user and survivor movements in mental health care (McLean 2010; Shakespeare 1993). These movements contained elements of rejection of professional expertise as well as the introduction of alternative conceptualizations of the meanings of disability and mental problems. Demedicalization rather than medicalization is the consequence of their demands.

RESEARCHING THE SERVICE USER'S PERSPECTIVE

This brings us to the leading question of my research: how is professionalism and professional intervention actually perceived from the service user's perspective? The question inspired an analysis of the statements and arguments raised in a study of the consultation process that was connected with the organizational restructuring of the specialized health services in Norway. This included somatic and psychiatric care, as well as the specialized treatment of addiction.

The Empirical Material

The resulting empirical material derives from a two-year process of service user involvement in the southeastern region of Norway. From consultations with service user spokespersons in relation to qualities of importance to patients that should be taken into consideration when outlining a reformed structure of specialized health care, I incorporated reports from focus group discussions taking place at a "dialogue conference." The conference had 87 registered participants speaking on behalf of organizations representing people with different kinds of health problems. These included mental problems, physical impairments, blindness/visual impairments, deafblindness, developmental disabilities, heart disease, cancer, lung disease, allergies, rheumatism, kidney transplants, diabetes, cerebral palsy, Parkinson's disease, muscular atrophy, and drug abuse. In addition, steps were taken to include spokespersons representing older people, immigrants, and ethnic minorities.

Representatives of the conference organizers also were present. These included the regional "user council" (ten participants) and four managers from the regional health authorities. The managers took part in the opening of the conference, where they introduced the aim of the restructuring process, and in the concluding part, where they listened to feedback from the conference participants.

For most of the participants, it was not their first time as a spokesperson. Many were "professional amateurs," so to speak (Alm Andreassen, Breit, and Legard 2014)—trained spokespersons familiar with the kind of setting they were attending and with its rules, norms, and expectations. They knew that they would be asked to share opinions from the service users' perspective and that they were expected not only to tell their own stories but primarily to convey experiences and speak on behalf of the constituencies they were there to represent.

The discussions were organized into ten focus groups, divided according to homogeneity in illness and disability into four different categories: (a) long-term illnesses, (b) acute and severe illnesses or trauma, (c) congenital impairments, and (d) complex, troubled youth (combination of mental problems and drug abuse). Members of the regional user council chaired the focus group discussions and recorded what the participants said. The groups were advised not to strive for consensus or unified conclusions but rather to report contrasting or contradictory viewpoints if such were present in the group. Highlights from each group discussion were introduced in plenary sessions so that participants from other groups could comment on and add to the views presented.

All group discussions were reported in writing, and altogether the reports totaled around 30 pages. In addition, I was present for the whole day, and I observed the conversations and took notes. My task as a researcher was to summarize the opinions and experiences presented at the conference and thus to provide documentation of the users' points of view concerning forthcoming service restructuring. I focus here on the discussion of which aspects of the health service are important from the service users' perspective when it comes to providing high-quality health services with good treatment outcomes and the efficient use of the resources. Many of the statements touched on facets of the issue of professionalism in service intervention.

The Analytic Process

My analytical interest was oriented toward the issue of what was advocated or asked for in relation to the research question. It was my intention to understand the frame of reference from which the users spoke: what do their requests tell us about their lives—the conditions and circumstances that give rise to these wishes, experiences, and statements?

Rather than condensing the empirical material, this analysis expands the material by adding semiotic interpretations of the data (Kvale 1996), inspired by a semiotic cluster analysis (Feldman 1995). In such an analysis, the researcher first registers "denotations" in the material (the primary

Semiotic analysis	Denotations	Connotations	Institutional concerns
The analysis of this material	The statements ➤	The frame of reference in which they are embedded ➤	The condensed messages and their implications for health services

FIGURE 2.1 Translation of the semiotic analysis of this empirical material.

meaning of statements or accounts), then investigates the "connotations" (the meaning within a specific setting), and finally considers the institutional concerns implicated. In my analysis, the denotations are the utterances and statements from the conference discussions. The connotations are the frame of reference in which the statements must be understood. This frame of reference is not the actual context in which the statements are produced; rather, it is deduced by the researcher from the content of these statements. Finally, the institutional concerns are the messages implied in the denotations and connotations. Figure 2.1 illustrates the translation of this form of analysis into an analysis that works for this particular empirical material.

With most statements, the process of framing and identifying implications was straightforward. Some demanded more reflection regarding their interpretations and inferences. The process is illustrated in Table 2.1, which shows the inferences from a sample of two statements contained in the reports from the group discussions. The first column at the left is the statement from a patient spokesperson; the two columns to the right of that are the inferences produced through the analysis.

This analytic process also allows the researcher to make sense of statements that, at the tangible level—the level of denotations—are incoherent. Table 2.2 illustrates this. All the statements are collected from the same discussion. Every statement asks for some parts of the health and welfare service system to be in a position to instruct the others, but, taken together, they demonstrate no consensus concerning which part of the system should be in charge. Instead, the report from the discussion gives the impression that the preference concerning who should be in charge is dependent on how supportive the individuals are of the patient's own view. At the level of connotations, the statements reveal common underlying experiences.

TABLE 2.1 Sample Statement Analyses Illustrating the Process of Interpretation

THE STATEMENT	THE FRAME OF REFERENCE	THE MESSAGE
"When acute hospital admission for mental problems is necessary, transportation should be by ambulance, not a police car."	(a) An experience of stigma—being seen as a criminal. (b) An experience of fear—being imprisoned instead of helped; feeling threatened instead of taken care of.	(a) Offended dignity—not treated the same way as patients with other kinds of diagnoses. (b) Ineffective, self-defeating treatment.
"When admitted to a psychiatric hospital, the patient should be only lightly medicated, to enable realistic observation of the mental illness."	(a) An experience that the patients' relatives have seen; they are familiar with manifestations and impacts of mental illness that the professionals fail to see because of heavy medication. (b) An experience that the next of kin has a kind of knowledge that the professionals do not have and that they do not obtain unless they actually ask for it from those who have it.	(a) Hospital practice might result in insufficient treatment. (b) The hospitals should listen to those who are involved in the patients' everyday life and everyday manifestations of their illness.

SERVICE USER CONCEPTUALIZATION OF CARE

Turning to the findings, I start with four messages formulated as headlines, each of them containing many statements and relating frames. From the experiences and opinions of the user spokesperson, four key messages were extracted, each of which I will discuss in turn.

1. Care is not only provided by health care services.
2. Interventions involve lives, not just illnesses.
3. Co-morbidity is common—health care is organized around single issues.
4. Interventions should be knowledge-based and respectful.

TABLE 2.2 Illustration of Incoherent Statements with Common Underlying Experiences

STATEMENT	FRAMING	MESSAGE
"Patients should be listened to and referred to specialized services by general practitioners when the GP's competence is insufficient." "The specialized services should listen to the GP and carry out the requests of the referral no matter what opinions the specialized professional might hold." "The Labor and Welfare Administration refers patients for specialized health care examination, and their conclusions are re-examined by the Administration's own physicians." "Recommendations given by professionals in specialized health care are not mandatory for local health care."	An experience that health professionals hold and act on diverse and conflicting opinions about the health problems of the patient and continuously override or overrule one another. Thus, even when the patients' wishes and understanding of their illness have been recognized by one professional or one part of the system, patients are still at risk of being disregarded by other professionals.	In the encounter with the health and welfare system, the patients are vulnerable. They are exposed to an unpredictable system, where trust and confidence acquired once could be replaced by distrust and doubt. The consequence will be a feeling of insecurity.

Care Is Not Only Provided by Health Care Services

The first message derived from the material was that care is not only provided by health care services, a message related to a metaphor introduced to user spokespersons by the manager at the opening session of the conference. A picture showed a pyramid with a base consisting of the widespread, local first-line service of primary health care (home-based care, general practitioners, and nursing homes). Above this, there was a higher and regionalized level of more specialized secondary (hospital) care, followed by an even higher level of increasingly specialized and centralized third-line services. The pyramid metaphor aimed to illustrate the significance of primary health care. The argument of the manager was that primary care is the foundation of health care; the patients are only "temporarily discharged to hospitals."

In the subsequent discussion, one participant immediately commented: "The ground level is missing from the health care pyramid. We, the next of kin, are the base level of the health care system." His statement was only one of many that emphasized the role of the patients themselves and their relatives when it comes to treating, mastering, and living with illnesses and injuries. All of these statements conveyed, directly or implicitly, that health problems have to be handled by those stricken by illness and injuries, and that the health care system should enable them to do so through patient education, information, and available discharge summaries. The statement that "where and how information is given affects the course of the illness" illustrates the importance of information in coping with illness.

It is important to underscore that the enabling resources referenced by the participant were not only knowledge provided by professionals but also experiential knowledge provided by fellow patients and service users. The importance of peer support was illustrated by this emotional utterance: "Peers are a tremendous resource. They give patients hope—they are shining examples." Moreover, the participants emphasized that it is necessary to enable not only the patients themselves but also their next of kin, and that relatives should not be seen merely as resources for the patients to provide them with support and care but valued in their own right as people who are hurt, burdened, and experience sequelae. An example underlining this point was the statement that "the next of kin needs adapted assistance and treatment, and the longer the primary patient is thrown back and forth between services, the larger are the needs of their relatives."

Interventions Involve Lives, Not Just Illnesses

The second message derived from the material was that interventions involve not only illnesses but also everyday life following professional intervention. It was emphasized that the effect of hospital treatment would be enlarged if systematically incorporated into, and considered to belong to, a course of recovery in which many other services contribute. The course of recovery should start at admittance to the hospital, as stated in the argument of a spokesperson that "planning for discharge should start at the time of hospital admittance." The process of recovery should include rehabilitation and systematic follow-up over extended periods.

The participants pointed out that specialized health services should reach out to primary care services and provide treatment closer to where patients live, through ambulant teams, mobile outpatient services, ICT, and telemedicine. They stressed the need for coordinated action across service levels and sectors, as illustrated in this statement: "Primary and secondary health care should either enter into predictable cooperation, or else there is a need for 'pilots' to accompany service users through the system."

They argued that for those living with chronic illness, opportunities for continuous contact with health care should be available, such as "patient-controlled services" initiated by patients when they feel they are in need. The following typical statement illustrates this message: "Frequent follow-up of patients is needed: an 'open door' to outpatient clinics, hospital beds to which the patients themselves control admittance, emergency telephone lines open to patients with long-term illnesses."

Co-morbidity Is Common—Health Care Is Organized Around Single Issues

The third message derived from the material emphasized that many patients have more than one diagnosis, that mental health problems could follow from physical problems or that mental health patients could also have physical problems (which are often ignored or missed), and that drug abuse could cause, as well as be caused by, mental and physical health problems. In short, many patients experience a version of the statement that "it never rains but it pours." The following comment illustrates this message: "Drug abuse and mental health problems are complex illnesses, often with concomitant somatic diseases, social deprivation and discrimination."

While patients have complex problems, the health care organizations deal with them problem by problem. They are geared toward single problems approached through sequential investigations, tests, and interventions, the participants argued. Because of this one-sidedness, health care institutions are seldom equipped to handle co-morbidity or multiple problems, as illustrated by these statements: "Healthcare institutions that treat bodily problems lack knowledge of and competence to treat concomitant drug problems"; "Hospitals have insufficient capacity and are not staffed to take care of patients with co-morbidity."

Participants' statements explained that although people with chronic illnesses and impairments are among the most frequent users of health care, the institutions neither have buildings adapted to impairments nor offer sufficient assistance with the everyday activities of life. The following statement is an example: "People in need of assistance with personal hygiene are excluded from several rehabilitation institutions because this kind of assistance is not offered." Thus, health services are at their most inadequate when it comes to the neediest and most troubled of patients.

Interventions Should Be Knowledge-Based and Respectful

The fourth message—the request for knowledge-based and respectful encounters—pointed to experiences of professional incompetence and insufficient professional expertise, as illustrated by the comment that "emergency wards should know that intoxication is an illness and that drug abusers are also protected by patients' rights legislation." The message also referred to experiences of demeaning encounters with the health care system. Participants told of service users not being seen and met with respect, experiences similar to those expressed elsewhere in this volume by Eriksson and Jacobsson (Chapter 13) and by Järvinen (Chapter 3).

Statements communicated that practices of ignorance and disrespect were present in the health care system, as indicated earlier in Table 2.1 by the experience of stigma and fear—of being seen as a criminal and feeling threatened instead of cared for—when transported to a mental hospital in a police car instead of an ambulance.

This message was voiced especially from spokespersons of drug abusers, mental-health patients, and people with "lifestyle diseases" or from immigrant and ethnic minority communities, summed up in statements such as this: "Discrimination against young people and ethnic minorities hinders early interventions. Taboos, prejudice and discrimination must be identified and counteracted."

The participants also requested up-to-date education and training programs, knowledge-based practices, elimination of ineffective practices, and supervision of primary health care from experts within specialized hospitals. In addition, they argued for research on service users' experiences and for research together with service users.

ORGANIZATIONAL SYSTEMS AND EXPERIENTIAL KNOWLEDGE

Two user-defined facets of professionalism come to light in this material. One is the effect of formal organizations on professionalism, and the other is the need for a broader and more comprehensive understanding of expertise that incorporates the everyday recovery work of the patients and their significant others.

Service Users Encounter Organizational Systems

The issues raised by the service user representatives demonstrate that when shedding light on the health care context within which their wishes can be understood, service user spokespersons emphasize a feature of medical intervention different from the dominant feature of the literature of the professions. From a service user perspective, these are interventions not by a professional but by a system of organizations. The intervention is not merely (or primarily) an act of a single professional but procedures and routines of professional organizations.

Two consequences are evident. First is that the code of ethics of the professionals does not protect people against demeaning practices inherent in organizational routines, as in the case of transporting acutely ill mental patients in police cars. The second is that the professionals are guided only to some degree by shared, consistent, and coherent professional knowledge and ethics. The professionals are also guided by the tasks of the organizations within which they perform their professional work. This is illustrated by the wishes expressed in Table 2.2 for professionals in a position to overturn opinions and decisions of other professionals, and by the emphasis on the problems in encountering a disunited health care system ill equipped to deal with co-morbidity and complex conditions. The professional understanding of the patient's problem takes shape from his or her organizational position.

The literature on professionalism often depicts organizations in opposition to professionalism and perceives professionalism and organization as intrinsically conflicting (Bourgeault, Hirschkorn, and Sainsaulieu 2011; Evetts 2013; Noordegraaf 2011). Freidson (2001) describes the ideal-typical logic of professionalism and the logic of organizations as two contrasting logics. The logic of organization implies a rational-legal bureaucracy, clear lines of authority, and hierarchical control by people in leadership positions whose education equips them to direct or lead specialists, consumers, or citizens. In contrast, in the logic of professionalism, professionals ostensibly control their own work and the work of colleagues independently of both managers and consumers, in order to be able to exercise discretionary judgment grounded in abstract theory and concepts (Freidson 2001). The result of combining them is a kind of "organizational professionalism" (Evetts 2013), which amounts to standardization of work procedures and practices, externalized forms of regulation, and accountability measures such as target setting and performance reviews.

On the other hand, some have depicted the relationship between organizations and professionals in more hybrid terms. The concept of "organized professionalism" spawns a different understanding of the relationship between professionals and organizations (Noordegraaf 2011). Here, organizational features are not opposed to professional features but import dimensions of professional work. "Organized professionalism" recognizes the multiproblem character of the situations professionals have to deal with—their "organizational embeddedness," if you will (see Gubrium, Chapter 1, this volume)—which requires multiprofessional forms of organizing. Within this conceptualization, professionalism must include the crossing of specialist boundaries and organizational borders in order to treat and support patients effectively. It is a professionalism that works through and across organizations, and through professionals that apply not only skills within their own particular specialized field of expertise but also communication and coordination skills.

From the perspective of service users, living with chronic illness and disabilities in particular implies that they continuously encounter an organizational system of professional services and are in need of assistance that cannot be met by single professionals or one professional service (see Solvang, Chapter 7, this volume). Rather, they are dependent on a range of coordinated assistance spanning specialized professions and service organizations. A consistent theme of their messages is the desire for professionalism that involves interdisciplinary and interorganizational collaboration. A conceptualization of professionalism that embraces organizational aspects and actions seems to be the consequence of this service user perspective.

User Recovery Work

From the issues voiced by the service users, an image of professional work is evident that is different from that envisioned by Abbott (1988) and others, where the core comes in the form of diagnosis—inference—treatment. While the theory of professions emphasizes professional intervention in the problems of clients, the issues advocated by the user spokespersons point to the recovery work performed by the patients themselves and their families, and to the role of professionals and professional expertise in managing everyday life with chronic illnesses, injuries, and impairments.

I found this divergent perception to be even more pronounced in a related study of service user involvement (Alm Andreassen 2004). In that study, individuals with brain injuries were engaged in discussions with professionals regarding an issue that occupied the professionals: which professional interventions had made a difference in the life of the injured person? The difference was palpable. The professionals talked about rehabilitation in the language of a professional bureaucracy: of goal setting, goal achievement, processes delimited in time, differentiation from acute treatment, and ongoing care. The people with brain injuries, in contrast, talked about rehabilitating themselves, about rediscovering themselves, and about insight more than interventions. To them, rehabilitation was an indefinite process, going on steadily, without an endpoint (see Eriksson and Jacobsson, Chapter 13, this volume).

These perceptions challenge the professionals' claims both to classify a problem and to take action on it. A different interpretation of the problem is introduced by the spokespersons. The problem is not merely an illness, injury, or impairment requiring intervention but is also about dealing with everyday lives affected by such health problems, indicating that the problem, in its narrow definition, has not been fully treated or taken care of when the patient leaves the institutional sphere of professional health care. Hence, because, according to Abbott, the definition of the problem also defines the responsibility of the professionals, an alternative definition of the problem implies an alternative definition of professional responsibility. To treat is not solely to intervene in the patients' problems but is also to provide assistance with the work undertaken by patients and their relatives in the matter of living with the problems. While the image of the pyramid described earlier leaves the patients and their relatives *outside* the health care system, implicitly regarding them as recipients—as receivers of services provided by the work performed by the services that make up the pyramid—the message of the service user spokespersons highlights the work of the patients themselves and their next of kin.

This also speaks of a perception of professional knowledge as being incapable of supplying the experiential forms of knowledge necessary in addressing the everyday lives of those coping with illnesses and impairments. The experiential knowledge of those in comparable situations, the cosufferers, is advanced as an additional source of expertise. In this respect, their message contains an impulse to demedicalization, a transformation of the problem from a problem to be handled by the medical profession and the health care system to a problem or trouble to be handled by those whose life it is a part of, and with the help of the experiential knowledge acquired through managing the problems. "Expert" knowledge, in other words, has to be complemented with knowledge derived from the experiences of the patients; that is, both the knowledge held by the individual patients about their own situation and the knowledge held by peers, by their "own" as Goffman (1963) puts it (also see Shakespeare and Collins, Chapter 12, this volume).

Also worth noting is that the messages do not imply denial of the significance of professional expertise. This is in line with findings from other studies in which patients call for trustworthy professionals (Allen, Wainwright, and Hutchinson 2011; Lupton 1997; see also Järvinen, Chapter 3, this volume). Professionalism is sought as a valuable asset, despite experiences that might otherwise give rise to distrust.

The message about the work of users themselves and their next of kin resonates with extensive "long-term conditions management literature" describing how people with chronic illnesses cope with their illness, recovery, and rehabilitation. Here, the impact of biographical interruption is described, as well as ways of mobilizing resources, maintaining usual activities, and establishing continuity in their daily lives (Bury 1982; Charmaz 1983; Kleinman 1988).

The patients' view is presented as a source of understanding, not merely a distortion, in the eyes of the doctor. Put differently, illness resides not only in bodily lesions but also in the mind and social relationships (Allen, Wainwright, and Hutchinson 2011; Armstrong 1984; Lupton 1997). As Arthur Kleinman (1988) emphasized, the explanatory models of illness episodes and progressions as described by patients and their families help professionals take the patient's perspective seriously in organizing strategies for clinical care. Applying patient-centered care and approaching the patient's view becomes not only a matter of respect and regard but also a means of enabling adequate care. The image that guides professional intervention still seems to be one of professional intervention as the remedy for illnesses and injuries. In this context, Robert Merton's image of the sick role and the concurrent position of professional expertise seems remarkably persistent (Lutfey 2005).

While the message of the service users to some extent complies with the sick role, as delineated by Parsons (a need for professional expertise and professional services to amend their problems), the passivity of the sick role misrepresents the everyday recovery work of the patients. While the message displays the service users' wish for expertise in which to place their trust, the message contains no visions of a life where illness could be entrusted to the health care system only (see Greener, Chapter 14, this volume).

The message of the service users instead links to descriptions of the recovery work of patients: how patients participate in the managing and shaping of their own illness trajectories (Strauss 1985). According to Strauss and his colleagues, patients' recovery work is part of the division of labor in hospitals. It is work that *mirrors* the staff's work, work that is *supplementary* to the staff's work, work that is a *substitute* for work that staff should have done or that the patients believe they should have done. It also comprises forms of work beyond what the staff might conceive of as the locus of their own responsibility, such as coping with highly personalized, deep-seated issues of identity precipitated by the illness. Analyzing the degrees of work as work "on" or work "with," Strauss delineates a continuum between two poles: (a) the person treated primarily as an object, as if he or she were non-existent, and (b) the person explicitly regarded as a member of the working team, as if the division of labor includes him or her as an essential element in getting the recovery project done.

Recent policy discussions envisage activated, responsible patients capable of self-management and self-care, meaning those who are able to monitor their own status and control the medication for their long-term conditions. New health technologies seemingly increase the space and tools for these forms of patient work. In Strauss's terms, this kind of work mainly mirrors or supplements the work of the professionals. It is professionally delegated work, offering opportunities to relieve professionals of standardized or "dirty" tasks (Rogers et al. 2011). It is not necessarily depicted as "work" but rather as "participation" in the work of professionals, who for their part have to engage in the "invisible" work—teaching, motivating, instructing—presumed necessary to produce active patients (Oudshoorn 2008).

The magnitude of this patient work is illustrated by Mrs. Alcott's story, which is a vignette of illness-as-experience described in Kleinman's (1988) book *Illness Narratives*. Mrs. Alcott is a married woman in her forties with two teenage daughters. She has early-onset and ever-worsening diabetes. Her patient work comprises treating herself with insulin and doing her own blood sugar and urine sugar tests, controlling the diabetes and working hard to control the risk factors, carefully regulating her diet, exercise, and relaxation to handle circulatory insufficiencies. These are part of every episode of new complications, such as visual problems (diabetes retinopathy), toe amputations, coronary artery insufficiency (angina), and amputation of the leg below the knee (due to gangrenous ulceration causing infection in the bone), as well as administering the treatment and work of her rehabilitation. Even more demanding, it seems, is the never-ending work of grieving for her many losses, and, for every new loss, fighting her way back and restoring her normal life as a mother and wife, still knowing that all she is facing is a long, downhill battle. This kind of work is what the health services seem to conceive of as outside the locus of their own work. It is "unending work and care" taking place not within the institutional context of health care but at home in the daily lives of the patients and their relatives (Corbin and Strauss 1988).

REIMAGINING THE PROFESSIONAL–SERVICE USER RELATIONSHIP

The policy of service user involvement has provided people living with chronic illnesses, disabilities, mental problems, and addictions with arenas in which to express opinions about the relationship between professionals and service users. Inherent in their messages is an experience-near conceptualization of professional intervention. It contrasts with the view more or less implicitly residing in presentations of professions and professionalism. Reimagining the relationship from a service user perspective, the essence of treatment and care is not just the work that the professionals do in relation to their clients' problems but also extends to and includes the work of patients in recovery. In this context, a signal ingredient of professional work is to enable the daily recovery work of patients and their significant others.

Oddly enough, this is a rather old story, seemingly told again and again. Among the participants at the conference, many concluded that everything had been said before. Why, then, are the messages being repeated again and again? After all, the recovery work of patients was outlined in research three decades ago (Corbin and Strauss 1988; Strauss 1985). The answer can partly be found in a sociocultural framework in which only paid work performed through occupations is regarded as "work." Thus, the observation of Strauss (1985:191), that because the patients are "not employees of the hospitals and have no status as health professionals or other kinds of health workers" they are not easily conceived of as actually working, still holds validity. Searches on Google Scholar for "work of patients" or "patient work" mostly reveal publications on the subject of "return to work" of patients with various diagnoses, as well as the patient work provided by health care professionals: the work with patients. The work of patients seems invisible, which extends significantly to the literature of professions and professionalism.

Better understanding of the role clients play is particularly critical in assessing the work of professions within service organizations where clients are directly involved in their mandate, argue Bourgeault, Hirschkorn, and Sainsaulieu (2011). Bringing the everyday experience of patients and their relatives into discussions about responsibility for health care immediately points toward an expansion of the medical domain. However, refocusing from the work of professionals to the work of service users implies no absolution from responsibility, as emphasized in the concept of medicalization. Rather, the service users' reformulation of professionalism seems to be based on the premise that patients and their next of kin do, and have to, take care of themselves, and also on a perception, derived from experience, that the work of controlling, caring, mourning, and restoring could never be handed over to professional services.

REFERENCES

Abbott, Andrew. 1988. *The System of Professions: An Essay on the Division of Expert Labor.* Chicago: University of Chicago Press.

Aberbach, Joel D., and Tom Christensen. 2005. "Citizens and Consumers." *Public Management Review* 7(2): 225–246. doi: 10.1080/14719030500091319.

Adams, Tracey L. 2015. "Sociology of Professions: International Divergences and Research Directions." *Work, Employment and Society* 29(1): 154–165. doi: 10.1177/0950017014523467.

Allen, Dawn, Megan Wainwright, and Thomas Hutchinson. 2011. "'Non-compliance' as Illness Management: Hemodialysis Patients' Descriptions of Adversarial

Patient–Clinician Interactions." *Social Science and Medicine* 73(1): 129–134. doi: http://dx.doi.org/10.1016/j.socscimed.2011.05.018.

Alm Andreassen, Tone. 2004. *Brukermedvirkning, politikk og velferdsstat: Dr. polit. avhandling ved Institutt for Sosiologi og samfunnsgeografi, Universitetet i Oslo.* Arbeidsforskningsinstituttets Skriftserie 13. Oslo: Arbeidsforskningsinstituttet.

Alm Andreassen, Tone. 2008. "'Asymmetric Mutuality': User Involvement as a Government–Voluntary Sector Relationship in Norway." *Nonprofit and Voluntary Sector Quarterly* 37(2): 281–299.

Alm Andreassen, Tone. 2009. "The Consumerism of 'Voice' in Norwegian Health Policy and Its Dynamics in Transformation of Health Service." *Public Money and Management* 29(2): 117–122.

Alm Andreassen, Tone, Eric Breit, and Sveinung Legard. 2014. "The Making of 'Professional Amateurs': Professionalizing the Voluntary Work of Service User Representatives." *Acta Sociologica* 57(4): 325–340. doi: http://dx.doi.org10.1177/0001699314552736.

Armstrong, David. 1984. "The Patient's View." *Social Science and Medicine* 18(9): 737–744. doi: http://dx.doi.org/10.1016/0277–9536(84)90099–6.

Ballard, Karen, and Mary Ann Elston. 2005. "Medicalisation: A Multidimensional Concept." *Social Theory and Health* 3(3): 228–241. doi: 10.1057/palgrave.sth.8700053.

Banaszak-Holl, Jane, Sandra Levitsky, and Mayer N. Zald. 2010. *Social Movements and the Transformation of American Health Care.* Oxford: Oxford University Press.

Barnes, Colin. 2003. "Rehabilitation for Disabled People: A 'Sick' Joke?" *Scandinavian Journal of Disability Research* 5(1): 7–23. doi: 10.1080/15017410309512609.

Barnes, Colin, and Geoffrey Mercer. 1996. *Exploring the Divide: Illness and Disability.* Leeds: Disability.

Barnes, Marian, and Phil Cotterell. 2012. *Critical Perspectives on User Involvement.* Bristol: Policy.

Barnes, Marian, Janet Newman, and Helen Sullivan. 2007. *Power, Participation and Political Renewal: Case Studies in Public Participation.* Bristol: Policy.

Beresford, Peter. 2002. "User Involvement in Research and Evaluation: Liberation or Regulation?" *Social Policy and Society* 1(2): 95–105. doi:10.1017/S1474746402000222.

Bourgeault, Ivy Lynn, Kristine Hirschkorn, and Ivan Sainsaulieu. 2011. "Relations Between Professions and Organizations: More Fully Considering the Role of the Client." *Professions and Professionalism* 1(1): 67–86.

Brante, Thomas. 2011. "Professions as Science Based Occupations." *Professions and Professionalism* 1(1): 4–20. doi: dx.doi.org/10.7577/pp.v1i1.147.

Brown, Phil, Racel Morello-Frosch, Stephen Zavestoski, Laura Senier, Rebecca Gasior Altman, Elizabeth Hoover, Sabrina McCormick, Brian Mayer, and Crystal Adams. 2011. "Health Social Movements: Advancing Traditional Medical Sociology Concepts." In *Handbook of the Sociology of Health, Illness, and Healing*, edited by Bernice A. Pescosolido, Jack K. Martin, Jane D. McLeod, and Anne Rogers, 117–137. New York: Springer.

Bury, Michael. 1982. "Chronic Illness as Biographical Disruption." *Sociology of Health and Illness* 4(2): 167–182. doi: 10.1111/1467–9566.ep11339939.

Charmaz, Kathy. 1983. "Loss of Self: A Fundamental Form of Suffering in the Chronically Ill." *Sociology of Health and Illness* 5(2): 168–195. doi: 10.1111/1467–9566.ep10491512.

Conrad, Peter. 2005. "The Shifting Engines of Medicalization." *Journal of Health and Social Behavior* 46(1): 3–14. doi: 10.1177/002214650504600102.

Corbin, Juliet M., and Anselm L. Strauss. 1988. *Unending Work and Care: Managing Chronic Illness at Home*. San Francisco: Jossey-Bass.

Crawford, M. J., T. Aldridge, K. Bhui, D. Rutter, C. Manley, T. Weaver, P. Tyrer, and N. Fulop. 2003. "User Involvement in the Planning and Delivery of Mental Health Services: A Cross-Sectional Survey of Service Users and Providers." *Acta Psychiatrica Scandinavia* 107(6): 410–414.

Dent, Mike. 2006a. "Disciplining the Medical Profession? Implications of Patient Choice for Medical Dominance." *Health Sociology Review* 15(5): 458–468.

Dent, Mike. 2006b. "Patient Choice and Medicine in Health Care." *Public Management Review* 8(3): 449–462. doi: 10.1080/14719030600853360.

Evetts, Julia. 2013. "Professionalism: Value and Ideology." *Current Sociology* 61(5–6): 778–796. doi: 10.1177/0011392113479316.

Faulkner, Alison, and Phil Thomas. 2002. "User-Led Research and Evidence-Based Medicine." *British Journal of Psychiatry* 180(1): 1–3. doi: 10.1192/bjp.180.1.1.

Feldman, Martha S. 1995. *Strategies for Interpreting Qualitative Data*. Thousand Oaks, CA: Sage.

Freidson, Eliot. 2001. *Professionalism: The Third Logic*. London: Polity.

Goffman, Erving. 1963. *Stigma: Notes on the Management of Spoiled Identity*. Harmondsworth: Penguin.

Gubrium, Jaber F., and Margaretha Järvinen. 2014. *Turning Troubles into Problems: Clientization in Human Services*. London: Routledge.

Haug, Marie R., and Marvin B. Sussman. 1969. "Professional Autonomy and the Revolt of the Client." *Social Problems* 17(2): 153–161.

Kleinman, Arthur. 1988. *The Illness Narratives: Suffering, Healing, and the Human Condition*. New York: Basic.

Kvale, Steinar. 1996. *Interviews: An Introduction to Qualitative Research Interviewing*. Thousand Oaks, CA: Sage.

Lupton, Deborah. 1997. "Consumerism, Reflexivity and the Medical Encounter." *Social Science and Medicine* 45(3): 373–381. doi: http://dx.doi.org/10.1016/S0277-9536(96)00353-X.

Lutfey, Karen. 2005. "On Practices of 'Good Doctoring': Reconsidering the Relationship Between Provider Roles and Patient Adherence." *Sociology of Health and Illness* 27(4): 421–447. doi: 10.1111/j.1467–9566.2005.00450.x.

Martin, Graham P. 2009. "Public and User Participation in Public Service Delivery: Tensions in Policy and Practice." *Sociology Compass* 3(2): 310–326. doi: 10.1111/j.1751–9020.2009.00200.x.

McLaughlin, Hugh. 2010. "Keeping Service User Involvement in Research Honest." *British Journal of Social Work* 40(5): 1591–1608. doi: 10.1093/bjsw/bcp064.

McLean, Athena. 2010. "The Mental Health Consumers/Survivors Movement in the United States." In *A Handbook for the Study of Mental Health*, edited by Teresa L. Scheid and Tony N. Brown, 461–477. Cambridge: Cambridge University Press.

Noordegraaf, Mirko. 2011. "Risky Business: How Professionals and Professional Fields (Must) Deal with Organizational Issues." *Organization Studies* 32(10): 1349–1371. doi: 10.1177/0170840611416748.

Oudshoorn, Nelly. 2008. "Diagnosis at a Distance: The Invisible Work of Patients and Healthcare Professionals in Cardiac Telemonitoring Technology." *Sociology of Health and Illness* 30(2): 272–288. doi: 10.1111/j.1467–9566.2007.01032.x.

Parsons, Talcott. 2005[1951]. "Social Structure and Dynamic Process." In *Medical Sociology, Volume I*, edited by Graham Scambler. London: Routledge. Original edition published as *The Social System*, London: Routledge.

Rogers, Anne, Sue Kirk, Claire Gately, Carl R. May, and Tracy Finch. 2011. "Established Users and the Making of Telecare Work in Long Term Condition Management: Implications for Health Policy." *Social Science and Medicine* 72(7): 1077–1084. doi: http://dx.doi.org/10.1016/j.socscimed.2011.01.031.

Rutter, D., C. Manley, T. Weaver, M. J. Crawford, and N. Fulop. 2004. "Patients or Partners? Case Studies of User Involvement in the Planning and Delivery of

Adult Mental Health Service in London." *Social Science and Medicine* 58(10): 1973–1984.

Schön, Donald A. 1983. *The Reflective Practitioner: How Professionals Think in Action*. New York: Basic.

Shakespeare, Tom. 1993. "Disabled People's Self-Organisation: A New Social Movement?" *Disability, Handicap and Society* 8(3): 249–264.

Smith, Elizabeth, Sheila Donovan, Peter Beresford, Jill Manthorpe, Sally Brearley, John Sitzia, and Fiona Ross. 2009. "Getting Ready for User Involvement in a Systematic Review." *Health Expectations* 12(2): 197–208. doi: 10.1111/j.1369–7625.2009.00535.x.

Strauss, Anselm L. 1985. *Social Organization of Medical Work*. Chicago: University of Chicago Press.

Tritter, Jonathan Q. 2009. "Revolution or Evolution: The Challenges of Conceptualizing Patient and Public Involvement in a Consumerist World." *Health Expectations* 12(3): 275–287. doi: 10.1111/j.1369–7625.2009.00564.x.

Trivedi, Premila, and Til Wykes. 2002. "From Passive Subjects to Equal Partners: Qualitative Review of User Involvement in Research." *British Journal of Psychiatry* 181(6): 468–472. doi: 10.1192/bjp.181.6.468.

Veronesi, Gianluca, and Kevin Keasey. 2013. "Patient and Public Participation in the English NHS: An Assessment of Experimental Implementation Processes." *Public Management Review* 17(4): 543–564. doi: 10.1080/14719037.2013.822526.

3

Expertise and Ambivalence in User-Focused Human Service Work

▸ MARGARETHA JÄRVINEN

IN THE PAST FEW DECADES, social work has become increasingly focused on client autonomy and empowerment, and shared expertise and decision making. Professionals in some parts of the human services field no longer regard themselves as experts who know what is "best for their clients" and who therefore play the leading part in setting up goals for client work (Baistow 1994/1995; Adams 1996; Gergen and McNamee 1992; Pease 2002). Rather, they define themselves as "facilitators" and "coaches," assisting the clients in choosing their own goals and guiding them in their process of change and self-development. In this view, the task of a facilitator or coach is not to solve the clients' problems but to create the best possible conditions for the clients to solve their own problems (Järvinen and Mik-Meyer 2012; also see Miller and Kontos, Chapter 8, this volume). In this chapter, I analyze the potentials and difficulties with which the new forms of client-centered social work may be associated by using the concept of *ambivalence* as my point of departure (see Eriksson and Jacobsson, Chapter 13, this volume).

In Denmark, new ways of working with service users have been especially prevalent in social work with young people (Nissen 2006; Vitus 2014; also see in this volume Solvang, Chapter 7, and Shakespeare and Collins, Chapter 12). The subfield that I will focus on in this chapter is work with young drug users at an addiction treatment center in Copenhagen. The center is regarded as one of the flagships of late modern social work in Denmark, functioning as a model for the development of addiction treatment and youth work in the country and attracting attention also from other countries. The chapter is based on qualitative interviews with clients and staff members at the center.

In a classic text from the 1960s, which is often regarded as the start of the sociology of ambivalence, Merton and Barber (1963) described relations between professionals and their clients as representing a core type of ambivalent relationship. In Merton and Barber's view, there is a large measure of incompatibility in the social definition of behaviors, attitudes, and feelings related to the roles of professionals (e.g., doctors, lawyers, social workers) and an equal incompatibility in the different aspects of the client role. A doctor, for instance, must balance between affective neutrality and compassion and between authoritative decisions and the recognition that diagnoses are often provisional (Merton 1976:68). Patients and clients, according to Merton, often navigate between respect for and dependence on the expertise of the professionals on the one hand and experiences of helplessness, inferiority, and frustration on the other because they feel the services they receive are insufficient (p. 19ff.). I will use Merton's insights on the relationships between experts and clients as inspiration in my analysis. Just like the professional relationships described by Merton, the relationships in the present study are characterized by ambivalence. However, today's social workers and therapists operate with an expert role that deviates from the (typical) professional role of the 1960s and 1970s. They work with the ideal that human services should be based on client autonomy and responsibility and on processes that act "on the choices and self-steering properties of individuals" (Rose 1999:xxiii; also see in this volume Greener, Chapter 14, and Newman, Chapter 16). This creates new potentials for the service relationships but also new types of controversies, contradictions, and frustrations.

THE INTERVIEWS

The analysis centers on interviews[1] with 24 young people enrolled at a treatment center for youths with drug problems in Copenhagen. The interviewees were recruited via staff members who told their clients about the research project; those who were interested provided their telephone numbers, after which they were contacted by the interviewers. The interviews were semistructured and based on a schedule consisting of four overall themes covering drug use development and drug "career," present drug use, expectations when seeking treatment, and experiences with being in treatment. In addition to the young drug users, eight staff members (psychologists, social workers, and social education workers) at the center were interviewed. These interviews focused on the center's general treatment approach, therapeutic traditions influencing treatment, staff members' conceptions of drug problems and of clients' treatment goals, and progression in treatment. The main part of this chapter consists of an analysis of the interviews with clients, whereas the staff interviews are primarily used to provide background information about the center (for a more thorough analysis of the staff interviews, see Järvinen and Miller 2015).

The ages of the young drug users, 14 males and 10 females, varied between 19 and 25 years (with an average age of 22 years). Most of them had sought treatment because of problems with cannabis, which they all used or had previously used intensely and on a daily basis, whereas six described use of other drugs, such as ecstasy, amphetamines, or cocaine, as their main problem. At the time of the interviews, six participants were enrolled in education, five were in regular jobs (typically part-time and/or temporary), and the rest received welfare payments (social welfare or sickness benefits). The time period during which participants had been in contact with the center varied from six weeks to two and a half years. Most interviewees visited the center once or twice a week.

THE CENTER'S TREATMENT APPROACH

The center offers outpatient treatment—group therapy and individual therapy—to young people (under 25) with drug problems. Although the psychologists, social workers, and social education workers interviewed say they are inspired by different therapeutic approaches (e.g., cognitive therapy and solution-focused therapy), most of them work with methods based on the tradition of narrative therapy (White and Epston 1990; White 1995; Payne 2006) or constructivist therapy in general. Another important influence is the tradition of person-centered therapy (Rogers 1989, 1995) challenging hierarchical relationships between professionals and their clients, and pronouncing nonjudgment, strengthening of clients' self-esteem, client empowerment, and self-development.

The center, as it is described in written material and by the staff members interviewed, may be said to rest on three main principles. The first is user democracy and user self-determination. The users are defined as the experts on their own lives and as rational and responsible individuals who know what is in their own best interest. Human development is seen as possible only if the goals for change are defined by the clients themselves and if they feel they have ownership of the methods used to solve their problems. This does not mean that staff members renounce their own expertise about drug problems and in addiction treatment. The "client as expert" approach described in the interviews means instead that the young drug users should be allowed to define what is good and bad in their lives (including what is good and bad in illicit drug use), what they want to achieve in treatment, and at what pace they want to work for changes—and that professionals should guide them in this.

The second principle is that treatment should focus on the clients' resources and not only (or even primarily) on their problems. This is a central aspect of the form of therapeutic thinking that dominates the center (White and Epston 1990; White 1995). Part of narrative therapy is to focus on the positive aspects of people's lives and to "externalize" the negative aspects (here, drug problems) by making the clients regard them as exterior "things" they can combat and learn to control (Järvinen and Miller 2015).

Third, the center works with a goal (explicit or implicit, varying with the interviews) of "destigmatizing" drug users. Hence, staff members say they avoid words such as "abuse" and "abusers" because they regard them as derogatory and because they see the boundary between "use" and "abuse" as relative and dependent on the individual's own perspective and circumstances. Most staff members say they do not want to take a stance as to whether drugs in and of themselves are bad for the users. Related to this, "controlled use" of illicit drugs is defined as a treatment goal that is just as good as cessation of drug use. Staff members describe graduated goals as especially important for young people. They think that many of their young clients are not yet ready to give up drugs altogether—if abstinence was a demand, this would frighten them off. Also, some therapists associate cessation (as a treatment goal) with a pathology approach to drug use, where users are comprehended as helpless and incapable of self-control. These therapists reason that if clients are defined as unable to control their drug use, they become unable to control their drug use.

Staff members are well aware that the center's approach to addressing drug problems is different from more conventional treatment forms and also that their noncondemning attitudes toward illicit drug use may be controversial. They say, for instance, that they sometimes use the terms "abuse" and "abusers" when communicating with the authorities, such as the City of Copenhagen and the Ministry of Social Welfare, because these are the terms used in legislation and other official documents in Denmark. They also say that they have to submit to "diagnostic language" (describing their clients' problems in terms of addiction, depression, or anxiety) when writing statements (e.g., to social security offices or the Prison Service) if this is necessary for the progress of the client's case. However, they never share client information with other parts of the system without the young people's permission, and they always write the statements that need to be written together with them.

In written material, the center identifies an "evaluation culture" as part of its profile, meaning that critical reflection, supervision, and a willingness to continuously change the center's practice are stressed. The center has also published reports, based on questionnaires to former clients, showing good treatment outcomes: three-fourths of the respondents said either that they had reduced their drug use or (more seldom) stopped completely. As stated by the center, however, these are not "scientific," external evaluations of the center but smaller reports saying something about (the self-descriptions of) some former clients. At the time of writing this chapter, a scientific, representative study of the center's treatment model is under way comparing the model to other forms of addiction treatment in Denmark.

POSITIVELY SURPRISED

Many interviews with the young clients at the center contain the expression "I was positively surprised." In some cases, participants were simply astonished by the center's interior and the services it has to offer: a beautifully renovated old building, comfortable furniture, candles burning, sandwiches and soft drinks for free, and fitness and computer rooms for the clients to use. Isabella, 23 years old, explains: "This place is very different from other treatment centers.... When they told us there is fitness and brunch for free, I thought 'What? Do[es] the tax-payers' money really go to[ward] this? It's a waste of money. I was indignant.'" Isabella soon changed her mind, though, when she realized that many of the users are "frail and in need of some positive elements in life, and these small things make people feel good and safe." The welcoming atmosphere and the generous offers are also mentioned in many interviews with staff members (see Järvinen and Miller 2015). They say they want the clients to experience something completely different from the "everything is grave" ambience at social security offices, job centers, and traditional addiction treatment centers, where clients "buy a cup of coffee at the vending machine and sit looking at the annunciator for their turn" (quoted from a staff interview).

Another type of "I was surprised by" answer concerns the communication forms at the center, with many interviewees mentioning that they feel staff members "talk with us rather than about us." Emma, 22 years old, has been in psychiatric treatment at a hospital and compares the center to her previous experience:

> It's very different from what I expected. . . . Normally when you see a psychiatrist or a doctor, they sit there writing things in your file, and I am always a bit worried because "what did I just say, what did you write down?" and they just say not to worry. But I do worry, I don't like it. Here they have a whiteboard, and you can keep up with what they write. It's like: "no, that's not what I meant"—"then what did you mean?"—"I meant so and so," . . . whereas at the hospital the psychiatrist was just writing without even looking at me. And then the file said: "the patient has difficulties with eye contact." Eye contact? He hardly glanced at me.

The whiteboard used during therapy sessions is commended by many interviewees, as are several other methods for making the therapy sessions more equal and democratic. Emma also mentions that staff members participate in the meetings "like human beings and not as employees at an institution": "Then suddenly, he [the therapist] said, 'Hey, I think I forgot to say that I am Eric and I live in [part of Copenhagen] and I have a wife and a little girl.' It was nice. It gives you something, it's not just me reeling off." Another thing the interviewees say they had not expected is that staff members are available to them without the clients having to register and without waiting lists. Lina, 20 years old, relates: "The center was closed but she let me in, and that makes you want to come back because you don't feel like a case. It feels like they are part of your life, they may text us and ask how we're doing even on days when we're not here."

All these things add up to giving the clients a very favorable view of the center and its staff. Almost without exception, the interviewees praise the center's ambience and facilities, the staff members' friendliness and "embracing" (a word used by interviewees) style, and say that, compared to other public institutions, this is a place where you do not feel like a "client" or a "case." The center is a place where the participants feel welcome and not "like a nuisance as I always feel elsewhere in the system"; it is "a good place to go to when you feel lonely and don't know what to do with yourself," and the visits at the center are for several participants "the high spots of the week" (quoted from interviews).

AMBIVALENCE: WHO IS THE EXPERT?

In their 1963 essay, Merton and Barber described the ambivalence of the client role as centered on the authority of the professional. On the positive side, authoritative expertise was something the clients expected, demanded, and longed for (and often also paid for). On the negative side, the client role was associated with subordination, acceptance of bureaucratic rules and categorizations, disclosure of personal weaknesses and shortcomings, and anxiety about one's fate. According to Merton and Barber (1963), this tension between different aspects of the relationship between clients and professionals was bound to create ambivalence among those subjected to it. The professionals were by definition the experts in problem solving, and this called for the clients' admiration and confidence. At the same time, the professionals had the institutionalized right to make decisions and prescribe action for the client, including unwanted action: "The client may be required to abandon favored practices or values. He may be required to live a more limited version of his former life" (Merton 1976:26). This, in combination with the client's experience that the relationship is much more important to him or her than to the professional—given that the expert has many clients and only participates with detached concern while the client may have his or her whole future on the line—makes the client–expert relationship into a core type of ambivalent relationship (Merton 1976).

In today's user-oriented human service work, professional authority may face challenges that are very different from those described by Merton. One of the few other studies I have been able to identify addressing democratization and authority in modern human services is Whooley's (2010) analysis of psychiatric practice in New York. Whooley focused on the therapists' use of the *DSM* (the *Diagnostic and Statistical Manual of Mental*

Disorders). He showed that the psychiatrists, although obliged to follow the *DSM* when dealing with insurance companies, for example, used "workarounds" that undermined the manual in practice. They negotiated diagnoses with their patients, used alternative diagnoses to those in the *DSM*, and employed a few standard codes on all patients, ignoring the hundreds of diagnoses of the *DSM*. On the one hand, these workarounds had the effect of creating good relationships between psychiatrists and their patients; they were part of a democratization of the expert–patient relationship and part of a fight against the formalization and bureaucratization of psychiatric practice. On the other hand, some psychiatrists in Whooley's study worried that negotiation with patients, and the questioning of absolute diagnoses that negotiation was associated with, might lead to a (problematic) forfeiture of expert authority: "the professional authority of the psychiatrist is expected by patients and useful for treatment" (p. 463). Hence, while the *DSM* system was originally intended to bolster psychiatry's scientificity and to validate psychiatrists' claim to expertise, the workarounds described by Whooley risk having the opposite effect: patients and other actors (in Whooley's study, hospitals, insurance companies, etc.) may lose respect for and confidence in psychiatric treatment.

In my study as well, there are accounts indicating that user-focused human service work may create ambivalence when it comes to professional expertise (see Barnes, Chapter 15, this volume). The young drug users do not describe feelings of subordination or being ill at ease about the staff members' authority and decision making, as was often the case in the traditional service relationships described by Merton and Barber (1963). Quite the contrary, what confuses them is staff members' cautious and noncontrolling approach to them, and the center's insistence that clients take the lead in problem solving. Some interviewees experience this as a signing away of expertise on the part of the staff members: "I thought they would tell me what I should do and what I shouldn't do to get rid of my problems, but there is not much of that here. . . . Sometimes I wonder if this is a treatment center at all," Isabella says (Isabella was also quoted earlier, where she praised the center for its ambience and services). In what follows, I describe client ambivalence related to conceptions of professional expertise (or lack thereof) using somewhat longer quotations from two interviews, in order to contextualize the clients' experiences.

Adrian, 19 years old, smokes cannabis on a daily basis but does not regard this as a problem. He contacted the center because of his use of cocaine and ecstasy, which he felt affected his life negatively. He says he likes the way his therapist relates to him: "She is not strict. She is the way a therapist should be. I don't want her to tell me what to do. . . . When I say to her that I don't have a problem with cannabis, she respects it." At the same time, he is unsure as to what his therapist has to offer: "It's a way of unburdening your mind. Otherwise, they can't help me much because I'm the one with drug experience. They can't teach me anything, it's just a question of me pulling myself together." Adrian is very attentive to, and reflective about, his relationship to the therapist, which he says is not just about "the therapist watching me but also me watching her." He explains:

> I know some things about psychology, or just about people's reactions when you say things. I told Marie [the therapist] I had been unfaithful to my girlfriend and the moment I said it, Marie started to fiddle with her wedding ring. And I was like, "Well, is there something *you* would like to talk about Marie" [laughs]. It was very, very sweet. . . . So yes, I like talking with her.

Adrian does not associate the therapist's role with authority—quite the contrary, he positions himself and Marie as equals, or even regards himself as being more knowledgeable than she is. This makes him proud but also confused. If the therapist, or the center in general, cannot teach him much new about his drug use, "it's just talk, Ping-Pong over the table." Adrian has difficulties in seeing how the treatment can help him. In consequence, and although he "really enjoys talking with Marie," he has recently decided to scale down his treatment attendance.

Another user who feels very well informed is Christian, 20 years old. Christian has been a daily cannabis smoker since he was 16, and he also uses other drugs (e.g., amphetamines, ecstasy, and mushrooms) occasionally but does not feel he has a problem with them. However, he wants to take a break from cannabis, whereupon he plans to "learn to control" his smoking. Just like Adrian, Christian describes himself as well informed about drugs—"I know all there is to know about these things because I look it up on the Internet." He is also knowledgeable about different treatment forms:

> I know what the psychologist tries to do. You can look it up, narrative therapy, that's what they do here, although they mix it with other things. He keeps on asking, "Do you find this important to talk about; should we talk about other things next time?" It's really after the book: "Ask the patient: do you think we focus on the right things or should we talk about something else instead?" . . . But I just told him: "No, it's fine. You're doing just fine."

Christian had tried other treatment forms before, which he compares to the center's services. He dissociates himself from "more strict treatment," where the therapists "decide too much, you must do this and that, bang, bang, bang—that would never work with me, I would do the exact opposite." He says he is happy about the treatment at the center, most of all because his psychologist is a "fantastic person, real open about things and genuinely interested in me, sometimes he forgets about time—'oops, one and a half hours, we overran time' [laughs]." Yet, when it comes to "actual change," Christian is hesitant. So far, he has only had four therapy sessions at the center, and although his psychologist is "very good at what he is doing," Christian says he needs more "structured help" if he is to solve his problems with cannabis in the long run. For now, however, the center's services are enough for him because his therapist supports him in reaching his immediate goal, a three-month break in cannabis smoking.

The interviews with Adrian and Christian (and several other participants) describe a certain demystification and "disenchantment" with treatment. The accounts do not express the combination of awe, fear, and admiration that Merton (1976) regarded as typical of client–expert relationships. They rather describe clients feeling that they can "see right through" the treatment at the center, and in some cases right through the staff members, and that they know "what the therapists are up to" (expression in interview). These are not hierarchical relationships, like the classical client–expert relationships; they are not even oppositional relationships, where the client–expert roles are clearly separated. They are relationships built on ideals of equality, democracy, and empowerment, and with the aim of helping the clients gain control over their own lives. The young drug users are not merely consulted about their plans and wishes; they are the ones defining the very framework for action. Although clients cherish their autonomy and self-determination in treatment, some interviewees (like Adrian, Christian, and Isabella) regard the center's treatment approach as too vague and nondirective. In these cases, the transfer of initiative and influence from professionals to clients seems to have caused bewilderment and a questioning of staff members' professionalism and ability to help.

It is important to note that Adrian's and Christian's positioning of themselves as having the upper hand in their meetings with therapists may be related to things other than the center's user-focused service approach. Adrian's account is clearly influenced by the fact that his therapist is a woman (to this may be added that the interviewer is also a young woman). By describing his therapist as "very sweet" when she "fiddles with her wedding ring" and himself as more knowledgeable than she is, he also presents himself as being a man in control, despite the fact that he has drug problems. Christian, in turn, refers to himself as "intelligent," "reflective," and "academically interested" several times during the interview, thereby also presenting himself as a worthy dialogue partner for an interviewer from the university. He is not just a client with drug problems but a person on top of the situation, collaborating with the interviewer (and his therapist) in critically analyzing user-focused treatment.

AMBIVALENCE: HOW DOES ONE FIGURE THE PROBLEM?

When Merton and Barber (1963) coined the term sociological ambivalence, it was an attempt to create an alternative to the individualist conceptions of ambivalence long employed in the psychological literature. Whereas psychological ambivalence is usually understood as subjective contradictions in emotions and cognitions, sociological ambivalence is a feature of structured sets of social relationships. Sociological ambivalence refers to social roles and institutions "patterned in terms of potentially conflicting pairs of norms" (Merton 1976:33). Smelser describes sociological ambivalence as institutionally conditioned and as communicated in dichotomies, such as freedom versus constraint and independence versus dependence, pointing out that neither pole is a separate state of condition: "Neither freedom nor dependence can be realized in a full or exclusive form, because one is part of the other" (Smelser 1998:13). Ambivalence, then, should be recognized as an expected part of human service relationships. It is not a question of individual clients having "mixed feelings" about individual therapists, or vice versa (although this may be an interesting research topic in more individually oriented research on ambivalence). It is a question of looking at ambivalence originating in structural, institutional conditions. And, as Hillcoat-Nallétamby and Phillips point out: "Whilst its manifestation may appear at the level of individual experience, its genesis stems from the embedding of this individual within figurations of relations with others which themselves form more or less extensive chains of interdependencies" (Hillcoat-Nallétamby and Phillips 2011:206–207). Ambivalence arises in concrete interaction but is conditioned on structural elements, including bureaucratic restrictions and factors defining the relationship between a specific service organization and the social environment of the organization (cf. Merton 1976:85).

As a case in point, when it comes to client ambivalence reflecting institutionally anchored conflicts, I will use the center's attempts at destigmatizing illegal drug use. Ambivalence on this front relates to the question of how to figure the problem. As mentioned earlier, staff members take care not to position their clients as deviants but to treat them as normal youths who have resources as well as problems. By all accounts, and as illustrated in the following quotations from client interviews, staff members are successful in these attempts. Mathilda, 22 years old, recalls her first visit at the center: "I was so nervous because coming to a treatment center is like getting a label in your face, 'abuser!' But it wasn't like that at all. . . . Susanne [the therapist] didn't exactly say that it was okay to use drugs but she said it's quite normal for young people to do it." Mathilda explains that the center's approach to addressing drug use has helped her accept herself and to feel that she "is not as bad a person as [she] always thought." Similarly, Caroline, 22 years old, seems to have understood and accepted the center's constructivist approach to drug use: "You don't feel different here. . . . If I feel wrong I just like to take more drugs, and if I take more drugs, people may start to think I am strange. And if somebody thinks you're strange, you'll start to feel even more strange." Caroline commends the staff members for focusing on the things she is good at (e.g., social relations) and for not criticizing her for taking drugs: "I always tell them everything and they're just cool; you never have to hide things here."

In an article about narrative approaches in psychotherapy, Skovlund (2011) discusses the problem that narratives generated in therapy—in my study, narratives normalizing drug use and drug users—may be challenged in contexts outside of therapy. In narrative therapy, a client's self is comprehended as a relational phenomenon, based on stories from different contexts in which the client participates. If positive, empowering narratives about a client are to be effective, they have to be transferred from therapy to other domains. Skovlund talks about "resistance from the surroundings," stating that social and cultural circumstances force restrictions on narrative therapy, and that the change of behaviors and identity aimed at in treatment is not always supported by the world outside of treatment (p. 190).

In the present study, resistance from the surroundings is most visible when it comes to the center's treatment goal: "controlled drug use" (see Jensen and Villadsen, Chapter 11, this volume). According to staff members, this treatment goal signals optimism and belief in the clients' resources; the young drug users are seen as normal youths who for some reason or other have come to "overuse" drugs and who should be gently guided back to recreational drug use if they do not want to stop completely. The traditional approach to treatment defining abstinence as a goal for all clients is a form of "overdiagnosing" and "pathologizing" them, staff members say. Stephanie, 23 years old, explains how she, together with her therapist, reasoned about treatment goals during her first months at the center: "I didn't want to stop completely because that would mean I had a serious problem, and I didn't, right? I would have been an addict if I couldn't smoke a little now and then, and I wasn't an addict." Stephanie, however, soon realized that other parts of the system (e.g., her case manager at the social security office and a social worker at a job center) were of the opinion that she was not able to control her use of cannabis, amphetamines, and cocaine. Coincidentally, she came into contact with Narcotics Anonymous (NA), where she started to attend weekly meetings. She says that NA has made her "realize that [she] is an addict" and that she needs to stop using drugs: "I know now that reduction wouldn't work for me. I would be unhappy for not being allowed to smoke enough and at the same time I would be unhappy because I still smoked, and so I would start to smoke more." Although the staff members at the center do not explicitly condemn Stephanie's association with NA, she says they are "extremely skeptical, they think NA turns us into chronically ill people." Our interviews with staff members confirm the negative attitudes toward NA at the center. It is described as a network for "hardened junkies" and an organization "focusing on people's problems rather than their resources" and "building on an illness model that deprives users of responsibility"—in other words, an organization that represents the exact opposite of what the center stands for. For Stephanie, this constitutes a problem: she thinks that both NA and the center have helped her, and she would like to continue visiting both, but she feels torn between the two approaches to drug problems they represent.

Another type of resistance from the world outside the center comes from parents thinking their children should stop their drug use altogether rather than just reduce it. One example of this is Alexander, 20 years old, who has been a daily cannabis user since he was 16 and dropped out of several schools because of his cannabis smoking. He is very pleased with the therapy sessions at the center because "it's support, it's kind of non-judging," and he says he has reduced his cannabis use so that he mostly smokes in the evenings and that he has "even had a few days without cannabis." Alexander explains:

> Before I came here I thought you either smoke or do not smoke—one day without a joint is worth nothing. But here it's a big thing, small things are big here. . . . The problem is my mother. She has been very supportive but I can't say to her . . . I don't know. . . . In here they're like "could you imagine not smoking for one day" and then praise me for doing it. But for my parents that's not enough.

Staff members are conscious of the differences between their own and (some) parents' views on drug use. The center invites parents, with or without their children, to meetings where they inform them about drug use and the center's treatment approach. The aim of these meetings is, according to the staff members interviewed, to "make parents relax," to "teach them to sit on their hands and not to dramatize," to tell them that "many young people experiment with drugs these days without getting addicted," and "to deconstruct the concept of abuse together with them" (quoted from staff interviews). Crucial to the contacts with parents is that the center never "makes deals" with them about their children. "We work for the young people, and nobody else, not the parents, not the municipality, not the schools, not the police," as one of the staff members put it. Hence, the aim of the meetings with the parents is not to involve them in the treatment process (e.g., as supporters in the young client's recovery). It is rather to make them "step back," "stop worrying," and realize that "focusing on their kids' drug use only makes things worse" (quoted from staff interviews).

A final example of actors who may resist the center's approach to addressing drug use is employers. As mentioned in The Center's Treatment Approach section, most interviewees were unemployed or held short-term (often part-time) jobs at the time of the interviews. In a few cases, interviewees were able to combine continued drug use with job attendance, while in others they were not. Jonathan's interview describes a situation where he and the center were content with the development of his drug use but his employer and colleagues were not. Jonathan, 24 years old, had a job as a substitute in a day care center, which he was very fond of. He had succeeded in reducing his cannabis smoking from "massive use, almost continuous" to "one joint in the morning and one or two joints in the evening to be able to sleep." This worked well for several months, until some of his colleagues confronted him and "accused [him] of looking after children while being under the influence of cannabis," which Jonathan said he was not: "My body is so used to cannabis, nobody notices any change in me. I don't get red eyes or anything, I'm just normal." At the time of the interview, he had just been called to a meeting with his employer, and he expected to be given the sack.

DISCUSSION

Professionalism has traditionally been seen as requiring the development and ownership of special knowledge in a field. Expertise is by definition the means by which professional groups claim jurisdiction over a set of problems (Abbott 1988). When clients seek professional help, they typically do it because they expect the professionals to know something they do not know themselves, something that may help them solve their problems. As Knapp (1999) points out, clients come to professionals in part because of the power the professionals have, or the power clients think they have. The professional role has typically included the right to define reality for clients, or at least the part of reality related to specific problems, and to decide the best way to cure these problems.

The center analyzed in this chapter works with a client-centered, narrative approach that to a considerable degree transfers initiative and responsibility to the clients. Staff members regard themselves as experts in young people's drug problems (in general) but take care not to be the dominant part in defining problems and setting up solutions for individual clients. Looking at drug use from a constructivist perspective, the therapists want to avoid having their clients' *troubles* with drugs turned into permanent *problems*. Gubrium and Järvinen describe troubles as existing "at the border of the acceptable and the unacceptable, the insistently normal and potentially problematic, the well-recognized and the murky" (Gubrium and Järvinen 2014:3). When human services work with troubles—here drug troubles among young people—they risk transforming them into "diseases, disabilities and dysfunctions," institutionalized categories that push the clients further into a deviant identity and a marginalized social status (p. 3). This is why staff members at the center resist "absolutist" understandings of drug addiction, such as the one represented by NA and the twelve-step treatment, defining addiction as an illness or illness-like condition, and why they are skeptical of tests, diagnoses, and labels such as "abuse" and "abusers." Taking an attitude toward drugs that is as neutral as possible, staff members point out that their clients are reasonable and resourceful young people capable of reflection and choice; that drugs have positive as well as negative effects on the users (if they only had negative effects, nobody would use them); and that nothing good comes out of defining clients as addicts who have "lost control" of their drug intake and of their life in general.

"The stronger the positive side of ambivalence, the stronger the negative," Smelser (1998:6) writes in a classical article on sociological ambivalence. It is quite clear that almost all the interviewed users appreciate the center and its services: they feel staff members understand, respect, and support them; they look forward to coming to the center and say that the visits "cheer them up"; they recommend the center to their drug-using friends; and so forth. It is also clear, however, that many interviewees are confused by the center's treatment concept and that some are frustrated because the center's treatment "is not thorough enough," "doesn't really work with my *abuse* although that is why I came here," or "doesn't give me directions or clear advice on what I should do and where I should go from here" (quoted from interviews). Ironically, these clients seem to call for a more traditional form of treatment—comprehending drug use as "abuse," focusing on explanations of "addiction," directing and governing clients in their problem solution—treatment that the staff members regard as inappropriate for young drug users.

Also, the center's openness and ideals of methodological transparency notwithstanding, many clients are puzzled by the role the professionals play in narrative therapy. Staff members seem to have the clients with them when trying to avoid stigmatization of drug use and drug users. They also possess their command when working with antiauthoritarian methods, user self-determination, and user empowerment. When it comes to the question of defining goals, describing directions, and giving instructions and advice, however, many clients seem to be less radical than their therapists. The center's approach to addressing drug use and drug problems is deliberately relativist: distinctions between "use" and "abuse" are avoided, and much of the traditional knowledge in the field (diagnostic systems, manuals, etc.) is described as oppressive. Therapeutic relativism is a stance where no knowledge claims are regarded as more objectively true than others, and where dominant expert discourses are seen as fixing clients in alienated positions. Client ambivalence arises when interviewees feel that truth is deconstructed and professional authority suspended without staff members offering them alternative understandings and directions in problem solving. Ambivalence also arises when clients define themselves as more knowledgeable than staff members and when they put themselves in the position of monitors and evaluators of their therapists' practices. Furthermore, ambivalence builds up when the center's relativist approach to treatment is confronted with the demands of bureaucracy and with more traditional, objectivist ways of thinking about drug problems among other professionals, parents, employers, and sometimes also among the young clients themselves.

This chapter analyzed user-focused therapy from the point of view of clients. If we had asked the therapists about individual clients (e.g., Adrian and Christian, who felt more knowledgeable than their therapists; Isabella, who questioned whether this is a treatment center; or Jonathan, who thought it was unproblematic to smoke before work, and indicated that his therapist agreed), we would probably have obtained different descriptions of the young drug users and their treatment progress. For reasons of confidentiality, we did not discuss named clients with professionals. However, from the general discussions in the staff interviews, it becomes clear that the professionals are aware of many of the therapeutic challenges presented in this chapter; for instance, the problem with clients asking for firmer therapist-steered treatment. It is also clear that staff members deliberately avoid such treatment—described in terms of "distinct directions," "detailed guidance," or "definitive answers" to the clients—because they think positive human change can only come about if it is anchored in the clients' own insights and decisions.

The starting point for this chapter was the idea that human service relationships are by necessity ambivalent because they are conditioned on contradictory elements. The ambivalence in user-focused human services is different from that in traditional client–staff meetings and has, in my analysis, centered on the division of labor between therapists and young drug users and on what happens when the center's noncondemning approach to addressing illicit drug use meets resistance from the world outside of treatment. The conclusion of the chapter is not that these ambivalences need to be solved, that staff members should give up their resistance to manuals, diagnostic systems, and objective truth doctrines, or that they should adapt their conceptions of illicit drug use to those of parents, employers, and other professionals. If anything, my advice would be that staff members embrace the ambivalence described by clients and work with it systematically in treatment. Ambivalence is an expected product of conflicting role expectations, norms and counternorms, and complexities and unpredictability in human relations (professional as well as others). Rather than being combatted by rules and regulations, ambivalence should be encouraged, respected, and used constructively in the further development of the center's treatment approach.

NOTE

1 The interviews were conducted by research assistants Ane Grubb and Maja Thorsteinsson, Department of Sociology, University of Copenhagen.

REFERENCES

Abbott, A. 1988. *The System of Professions: An Essay on the Division of Expert Labor.* Chicago: University of Chicago Press.

Adams, R. 1996. *Social Work and Empowerment.* London: Macmillan.

Baistow, K. 1994/1995. "Liberation and Regulation: Some Paradoxes of Empowerment." *Critical Social Policy* 14(3): 34–46.

Gergen, K. J., and S. McNamee, eds. 1992. *Therapy as Social Construction*. London: Sage.

Gubrium, J. F., and M. Järvinen, eds. 2014. *Turning Troubles into Problems: Clientization in Human Services*. London: Routledge.

Hillcoat-Nallétamby, S., and J. E. Phillips. 2011. "Sociological Ambivalence Revisited." *Sociology* 45(2): 202–217.

Järvinen, M., and N. Mik-Meyer. 2012. *At skabe en professionel: Ansvar og autonomi i velfærdsstaten* (Creating a professional: Responsibility and autonomy in a welfare state). Copenhagen: Hans Reitzels Forlag.

Järvinen, M., and G. Miller. 2015. "Social Constructionism Turned Into Human Service Work." *Qualitative Sociology Review* 11(2): 198–214.

Knapp, S. J. 1999. "Analyzing Narratives of Expertise: Toward the Development of a Burkeian Pentadic Scheme." *Sociological Quarterly* 40(4): 587–612.

Merton, R., and E. Barber, 1963. "Sociological Ambivalence." In *Sociological Theory, Values and Sociological Change: Essays in Honor of Pitirim A. Sorokin*, edited by E. A. Tryakian, 91–120. New York: Free.

Merton, R. K. 1976. *Sociological Ambivalence and Other Essays*. New York: Free.

Nissen, M. 2006. "Wild Objectification: Social Work as Object." *Outlines: Critical Practice Studies* 6(1): 73–89.

Payne, M. 2006. *Narrative Therapy*. London: Sage.

Pease, B. 2002. "Rethinking Empowerment: A Postmodern Reappraisal for Emancipatory Practice." *British Journal of Social Work* 32(2): 135–147.

Rogers, C. R. 1989. "A Client-Centered/Person-Centered Approach to Therapy." In *The Carl Rogers Reader*, edited by H. Kirschenbaum and V. L. Henderson, 135–152. Boston: Houghton Mifflin.

Rogers, C. R. 1995. *On Becoming a Person: A Therapist's View of Psychotherapy*. Boston: Houghton Mifflin.

Rose, N. 1999. *Governing the Soul: The Shaping of the Private Self*. London: Free Association.

Skovlund, H. 2011. "Overcoming Problems of Relativism in Postmodern Psychotherapy." *Journal of Contemporary Psychotherapy* 41(3): 187–198.

Smelser, N. J. 1998. "The Rational and the Ambivalent in the Social Sciences: 1997 Presidential Address." *American Sociological Review* 63(1): 1–16.

Vitus, K. 2014. "Wild Girls and the Deproblematization of Troubled Lives. In *Turning Troubles into Problems: Clientization in Human Services*, edited by J. F. Gubrium and M. Järvinen, 85–101. London: Routledge.

White, M. 1995. *Re-authoring Lives: Interviews and Essays.* Adalaide: Dulwich Centre Publications.

White, M., and D. Epston. 1990. *Narrative Means to Therapeutic Ends.* New York: Norton.

Whooley, O. 2010. "Diagnostic Ambivalence: Psychiatric Workarounds and the *Diagnostic and Statistical Manual of Mental Disorders.*" *Sociology of Health and Illness* 32(3): 452–469.

4

Flipping the Script

MANAGING AND REIMAGINING OUTPATIENT ADDICTION TREATMENT

▸ E. SUMMERSON CARR

I FIRST HEARD THE TERM "FLIPPING THE SCRIPT" one summer afternoon at Fresh Beginnings, an intensive outpatient drug treatment program for homeless women in the midwestern United States. It was ten months into my formal fieldwork in and around the program, which was affiliated with a network of local social service agencies (the Homeless Families Consortium, or HFC) that referred clients there.[1] Clients' participation in Fresh Beginnings programming was loaded. Like many "wraparound services" that include substance abuse treatment, the subsidized housing, child care, and other resources clients could receive from affiliated agencies was contingent on attending group therapy four days a week and complying with therapists' rules and regulations, including, of course, abstaining from drug and alcohol use. I would soon learn that "flipping the script" was a strategy clients used to cope with these laden circumstances.

On the afternoon in question, clients Nikki and Shauna were engaged in an intensive, hushed, but clearly entertaining exchange as the rest of us quietly lounged against the cool stone steps of the porch of the frame house on Cliff Street, where the program stood as unassumingly as possible amid the residences where students and young families lived. I gathered little about the conversation at the time, except that it seemed to involve an encounter Shauna had with an HFC social worker and that "flipping the script" was the reported tale's leitmotif. A couple of months later, I had the opportunity to interview Shauna (S), who was no longer a client at Fresh Beginnings, an extract from which follows.

1 I One time you said something and I, I wondered, I thought it meant, or had to do
2 with . . . like, "talking the talk." You said "*flipping the script*" in the treatment,
3 like, 'cuz you had, like, if you were/
4 S Oh, I did that *good*. Oh yeah, I had *that* down to a *science*.
5 I So whadaya mean you had it down to a science? Like, how'd you do it?
6 S When you've been to more than three treatment centers you learn how to say
7 *exactly what* they want ta hear, ya know.
8 And that, that's what kept me fucked up, [not] being able to do that, ya know,
9 bein' able to know what a person wanna hear and tell 'em exactly that.
10 I Mmmm.
11 S You forget, I'm a prostitute, that's what I do [with johns/customers].
12 I Um hm/
13 S I tell people what they wanna hear.
14 I And you had to be pretty convincing about it, how you said it, right?
15 S Well, yeah. You have to um . . . kinda, it's really hard to explain you have ta . . .
16 You have to almost be a fly on the wall to understand.

Trying to give me a quick lesson on script flipping, Shauna laid out some of the premises of the skill. She described an anticipatory practice of telling people—like johns (line 11) or professionals in treatment centers (line 6)—"what they want to hear" (lines 7, 9, 13). Shauna further implies that this requires acute analytical and rhetorical skills: discerning "*exactly*" (line 7) what is wanted by listeners and satisfying those desires "exactly" (line 9) in speech. Significantly, this mode of communication was quite at odds with how Fresh Beginnings therapists urged clients to speak as part of their treatment, which is to express their own inner states with "Honesty, Openness, and Willingness" (HOW) and without reference to the circumstances of speaking or specific interlocutors (see Carr 2006, 2011).

If Shauna's first lesson on script flipping is that it requires knowing how to use language to respond to social expectations rather than divulge personal inclinations, her second point is that script flipping is a matter of practice. Shauna explains that she "learned"—over time and across particular institutional contexts (line 6)—how to "know what a person wanna hear" (line 9) as well as how to calibrate her speech accordingly. She even goes so far as to liken script flipping to a "*science*" (line 4). And while Shauna emphasizes the science inherent to the profession of prostitution (line 11), she underscores that anyone who "has been to more than three treatment centers" (line 6) can learn to flip the script. As I would later learn, only those clients who had accrued ample experience in social service agencies knew how to effectively "flip the script," and they reaped the rewards and risks of the practice accordingly.

While I have described elsewhere what script flipping reveals about the social life of language (Carr 2011), this chapter is focused on what the practice suggests about social service clients' ability to manage their interactions with social service professionals and thereby control their fate in social service agencies (see Foley and Timonen, Chapter 6, this volume). Whereas prominent scholars of social service organizations have commonly assumed that "clients, especially when they lack power, become dependent on workers to construct their case in moral terms, and they have little recourse to address such constructions" (Hasenfeld 2009:419; see also Handler 1986; Lipsky 2010), I begin from the premise that social service professionals *depend on clients* when carrying out their evaluative (or "moral") charge. In general, whether in shelter intakes and clinical assessments, in-group or individual therapy, or even in administrative venues where decisions were made in conversation with "client representatives" (see Carr 2009, 2011), HFC professionals heavily relied on what clients said about themselves and their problems to do their work. As we will see, flipping a script effectively manipulates—or at least troubles—the practice of professional evaluation.

To the extent that script flippers influence the evaluative dimensions of social service professionals' labor, they can also influence their distributive work. Within HFC, as in many social service sites, the distribution of material resources (like housing, psychotropic medication, subsidized child care, or court advocacy) hinged on the flow of symbolic resources (like diagnoses and labels). It was not only that the evaluations made during ostensibly clinical exchanges—assessments, group and individual therapy sessions—served as the basis by which professionals allocated basic but scarce goods and services, including who was required to attend what kind of treatment. It was also that social workers continually deployed labels for people and problems in order to rationalize, post hoc, the way they distributed resources. So whether or not script flippers themselves believed that they were "abused," "drug dependent," "working the steps," or "in recovery"—at least in the same way professionals understood those terms—these clients knew that by managing these professional labels, they could both pave their own way to needed resources and potentially avoid punitive policies and sanctions.

For these reasons, an analysis of script flipping allows us to reimagine power dynamics of social service administration in the following ways (see Jensen and Villadsen, Chapter 11, this volume). First and most obviously, clients in human service organizations can exercise more agency than is typically assumed, with agency understood here as the capacity to effectively or meaningfully act. Second, clients' ability to manage human service relationships and organizations relies heavily on their ability to manage their own speech. This suggests that once students of social service organizations attend to the linguistic interactions between social workers and clients, our assumptions about professional control and client dependence may be concertedly challenged. Third, and as Shauna highlights, as clients accrue experience in social service agencies, they can also develop an acute—almost (social) "science"-like—awareness of how to manage human service relationships, an awareness without which flipping the script would be impossible. In other words, those who flip the script themselves reimagine the human service relationship in order to manage the dynamics of care and control that relationship inevitably entails.

With these points in mind, this chapter proposes that flipping the script is a *political* act not only because script flippers develop an acute awareness of how to speak efficaciously or even simply because they influence the professional work of distributing basic goods and services through this highly reflexive mode of communication. As we will see, there were limits in clients' ability to reap what they sowed in flipping the script. Rather, I emphasize that flipping the script is political because it denaturalizes and destabilizes the very ideology on which addiction treatment is premised, an ideology on which mainstream American addiction professionals typically depend both to care for and to control their clients.

LEARNING THE LINES OF ADDICTION TREATMENT

In their elicited explanations of script flipping, Fresh Beginnings clients appealed to the definition of "script" as a particular kind of text, one that is produced so that it can be performed. Shauna described a dramatic practice that is like learning lines appropriate to a stage (i.e., "a treatment center") and expected by an audience (i.e., social service professionals). In Erving Goffman's terms, a script is also a kind of text whose "author" (the one who selects the ideas and sentiments expressed) is not necessarily the same person as its "animator" (the one who actually utters those ideas and sentiments) (Goffman 1981). One's verbal rendering of a script is never true or false but rather more or less successful, faithful, or believable (Austin 1962). It is perhaps for this very reason that, in the contemporary United States, the term "script" commonly carries a pejorative meaning. To say that a particular strip of speech is "scripted"—take a public apology, for instance—is to indicate that it is out of line with the speaker's true thoughts, beliefs, and feelings or has been authored or orchestrated by another.

The idea that what one says should match what one already feels and believes—and the attendant disparaging of scripted speech—is especially potent in American addiction treatment, where addicts are thought to suffer from "denial," which is the inability to see one's inner self clearly and effectively render that self in words. Treatment is accordingly focused on getting clients to align what they say with preexisting inner states—that is, to use language as a mode of inner reference (Carr 2006, 2011). Thus, in flipping a script, clients circumvent a highly valued clinical and cultural goal. In this sense, flipping the script is risky business, for it is not simply a culturally disparaged way of speaking (even though there are very few of us who do not recognize the ways we use speech to influence others, rather than simply self-express, and the occasions that call for this kind of communication). In the context of mainstream American drug treatment, those who flip the script—or, as professionals put it, "talk the talk"—risk not only having their sincerity questioned but their sobriety doubted as well.

Still, while there were certainly risks to flipping the clinical scripts that Fresh Beginnings therapists prescribed, it could be equally dangerous to sincerely abide by them. After all, what clients said about themselves and their problems during therapeutic encounters was hardly insulated from program policies, and had far-reaching, often dramatic consequences. For instance, if a client confessed to a recent relapse during group or individual therapy, therapists generally informed the relevant case manager within HFC, who might take a hard line, strictly interpreting the reported drug use as a violation of program rules and terminating the client from housing or shelter.

Interlocutors that were more distant also were implicated in the therapeutic exchanges on Cliff Street. Fresh Beginnings clients were particularly incensed by one such instance in which a client named Monique—in an effort to follow the therapeutic injunction that she speak with "Honesty, Openness, and Willingness"—described various attempts to control a ten-year-old child using prescribed parenting skills, her mounting frustration at their apparent ineffectiveness, and her eventual use of a "good, old-fashioned whuppin'" when all else had failed. During the group, therapists offered alternative endings to the family struggle in cognitive-behavioral terms, and clients offered words of sympathy and support. Shortly thereafter, the very same therapists came to the dreaded decision to report Monique to Child Protective Services. In interviews conducted months after the event, clients' astonishment at the consequences of Monique's self-description hardly abated. At issue was not only that therapists had interpreted the reported "whuppin'" as "child abuse" but, moreover, that they had reported it accordingly. A client named Keisha recalled:

> It was like, *why* did it go out and she actually *wrote*, wrote her up and reported it, I think, to Protective Services . . . we were like *wow*, you know, it kind of made it feel like, *dang*, you know, we can't *share* (laughter) some things because we don't want to go to *jail* just for sharing things that we thought we were just honestly speaking on.

In light of such incidents, most clients eventually learned that to manage their housing, kin relations, and their very freedom, they had to manage what they said in group therapy. Indeed, clients could be, and often arguably were, quite earnest about their investment in recovery and still flip therapeutic scripts. Since speaking with "Honesty, Openness and Willingness," as therapists urged and expected, could lead to going to jail or losing one's children, clients were eager to find and make use of other options.

On the other hand, most Fresh Beginnings clients continued to struggle *within* therapeutic scripts by either hiding or sharing the information that clients were clinically urged to reveal. Yet especially astute clients, as they gained more experience in the program, eventually learned that overtly resisting therapeutic scripts—either by sitting in silence or challenging their terms—was not an effective option. After all, therapists readily detected this resistance and interpreted it as a clinical sign of denial or deception, and—by extension—unabated addiction. Furthermore, those who refused to "learn the lines" may have resisted the therapeutic scripts they were given, but they did nothing to challenge or destabilize their ideological bases.

By contrast, script flippers actively seized on and animated the prescribed language of self-revelation, without necessarily referring to the inner states so expressed. In doing so, they deployed authoritative scripts toward institutionally unauthorized ends. As these script-flipping clients garnered positive evaluations from their therapists, they also gained any number of resources: referrals for respite child care or free legal advocacy; exonerating phone calls to parole officers by protective service workers; and the benefit of the doubt when they did not show up for group therapy. Yet, as we will see, as a political act, script flipping achieved something far more powerful and enduring: it denaturalized and destabilized ideologies that aligned professional power and truth.

SITUATED PRACTICE MAKES PERFECT

Although all Fresh Beginnings clients were interested in managing the potentially far-reaching consequences of what they said during group therapy, the difference between those who could flip scripts and those who simply followed them boiled down to their relative experience. For instance, Shauna—who had spent many years in treatment programs and other social service settings—had considerable experience analyzing and manipulating the circumstances within which she spoke. By contrast, clients like Monique, who had little experience in social service settings, lacked the knowledge necessary to strategically deploy prescribed ways of acting and talking to their own ends. As in any performance, practice makes perfect when it comes to flipping the script.

However, flipping a script is not simply a matter of practice. Successful script flippers were engaged more specifically in keenly attuned, highly observant, situated practice (Lave and Wenger 1991). Fresh Beginnings clients accrued the knowledge required to flip the script through an apprentice-like participation in group therapy (see also Fox 2001; cf. Cain 1991). It was there that they learned the formal features and content of prescribed ways of speaking, and watched clients who were more experienced speak accordingly (see chapter 4 in Carr 2011). Thus, in addition to "learning the lines," fledglings strived to understand the local expectations of their professional audience and how a specific institutional stage was set. Notably, even those clients intent on actually abiding by the tenets of HOW—by transparently revealing what they already really thought, truly felt, or actually did in words—needed to persuade therapists that their investment in the script they spoke was earnest. So whether flipping or following the script, new clients at Fresh Beginnings acted very much like understudies, watching script flippers persuade therapists and reap the rewards of professionals' positive evaluations.

Given this necessary attunement to context-specific cues, even the most experienced script flippers did not succeed when they were unfamiliar with their institutional surroundings. This first became evident to me during an interview with Nikki, a veteran client and consummate script flipper, who contended that Fresh Beginnings therapists "didn't have a clue" about her continued use of cocaine, despite her frequent and loquacious contributions to group therapy. Nikki was determined to graduate from the program (and at one point was very close to doing so) in order to resume working during the days that she now spent in group therapy on Cliff Street. This, she figured, was the only viable way to secure her current housing arrangement and gain some measure of independence from her frequently incarcerated, common-law husband, which was all the more important once she became pregnant with her third child.

Yet, while Nikki was a master at persuading professionals, she was in no position to deploy her rhetorical skill set immediately after delivering a healthy baby boy in a local hospital. Operating in a relatively foreign institution, with unfamiliar rules, regulations, procedures, and personnel, she had not acquired the wherewithal to know *what* to say to whom. It was not surprising, then, that hospital nurses quickly procured evidence of her continued drug use, though that evidence did not derive from Nikki's body, and certainly not by way of her words. Rather, a test administered (without Nikki's consent or knowledge) determined that her newborn son had traces of drugs in his bloodstream, a discovery that quickly precipitated a

Child Protective Services report and another six-month stint at Fresh Beginnings.[2]

Of course, drug tests were also regularly and randomly administered at Fresh Beginnings, raising the question of how Nikki eluded detection throughout her tenure there. One might most readily point to the relative degrees to which clients could alter the evidence that the tests procured in the hospital on the one hand and the treatment program on the other, for even during the periods in which Fresh Beginnings instituted monitored screenings, some clients responded with increasingly ingenious strategies to produce "clean" urine, only some of which could be deployed at the hospital. However, alongside the various ways to substitute or chemically alter their urine—by adding water, salt, or sweetener, for example—script flippers also had ways to manage whatever came from their body with their words, if only when operating on well-studied institutional grounds and with familiar professional interlocutors.

Once released back into familiar discursive territory at Fresh Beginnings, Nikki spent the next six months doing just that. Now subject to significantly increased scrutiny, including monitored urine screening, she had to be even more persuasive—a challenge she seemed to savor. As she boasted during one of our later interviews, Nikki (N) was so good at flipping the script that she could "play off" and "explain away" inconclusive, or even positive, urine results:

1 I How did you do it? Whaddya mean "play it off"?
2 N Ya know, explain it away—talk 'em *through* it.
3 I shifted things around until they left me alone.

Considering that there are few discourses that enjoy a more "durable locus" (de Certeau 1984) than modern scientific ones, Nikki's ability to strategically "shift" (line 3) the results of urinalyses from the bifurcated grounds of positive/negative and true/false seems particularly noteworthy. And while urine screening may appear to be an extradiscursive element of the otherwise heavily talk-dependent treatment regimen at Fresh Beginnings, Nikki clearly suggests otherwise. According to this veteran client, evidence from the body could be "talked through" and ultimately "explained away."

Like many of Nikki's fellow clients, friends, and therapists, readers may understandably worry about the consequences of Nikki being "left alone" (line 3). It is nevertheless important not to miss the institutional and sociological significance of what she manages to do. Strategically acting as she does, Nikki exercises a kind of agency that is too easily overlooked or dismissed, in part because of the common tendency to pathologize it. After all, Nikki does not simply explain her own drug use away (line 2); she also, and more significantly, disables her therapists' primary means of monitoring and controlling her behavior, all while seeming to abide by their terms.

THE DISCURSIVE DEMISE AND RESURGENCE OF URINALYSIS

Consider the following two framings of urinalysis at Fresh Beginnings. The first was issued to every incoming client in a small packet of orientation materials. It reads: "Treatment is structured as three phases of treatment based upon each woman's progress, and includes regular random urinalysis, required recovery support meeting attendance (e.g., 12-Step and Women for Sobriety), and aftercare services." This rather straightforward rendering of urinalysis as an integral part of the program's treatment regimen betrayed none of the institutional troubles with urinalysis to which a second framing, recorded in the minutes of an advisory board meeting and distributed to professionals affiliated with the treatment program, alludes. There it is stated that, "[Therapist Laura] suggested the use of chemical tests to judge the validity of the clients [*sic*] voice. Empowerment is the key part of the efficacy of a treatment program."

In this latter case, urine tests are exposed as a necessary corrective to therapists' main method of treatment—the honest, open, and willing talk that group therapy was meant to elicit. Indeed, by indicating that urinalysis is, fundamentally, about the "validation" of clients' speech, the meeting minutes reveal the lead therapist's awareness that scripts are being flipped on her. Even more tellingly, the meeting minutes, which Laura herself authored, represent "chemical tests" as a "suggested" rather than required part of treatment, quite unlike the program description distributed to clients. The meeting minutes go on to mysteriously frame these tests as a matter of "empowerment," implying that they are a way to honor rather than hem in clients' agency.

Although Fresh Beginnings clients were not formally privy to Advisory Board meeting minutes, veteran clients probably understood why their therapists had to so carefully frame urinalysis when communicating with their colleagues. After all, script flippers, as established earlier, were keen ethnographers of their institutional surroundings. Indeed, for several months, a controversy had been brewing among the professionals who sat on the Advisory Board—which included HFC case managers and program directors, Laura's and Susan's clinical supervisor, and direct service staff from Fresh Beginnings. The troubles began when Laura and Susan, who were continually dogged by clean drug screen results from bodies they suspected were decidedly drugged, quietly instituted a policy of monitored urinalysis. In practice, this meant that one of the two therapists stood in the cramped Cliff Street bathroom, watching to make sure each initialed vial was filled by the appropriate client body.

Significantly, one of HFC's programs, a large, state-of-the-art domestic violence shelter, had objected long and loudly to urine screening, on the grounds that it could retraumatize those who had been victimized. And while they refused to conduct drug tests on-site, they allowed their clients to be screened at Fresh Beginnings once they had been admitted to the program. Quite aside from this long-standing tension, Laura and Susan could not help but be aware that professional affiliates of the program would object to *monitored* urinalysis in principle. And, indeed, when the issue was directly addressed at another Advisory Board meeting, the reaction was swift and blunt. According to the minutes, recorded by the HFC director's assistant, "The group discussed the use of urine screens. It was agreed that monitored screening brings shame and is demoralizing."

Administrators' reference to the shame-inducing quality of a therapeutic practice is especially striking. It was a reframing that struck at the heart of the frequently embattled Laura's well-known conviction—which has ample support in the clinical literature—that shame is the primary psychological cause of women's drug use. HFC professionals, who tended toward more structural than psychological explanations for their clients' behavior, hit on an effective way to cannily redirect the clinical discourse of shame to an institutional critique of a practice they long felt was unethical. Yet, while we might readily take this as a case of ideologically opposed *professionals* strategically reframing a practice in line with competing institutional goals, it appears that script-flipping clients had a hand in this recasting of monitored screening. After all, Fresh Beginnings clients certainly were very familiar with their therapists' theories of women's addiction, which drew causal links between sexual abuse, ensuing shame, and numbing drug use (see Carr 2011, chapter 3). Indeed, in group therapy, script flippers highlighted histories of child abuse, relegating the other significant traumas they had suffered, knowing it was an expected and sympathy-inducing way to explain their drug use as adults. As one veteran client once told me, "You've got to be [sexually] abused there, or they be thinkin' there is something wrong with *you*."

Whether they caught wind of their case managers' established critiques of their therapists' clinical reasoning or in fact helped author those critiques, clients were clearly involved in flipping the script of shame. According to the clients I spoke with directly and case managers who offered secondhand reports of what clients had said, monitored screening was "embarrassing," "traumatizing," and even "violating." And interestingly, not long after Nikki returned from the hospital, some clients began to elaborate as well as flip the script of shame. They claimed that being monitored by those who were supposed to care for them induced shameful memories of childhood sexual abuse, which in turn triggered intense urges to get high and sometimes, by extension, dirty drug screen results.

Perhaps, in citing the shame evoked by monitored screenings, Fresh Beginnings clients were flipping scripts. Or perhaps they were simply referencing what they actually felt and believed. The very point of script flipping was to raise the definite possibility that either could be the case, and the latter was too serious to be ignored by professionals, considering the threatened consequences. In either case, by flipping the script of shame, clients contributed to and sustained some HFC professionals' objections to monitored screening. They also effectively suspended the practice of monitored screenings as professionals debated its ethics.

Months after the Advisory Board halted the practice of monitored screenings, well-substantiated rumors surfaced that Fresh Beginnings clients who were staying at the domestic violence shelter were using drugs rampantly on-site. With this drug use considered a "crisis" by shelter and Fresh Beginnings professionals alike, Laura and Susan convinced the shelter to institute on-site testing, which it had adamantly resisted up to that date. Fresh Beginnings therapists also took the opportunity to persuade the Advisory Board that monitored screening should be reinstituted. At a particularly momentous Advisory Board meeting, therapists directly referenced the skillful work of "creative clients" (lines 4 and 7 in the following list) in defending the reinstitution of monitored screenings. The minutes read:

1 Drug Screens: [The domestic violence shelter] will not do drug screens on site.
2 However the [Fresh Beginnings] staff can do the screenings.
3 [Fresh Beginnings] has gone to observed urine screenings for everyone due to the fact
4 that some clients have found a way to creatively get around the drug testing.
5 A question was raised about the concern that some women may have about sexual abuse?
6 Most consumers understand and are not having a problem with the observed testing. The ones
7 that are having a problem with the testing are the ones who are being creative.

Note the collective assent therapists are able to secure in relation to what most Advisory Board members, HFC staff, and clients had all once agreed was a decidedly "shameful" practice. While that critique is referenced and raised in interrogative form (line 5), the long-standing objection is quickly resolved, recontextualized by pitting it against the wily workings of "creative clients" (lines 4, 7). Thus, script flippers eventually lost what they had gained in mobilizing the script of shame; that is, temporary relief from an intrusive and discerning means of detection. They also arguably lost their status as legitimate speakers—if they ever had it—in the eyes of Fresh Beginnings therapists and HFC professionals alike, who now disparaged their "creativity" against the cultural and clinical expectation that sincere and sober thinkers use language to simply self-refer.

Against these losses, however, clients developed their skills in institutional analysis, which allowed them to intervene in how institutionally powerful people, such as their case managers and therapists, engaged in evaluations of relatively less powerful ones, such as themselves (see Järvinen, Chapter 3, this volume). And although clients did not always get to keep what they earned in flipping the script—whether the suspension of an onerous treatment requirement or ancillary services such as respite day care—they were able to effectively influence policy debates that would have otherwise been off-limits to them. Script flippers' political efficacy was demonstrated all the more powerfully when they took on the policy that required them to attend Alcoholics Anonymous (AA) meetings. In this case, they troubled not just a policy but the ideological grounds on which it was premised.

FLIPPING FEMINISM AND AA ACROBATICS

From the inception of Fresh Beginnings in 1995, AA meetings were formally incorporated into the treatment regimen. After each Thursday afternoon therapy session on Cliff Street, the program van was reserved to transport clients to a community meeting held in the basement of a large church nearby. Although all Fresh Beginnings therapists acknowledged that their clients had little in common with the majority of local AA attendees—predominantly white, middle-class, professional men and a smattering of their female counterparts—all clients were nonetheless encouraged to find a "sponsor" and attend meetings on their own time as well. Significantly, Fresh Beginnings therapists also used AA as a sanction: clients who were determined to have relapsed were signed to stringent treatment contracts requiring them to attend 90 AA or NA meetings in ninety days (known as "90/90s") in addition to their hefty weekly schedule at Fresh Beginnings. The stated consequences for not complying with 90/90s were hefty: termination from the Fresh Beginnings program and loss of ancillary HFC services, including shelter, child care, and transitional housing.

Whether or not they were subject to these special contractual terms, many clients came to consider AA less like therapy and more like probation or punishment. Clients claimed that the Thursday afternoon AA meeting felt tedious, even intolerable, after a long week of meeting-filled days at Fresh Beginnings. Along with that, there was work and housing to find, family obligations to meet, and legal and bureaucratic matters to handle. With few exceptions, clients consistently complained of having too little time and far too much to do, especially when newly instituted state welfare policies added work requirements, which did not make exceptions for those in intensive outpatient treatment as they had in the past. Thus, from the early days of the program, it was not unusual for an individual client, complaining of illness or citing a domestic emergency, to cajole an AA-bound van driver into taking her straight to her home or shelter, thereby circumventing yet another round of therapeutic talk.

When Laura and Susan learned of these tactics, they tried to control them by requesting "rider logs" from van drivers. However, with little faith in and cooperation from the drivers, therapists soon loosened their monitoring of clients' participation in Thursday meetings. And while both therapists continued to give "90/90s" to clients who had relapsed or who, by not showing up for therapy sessions at Fresh Beginnings, were suspected of doing so, Laura subtly made it known that she was not wholly unsympathetic to her clients' attempts to avoid AA, in large part by offering an on-site alternative.

Laura was a longtime member and moderator of "Women for Sobriety" (WFS), a self-help group launched in 1976. Its founding had been spurred by charges that AA is insensitive to the gender-specific issues of alcoholic women, ideas that Laura largely shared. In an interview with me, Laura (L) explained her rationale for instituting WFS meetings on-site:

1 L: It's sort of like a self-help support group corollary for people who did not find
2 12-step programs that helpful. A *lot* of 12-step programs are not welcoming for
3 women, because it is a program that was started by middle-class, white males and
4 there's more *men* in attendance than there are women, and it's not a place where a
5 lot of women feel *safe* talkin' about their feelings or their sexual abuse issues.
6 I Uh, hmm/
7 L And in a lot of areas, [AA] is a place that's kinda like a meat market where
8 women are preyed upon as sex objects . . . that makes it feel unsafe to open up.

Laura explained that because AA is both *for* men, with more of them in attendance (line 4), and *by* men, founded by "middle-class, white males" (line 3), it is not welcoming for women (lines 2–3), or "their feelings" and "issues" for that matter (line 5). Appealing to the tenet of therapeutic "safety" (lines 5, 8), Laura cites two interrelated, androcentric dangers of AA. First, women are the "meat" of the AA marketplace, preyed on as "sex objects" (lines 7–8). Second, and perhaps partially as a result, women attending AA feel inhibited from "opening up" (lines 5, 8), particularly regarding their "issues," which, as was typically assumed, revolved around sexual abuse (line 5).

Held in the Fresh Beginnings building, conducted by Laura, and involving the same clients as with other therapy groups, WFS groups were much more convenient, if not "safer" for clients. When I inquired about them in the weeks after Laura launched them, clients suggested that the weekly WFS meetings were almost indistinguishable from their other activities at Fresh Beginnings—just another round of talk. However, clients' rather agnostic acceptance of Women for Sobriety shifted dramatically when Laura resigned from her position at Fresh Beginnings and a decidedly pro-AA therapist, Lizzy, took the helm.

Clients who survived the transition between therapists swiftly took up Laura's feminist critique of AA, adopting it with striking similitude. No longer was AA inconvenient, troublesome, or just plain "stupid, *embarrassing*, people cryin' all over themselves and telling all their *business*," as a particularly recalcitrant client once put it. Instead, well-schooled clients began to insist that AA was started and run by men, not welcoming of women, and therefore an "unsafe" place for women to "open up," especially about sex. During an interview with me conducted soon after Laura left Fresh Beginnings, one client (R) made the following claims:

1 R AA is for men. And it's *obvious* that you don't speak about some things
2 that you would when you're just females, you know.
3 I Like what?
4 R Okay. Like, when I went to, um . . . to AA one week, that one time I went,
5 it was an *all-male* group and it made me extremely nervous. And there's just some
6 things that you *won't* talk about, you know. Like your sex life, for instance.

Of course, what this client casts as "*obvious*" was also obvious to her departed therapist, as we saw. However, notice that the client does not simply parrot Laura's criticism of AA but also weaves in the fundamental therapeutic lessons that she learned at Fresh Beginnings. Drawing implicitly on the tenets of HOW (Honesty, Openness, Willingness), the client echoes Laura's portrayal of AA as an unsafe venue for verbal disclosure, particularly when that disclosure relates to one's sex life (line 6). Although we might suggest that this client came to this conclusion independent of her therapist, also notice that she refers to "that one time" she attended an AA meeting—a scant experiential base from which to launch such a critique (line 4). With this said, the fact that it is difficult to discern whether this client or clients *really* believe that it is obvious that AA is uncomfortable for women or whether she is flipping Laura's critical script is—again—precisely the point and power of flipping the script.

As a strong AA advocate, the new therapist Lizzy promptly wrote the Thursday AA meeting back into the weekly treatment schedule after Laura's departure and advised clients to attend additional meetings on their own time. She also began to dole out 90/90s to those who relapsed or broke the other conditions of their treatment contracts. In reaction, clients started working together to scaffold the feminist critiques of AA that they had acquired from Laura, effectively piecing together the critical content of Laura's feminist script in what at least appeared to be their very own words.

True to the feminist script, filled with compelling clinical content, and delivered with adamancy, clients' objections to AA posed a formidable conundrum for the new therapist, for although Lizzy doubted that her clients really believed that they could not "open up" in AA meetings, especially for the gender-based reasons they cited, she nevertheless had no proof to the contrary. In an interview with me, several months into her tenure at Fresh Beginnings and seemingly exhausted by clients' protests, Lizzy (L) rehearsed what had already come to be a canned response:

1 L And the way that I feel about AA is that AA has been more successful than
2 *any other treatment ever* for alcoholics, *including women* (sarcastic tone).
3 And for me to not recommend AA is un*ethical.*
4 Because it is the best treatment ever.
5 The best treatment is AA combined with treatment. (pause)
6 Research has proven this over and over.

7 And it is oriented towards *men*, but that's what we have and I think sucks too,
8 you know, um, but [it has] the highest rate of success.
9 And the reason you'll hate it is 'cause people are telling, you know,
10 pouring out their *guts* and that's *weird*.
11 I Uh-huh.
12 L *We* don't do that, I mean, in this society people just don't go up and say:
13 "My name is [Lizzy] and I am an alcoholic and I beat up my wife and I . . ."
14 It's very peculiar.
15 Now what happens is that a lot of women grab onto the idea that "it's not good for
16 me because I'm a woman and men created it" and "doctors, white male *doctors*!"
17 And those are all *true* things and I'm not going to *disagree* with that,
18 but I'm saying: it *works*, including with women, better than treatment.
19 I cannot treat you alone and be very effective.

In defense of AA and its role in her new clients' treatment, Lizzy pulls science onto her side (lines 1–5), constructing a frame that demotes the societal indexes of clients' objections (lines 11–13) in relation to ethical qua scientific claims (line 3–6). Conceding that there is some sociological "truth" in clients' criticisms (line 17), the new therapist nevertheless questions the validity of their protests, suggesting that they had "grab[bed] onto" an exogenous, feminist "idea" (line 14). Embellishing her recitation of clients' critiques with doses of sarcasm (lines 2, 12–15), Lizzy ultimately suggests that while the truth of science and society can be confirmed by research, the truth of the client remains tenaciously evasive.

Here, we should recall that the idea that one can clearly identify and verbally relay inner truths is the very ideological core of mainstream American addiction treatment. Tethered by a treatment philosophy to the ideology of inner reference, Lizzy faced a formidable epistemological bind, as her new clients had successfully pulled her into a guessing game with their words. Indeed, when I proposed later in our interview that perhaps clients "really *didn't* like AA" precisely for the reasons they stated, an inner referential premise of my own, Lizzy responded with a strikingly elaborate sociolinguistic analysis:

1 L *But* they would be talking and I would *see* their interactions and the way that
2 they were. And I would *hear* things that they said. But when they started talking
3 about AA, they were using someone *else's* words. It *felt* very different to me.
4 Um, because they were saying things *like* "Doctors developed AA, and that's
5 not good for women, and and and" (sarcastic).
6 And they would use all kinds of things that were not their ordinary way of *talking*
7 or relating to the world.

Rather than relying on the therapeutic ideology of inner reference, which allows one to connect the "things that they said" (line 2) with "the way that they were" (lines 1–2), Lizzy is now forced to consider a number of other possibilities about what her clients' words really mean. For instance, Lizzy accounts for observed "interactions" between clients (line 1), including the generic features of their "ordinary way of talking or relating to the world" (line 6) in relation to the feminist critiques of AA that they voiced directly to her. Furthermore, when Lizzy notes that "when they started talking about AA, they were using someone *else's* words" (lines 2–3), she acknowledges the existence of a group of possible, nonimmediate interlocutors, including the clients' former therapist. Unable to "*see*" (line 1) or monitor clients' interactions with these parties, a defeated Lizzy suggests that these unknown interlocutors will continue to exert force on clients' words: in closing her quotation with an exasperated "and and and," Lizzy indicates that she was prepared for the criticism of AA to keep coming in a number of skillfully deployed versions.

In much the same way as they destabilized the idea that one could find truth in urine, script flippers now troubled the central therapeutic principle that professionals could discern inner truths from words. Now unsure of what the truth was, Lizzy lost the very basis of her institutional authority; that is, her ability to assuredly align herself with the real. Thus, in flipping feminist scripts, Fresh Beginnings clients not only influenced the course of program policy. Nor did they simply influence the professional evaluations and in so doing redirect the flow of benefits, sanctions, and resources. As Lizzy makes clear, clients ultimately challenged and forced professionals to explicitly reckon with the entire ideological basis on which treatment was premised.

REIMAGINING THE WORK OF CLIENT AGENCY

In describing the everyday work of script flippers, I seek to challenge the very common assumption that clients are at the mercy of professionals, both because they are evaluated by those professionals and because resources are distributed on the basis of those evaluations. Consider the related research of anthropologist Robert Desjarlais, who in studying a Boston homeless shelter draws on Michel de Certeau's famous distinction between "strategies" (as the province of the powerful) and "tactics" (as the weapons of the weak) to analyze professionals' and clients' respective abilities to effectively act (Desjarlais 1997; see also Scott 1987). Desjarlais differentiates this "strategic" language of staff from the "tactical" language used by shelter residents—language characterized by questions, pleas, complaints, and entreaties. From this difference, Desjarlais draws a clear conclusion: clients' verbal tactics did not stand a chance in relation to the linguistic strategies of staff, grounded as the latter were in a durable locus of reason (cf. de Certeau 1984). More specifically, Desjarlais explains that residents' tactics were enfeebled by their tendency to locate agency in the staff listener, thereby providing an opportunity for a rationalized, strategic response.

In contrast, as the examples presented show, the script flippers at Fresh Beginnings were not destined to use the weak weapon of a "tactical" language, nor did they leave professional and institutional strategies intact. Rather, script flippers seized on the reason and agency of their professional audience, using them to their own ends. In doing so, they showed that there is necessarily nothing durable about social service professionals' locus of reason, even when culturally and institutionally reinforced.

In his brilliant early field study, long before he took a concerted interest in linguistic practice, Goffman (1961) suggested that while the inmate of his book titled *Asylums* might engage in prescribed activities, including authorized ways of speaking, his "capacities" may have migrated—that is, he does not believe or invest in what he dutifully does (see Newman, Chapter 16, this volume). Not only can an inmate be "an absentee" of his own activities, Goffman further explains, he can also conceal his own leave-taking. In doing so, the inmate does not shirk authorized ways of acting and speaking but instead plays with prescribed ways of being (Goffman 1961:188). Goffman wisely ends this section of *Asylums* with a methodological warning, which I have worked to heed throughout this chapter. Specifically, while acknowledging that "absenteeism" could be analyzed as a psychological phenomenon, I follow Goffman in holding the question of just what an individual "gets out of" a practice at bay. Indeed, if we are to reimagine social service interactions, the initial question should be not what a particular practice means to and for the practitioner. Instead, we should critically inquire into the nature of the social and institutional relations that require the acquisition and maintenance of practices like flipping the script (pp. 200–201). And rather than trying to reinforce professional and institutional control, we might join script flippers in reimagining and reworking the typical power relations of social service encounters.

NOTES

1 The names of the institutions and individuals involved in this ethnographic study, which included over three years of participant observation, dozens of interviews with program staff, clients, and affiliates, and extensive archival work and document review, have been altered to help guarantee their anonymity.

2 One might suspect a case of racial profiling in here, given that—at least according to Nikki—the baby showed no signs of ill health or distress. And while readers may readily count this case as illustrative of one of the most salient risks of flipping the script, they should do so in light of the now well-documented, dramatically overstated effects of in utero exposure to cocaine (Chavkin 2001).

REFERENCES

Austin, J. L. 1962. *How to Do Things with Words*. Cambridge, MA: Harvard University Press.

Cain, C. 1991. "Personal Stories: Identity Acquisition and Self-Understanding in Alcoholics Anonymous." *Ethos* 19:210–153.

Carr, E. Summerson. 2006. " 'Secrets Keep You Sick': Metalinguistic Labor in a Drug Treatment Program for Homeless Women." *Language in Society* 35(5): 631–653.

Carr, E. Summerson. 2009. "Anticipating and Inhabiting Institutional Identities." *American Ethnologist* 36(2): 317–336.

Carr, E. Summerson. 2011. *Scripting Addiction: The Politics of Therapeutic Talk and American Sobriety.* Princeton, NJ: Princeton University Press.

Chavkin, Wendy. 2001. "Cocaine and Pregnancy—Time to Look at the Evidence." *JAMA: Journal of the American Medical Association* 285:1626–1629.

de Certeau, Michel. 1984. *The Practice of Everyday Life.* Berkeley: University of California Press.

Desjarlais, Robert. 1997. *Shelter Blues: Sanity and Selfhood Among the Homeless.* Philadelphia: University of Pennsylvania Press.

Fox, Kathryn J. 2001. "Self Change and Resistance in Prison." In *Institutional Selves: Troubled Identities in a Post-modern World*, edited by J. Gubrium and J. Holstein, 176–192. Oxford: Oxford University Press.

Goffman, Erving. 1961. *Asylums: Essays on the Social Situation of Mental Patients and Other Inmates.* New York: Doubleday.

Goffman, Erving. 1981. *Forms of Talk.* Philadelphia: University of Pennsylvania Press.

Handler, Joel. 1986. *The Conditions of Discretion.* New York: Russell Sage Foundation.

Hasenfeld, Yeheskel. 2009. "Worker Client Relations: Social Policy in Practice." In *Human Services as Complex Organizations*, edited by Yeheskel Hasenfeld, 405–426. Thousand Oaks, CA: Sage.

Lave, Jean, and Etienne Wenger. 1991. *Situated Learning: Legitimate Peripheral Participation.* New York: Cambridge University Press.

Lipsky, Michael. 2010. *Street-Level Bureaucracy.* New York: Sage.

Scott, James. 1987. *Weapons of the Weak: Everyday Forms of Peasant Resistance.* New Haven, CT: Yale University Press.

5

Service Users' Negotiated Identity in a Social Enterprise and the Opportunity for Reflection in Action

▸ EVE E. GARROW

CAN VULNERABLE AND POWERLESS SERVICE USERS influence the practices of human service organizations to better meet their preferences? We want human service organizations to be responsive to the needs of the people who seek their services. We hope that service providers, as members of a helping profession, reflect on the lived experiences, interests, and preferences of their users and build these insights into their practices. Yet, as Michael Lipsky (1980) observed, when service users are powerless, they are unlikely to have an active voice in determining the systems under which they are the objects of intervention. A large body of street-level research has confirmed this observation (e.g., Brodkin 1997; Lin 2000; Maynard-Moody and Musheno 2003). Service providers have great discretion in their daily interactions with service users and may use it to ignore service user preferences that do not align with organizational ideologies concerning the deservingness of potential users for organizational services, the nature of their problems, and appropriate solutions.

According to Lipsky (1980), these power asymmetries derive from workers' control of resources that service users need, and are magnified under conditions of chronic resource scarcity as demand for services exceeds supply. Teresa Gowan's (2010) ethnography of the homeless services field in San Francisco is illustrative of this point. Faced with demand that far outpaced the availability of services, the homeless people she studied found that they had to take the services that were offered to them without complaint or go without them altogether.

But are vulnerable and marginalized service users always powerless under conditions of chronic resource scarcity? The street-level contexts that Lipsky (1980) explored, such as schools and welfare offices, were characterized by power arrangements that were highly institutionalized and self-reproducing. Yet, increasingly, human service organizations operate in multiple institutional fields, exposing these organizations to institutional pluralism (Kraatz and Block 2008). The proliferation of organizational forms that straddle the market and social services sectors, for example, is encouraged by a rising neoliberal ideology that promotes market solutions to social problems (see Jensen and Villadsen, Chapter 11, this volume). As institutional theorists have noted, pluralism begets institutional conflict, especially when competing institutional prescriptions are at odds. In turn, institutional conflict has a destabilizing effect on the organization of power (Seo and Creed 2002). When organizational power structures are unstable and contested, relations between service providers and users may look very different from those in the street-level bureaucracies depicted by Lipsky (1980) and other street-level researchers.

In this chapter, I suggest that the destabilization process resulting from institutional pluralism may generate praxis—political action embedded in multiple contradictory institutional arrangements (Seo and Creed 2002). Institutional contradiction produces political opportunities that otherwise powerless service users can exploit to advance their own interests (see in this volume Carr, Chapter 4; Järvinen, Chapter 3). In doing so, it can provide the scaffolding for a dialectical framework of social work practice that enables service users and providers to challenge the underlying assumptions of practice and dynamically experiment with and modify human service technology accordingly. That is, it provides the opportunity for service providers to engage in what Donald Schön calls "reflection in action" (Schön 1983). Such reflection brings to the surface—makes visible—and tests the tacit norms that inform professional judgment and guide organizational practices, taking into account the wholeness of the experiences of service users (see Newman, Chapter 16, this volume). As a result, service providers can develop new frames for the problems they are trying to solve and with them new strategies of action that more closely reflect the interests of their service users (see Greener, Chapter 14, this volume).

THE CASE STUDY

To build this argument, I present findings from an ethnographic case study that focuses on a hybrid organizational form at the intersection of the market and social services sectors. Work integration social enterprises (WISEs) aim to integrate hard-to-employ persons into the labor market by providing them with employment opportunities within a social service context while also producing and selling products or services in the market (Garrow and Hasenfeld 2012). Consequently, WISEs assume a dual institutional identity as human service organization and commercial enterprise. Correspondingly, clients assume identities as service users and workers, and service providers assume identities as social service workers and employers. I demonstrate how the presence of these contradictory identities can generate political conflict, praxis, and a dialectical model of service provision that stimulates reflection in practice.

The following analysis draws from data collected from early 2006 through 2008 in an organization I called "Employment Services." The data include (1) direct observation of board meetings, staff meetings, teleconferences, and email exchanges, (2) casual discussions with organizational members both before and after meetings, and (3) loosely structured interviews with current and previous organizational members at all levels. To reconstruct the history of the organization, I interviewed the founder, two original board members, and two staff members who worked in the organization during the decades between the founding and the study period. I also collected archival data, which included (1) ethnographic data collected over a three-year period in the mid- to late 1990s from an unpublished dissertation on the organization (Hill 2004), and (2) a variety of documents, including brochures, articles about the organization, balance sheets, financial reports, minutes and agendas of board and staff meetings, lists of board directors, strategic plans, market analyses, IRS tax returns, and client application and referral forms. The ethnographic approach is distinctly relational in that it focuses on the interplay of shifting logics that structure two separate but interrelated social worlds—the field of social services and the business sector (Desmond 2014). The research design was particularly useful for a relational analysis because it allowed me to trace the struggle of two competing fields over time, to explore how actors differently positioned in the organization (i.e., case managers, service users, and staff on the business enterprise side) channeled this struggle, and to examine the implications for the evolving relationship between service providers and users.

I conducted individual interviews with respondents representing the full range of positions within the organization, from board members and the executive leadership to frontline staff who worked with clients on a daily basis. Interviews typically focused on the backgrounds, attitudes, and experiences of respondents with regard to their own role and identity in the organization, their relations to individuals in other organizational positions, and the evaluative developments as they related to organizational dynamics and identity. The research proceeded iteratively, going back and forth between problem formulation, data collection, and data analysis.

HYBRID ORGANIZATIONS AND INSTITUTIONAL CONFLICT

From an institutional perspective, the organizational field is defined as a network of organizations that "partakes in common meaning system and whose participants interact more frequently and fatefully with one another than with actors outside the field" (Scott 1995:56). The human services are characterized by a diversity of organizational fields, including areas such as health care, homeless services, mental health, domestic violence, and child care. A key characteristic of the field is the powerful isomorphic pressures it exerts on its members. These pressures take the form of institutional logics—sets of symbolic constructions and material practices (Friedland and Alford 1991) that define the "interests, identities, values, and assumptions of individuals and organizations" (Thornton and Ocasio 2008:103) that constitute a given field. Logics provide prescriptions that guide the interpretation of reality and instruct organizational members on how to proceed in a given context. Beliefs and cognitive structures that organize the field are thought to deeply influence the internal decisions about the organization's reason for being, basic organizational identities, appropriate practices, and who should be in control (Friedland and Alford 1991; Greenwood and Hinings 1996). For human service organizations, a key structuring logic is expressed as a bundle of beliefs and material practices regarding the construction of the clients' problems, the causes or diagnosis of the problems, the desired outcomes, and the prescribed means to attain them (Garrow and Hasenfeld 2012).

Institutional logics define not only organizational practices but also the internal organizational hierarchy among the organizational members involved in implementing practices. The health care field, for example, privileges the forms of expertise monopolized by physicians over the skills and knowledge of nurses and social workers or the perspectives of patients and families, and this hierarchy is reproduced in the internal structure of hospitals (Heimer 1999). Structural patterns of relations in organizations tend to become settled when the logic is well institutionalized and taken for granted (Bourdieu 1989; Bourdieu and Wacquant 1992).

The taken-for-granted presuppositions that determine power relations and guide action within the field are undermined by the presence of institutional contradiction. As noted by Kraatz and Block (2008), organizations in pluralistic institutional environments are exposed to the demands of multiple institutional logics and are constituted by multiple legitimating identities that operate at the field level. When multiple and conflicting logics are "represented" by actors in organizations (Pache and Santos 2010; Zilber 2002), it is typically assumed that those actors are likely to engage in political struggles in ways that are aligned with their institutionally defined interests and identities (Greenwood et al. 2011). Institutional contradictions are especially likely in hybrid organizations that develop interdependencies in more than one organizational field, because they are by definition exposed to potentially disparate field-level institutional logics and, correspondingly, are defined by multiple organizational identities.

Scholars have argued that institutional contradiction and conflict set the stage for praxis—political action geared toward the reconstitution of social relations that takes place at the intersection of conflicting institutional arrangements (Friedland and Alford 1991; Seo and Creed 2002). Institutional contradiction provides the cultural material for praxis by challenging previously hegemonic logics, thus generating a reflective shift in consciousness. Political conflict plays out in the struggle over multiple logics that are encoded in the identities of the organization and its members, leading to political instability and change. In human service organizations, this struggle may create a space for otherwise powerless service users to express and advance their preferences. In part, they can do so by aligning themselves with those factions in the organization that uphold the organizational and service user identities that resonate with their interests. This chapter explores the institutional conflict experienced by one hybrid organization and shows how such conflict provided opportunities for praxis, which in turn stimulated reflection on the part of service providers that incorporated the experiences and preferences of service users.

EMPLOYMENT SERVICES AS SERVICE PROVIDER AND BUSINESS ENTERPRISE

Employment Services originated in the field of homeless social services but soon entered the market sector. It was founded in 1984 by a 22-year-old Jesuit volunteer in a "skid row" neighborhood characterized by concentrated homelessness. The early members developed a service model that involved a range of employment-readiness services for homeless clients, including the distribution of fresh clothing for job interviews; workshops on topics such as hygiene, résumé writing, and the interview process; and self-directed job searches aided by the support and guidance of case managers. As recounted by a founding board member,

> We decided to teach classes. The basic thing's to get a job. Cleaning yourself. Get a haircut. Make sure they are shaving. Make sure they look good so we can send them out on interviews. I remember teaching the first class at an office at city hall the mayor made available to us. The class was basic information. Show up on time. Shower, brush teeth, put a resume together. We'd get people to come in and do specific parts of the classes.

The organization's model was premised on the assumption that poverty and homelessness are caused by individual-level employment barriers such as ineffective résumé writing, lack of job search skills, and an unprofessional self-presentation during job interviews. Members expected that, once the organization addressed these deficits, service users would quickly secure employment in the labor market. Yet many service users, facing structural barriers to employment, such as discrimination based on race, criminal history, or scant employment experience, as well as personal barriers such as substance abuse and physical or mental health issues, were unable to retain employment despite their participation in the program.

Frustrated with the low employment rate of their service users, upper management augmented the service model by connecting users to day labor opportunities—an innovation that also failed to achieve the desired results. As one founding board member put it in an interview,

> To the extent that we had a defined mission—helping the homeless find jobs and become self-sufficient—we were doing case work. How to get your messages; how to write a resume. As [service users] crossed all these hurdles, not having a job history was a big problem. It was Steve [staff member] who said, "we can get these guys day labor jobs at least." He got commitments from companies to call Employment Services if they needed day laborers instead of just going to the street corner. Then their complaint was: these guys aren't dependable, they're not clean. The companies wanted to keep an arm's length. They didn't want to deal with the social problems of these guys.

In response to the failure of the day labor program, Employment Services developed an in-house work experience component. It created a business enterprise that provided transitional paid work experience opportunities in the janitorial field to service users who, despite having availed themselves of the usual repertoire of case management and directed job search services, were unable to obtain employment in the labor market. These work experiences, meant to last between three and six months, functioned to enhance soft skills such as punctuality and work ethic and, in the words of a previous manager who was interviewed, to "give our clients some income, keep them busy, and keep them motivated. Plus, for people who didn't have much of a work history, we could give them a track record." For organizational leaders, the businesses were a social service that also happened to double as a funding source—a perfect alignment of financial and programmatic goals. As a founding board member recounted in an interview:

> We could hire our own clients. They could get work history. Those with more potential could become supervisors. The businesses started becoming a funding source . . . but the best part of it is that it tied fundraising to the mission of the organization.

INSTITUTIONAL PLURALISM AND CONTRADICTION

As the addition of transitional work experiences moved Employment Services into the business sector, the organization could be understood as straddling two distinct fields—homeless services and market enterprises—leading to organizational hybridity. Employment Services started with small business contracts but quickly gained market share in the burgeoning

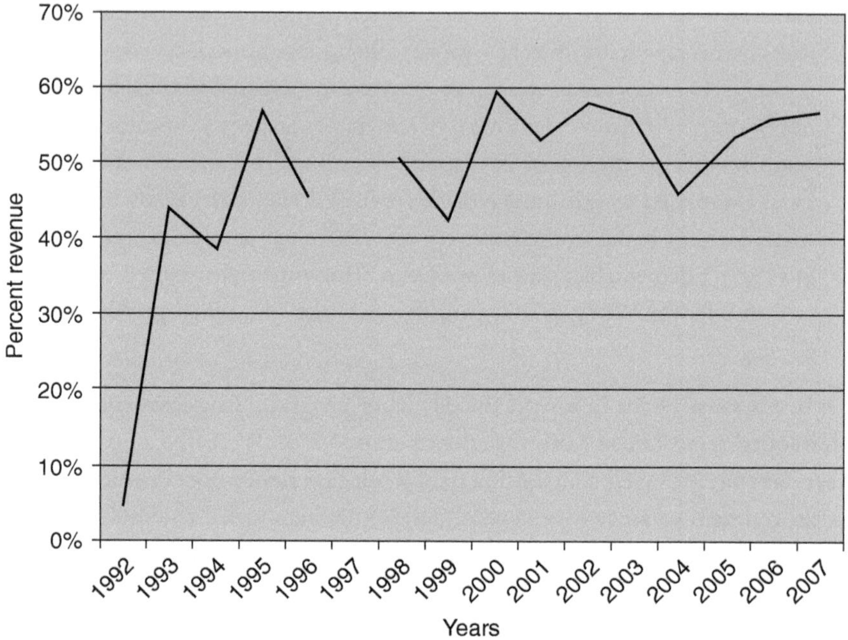

FIGURE 5.1 Commercial revenue as a share of total revenue.

field of street cleaning for Business Improvement Districts (BIDs)—associations comprised of businesses in a specified area that tax themselves and buy services intended to improve the district. As described by a previous manager in an interview, "We spent a year and a half in the [name of a BID] learning how to do the business, and then we went after all those other [BID] contracts." As shown in Figure 5.1, income from the commercial enterprises jumped from around 5 percent during the organization's early years to around 50 percent of total revenue when Employment Services began competing for more BID contracts during the early to mid-1990s.

Now, Employment Services was positioned in a highly pluralistic institutional environment. To adhere to the competing demands of the two fields in which it was positioned, it assumed dual organizational identities as human service organization and commercial enterprise, each represented by a distinct organizational unit. Case managers in the social services unit upheld the organization's identity in the homeless services field by providing case management for directed job search and service plans, while an enterprise unit provided contracted street cleaning services to

BIDs that doubled as transitional work opportunities for service users. According to the service model, service users were to complete an array of mandatory classes before engaging in a directed job search. Case managers were to use their professional judgment to selectively refer service users to the work experience opportunities once they had completed the service component of the program. Service users were expected to continue engaging in a directed job search while waiting for a position to open up in the enterprises, and to a more limited degree, while working in the enterprises. After gaining some work experience in the enterprises, the service users were supposed to return full-time to a directed job search with the guidance and support of their case managers.

Facing isomorphic pressures from both fields, the organization began to experience tension and conflict between the business and social services units. Staff members on the business side needed to respond to the demands of BID customers, who, consistent with a market logic of productivity, quality control, and cost savings, often expected prompt, efficient, high-quality street cleaning services despite the employment barriers of the Employment Services client-workers. This pressure was sometimes applied through direct interactions with service users, as noted by a former manager of the businesses in an interview:

> One guy who ran a BID was like an old county sheriff. He ran a great BID. His area was clean, safe. But he was a demanding customer. He wanted his crew on time, no absenteeism. He even did inspections of the crew, to make sure they were all in uniform. He would say, "I want the cream of the crop." He didn't want anyone on his contract until they were tested on a lesser contract.

Thus, for the business staff interacting with BID customers, the transitional work experiences were not only work therapy but also production jobs, and service users were not only clients but also production workers. If the business failed to meet the expectations of BID customers, it could (and sometimes did) lose lucrative contracts in the highly competitive BID market. Indeed, given the employment barriers experienced by their service users, the business staff often had difficulty fulfilling the work contracts. Service users would sometimes fail to show up for work, crash the cleaning trucks, or otherwise slow down the efficiency of the work crew. The WISE managers would pull service users from the labor pool to manage these exigencies, chip in with their own labor, and smooth things over with the BIDs. Service users became more valuable as labor once they were trained, and the enterprises tended to retain them well past the three- to six-month deadline.

At the same time, the organization continued to be highly dependent on stakeholders in the field of homeless social services. The organization's links to its key supporters, including elite donors and prestigious foundations, hinged on proving that their homeless service users could be placed in the job market and thereby increase their self-sufficiency. This was a widely appealing belief that had defined the organization's identity from its founding and, according to the executive director, was central to its ability to garner donations and foundation gifts. The social services unit upheld this belief by providing social services and case management designed to help homeless individuals obtain employment in the labor market. The belief was also enacted through institutionalized ceremonies such as service user testimonials prominently displayed on the organization's webpage, the display of photographs of service users who had obtained jobs, the ringing of a bell when a service user who was engaged in a directed job search was offered a job, and donor meetings, where service users talked about how the organization had changed their lives by helping them to become self-sufficient (field notes).

Perhaps inevitably, the goals of the business enterprise and social services units began to conflict. In response to occasional labor shortages, for example, managers on the business side of the organization rerouted service users engaged in a job search to the labor positions in the business enterprises in a practice organizational members referred to as "sweeping the lobby." As a manager of the enterprises explained in an interview, "You might get a call from one of the supervisors—two people didn't show. So, you go to the lobby to see who you can find to fill the spots. If people were in the lobby, whether they had gone through the process [of receiving services from the social services unit] or not, they would be put to work."

Sweeping the lobby was a symbolically forceful power play because it gave priority to business imperatives over social services, thereby legitimating the primacy of the market logic that structured the business field and the subordination of the service logic drawn from the field of homeless services. The impetus to sweep the lobby grew stronger as business contracts became larger. As a previous manager observed in an interview, "We had a couple of big customers once and the shock was enormous. They needed thirty people for one week and it sucked up [service users] from everywhere and became the only focus for everybody."

Case managers challenged these practices by complaining that the business's need for labor diverted service users from a trajectory toward permanent employment in the labor market. In an interview, a former manager on the business side of the organization said that "sometimes the case managers would get angry, because [sweeping the lobby] subverted their job and the process the clients were supposed to go through." Yet, to maintain good customer relations with the BID customers, upper management tacitly allowed the business needs of the enterprises to subordinate the service side's goals. As the executive director put it in an interview:

> The thing about our model is that it either works great as a business but bad as a program or great as a program but bad as a business. What happened was that the program was broken entirely.... [T]o make the businesses work, the businesses killed the program.... [T]he pendulum was swinging too much to the business side.

SERVICE USERS AND PRAXIS

How did service users respond to the organization's emerging hybrid identity as both a social service agency and a business? Financially destitute, socially excluded from the labor market, and desperate for work, they began to reconstitute the service organization as a potential employer, the work experiences as production jobs, and their roles as paid employees. In my discussions with residents in the skid row area in which Employment Services is located, homeless men often referred to Employment Services as one of the only "employers" in the area willing to hire them, although they recognized that the demand for the jobs at Employment Services far outpaced the supply. This account of a case manager highlights the sense of urgency felt by service users as they attempted to obtain the paid work experiences:

> I think in some instances, because of [the business enterprises], case managers are posed with a lot of people that come in here, and want a job. They want a job now, they heard that we're giving out, away jobs, which is great, you know, these people want to work, you might say. But then it's hard to

> get them away from that idea. Um, even if we don't have positions open. (Hill 2004:323)

As service user demand for paid work experiences in the business enterprises grew, case managers advanced ideas, consistent with the organization's mission, that constructed the organization as an employment-readiness program as opposed to an employer. The tension between claims and counterclaims is captured in the following narrative of one case manager, who, during an orientation for potential service users, builds a representation of the organization based on its historical identity as a homeless services organization:

> Let me start by saying that anybody who came in here today thinking that, uh, they walk into these doors and they'll have a job as they leave those doors, that's not the case. We don't give out jobs. We help people find jobs. Okay? And there's a big difference there. (Hill, 2004:162)

In response, service users exploited the political conflict between the service and enterprise units to express their preferences. They began actively avoiding their case managers once they had finished the repertoire of classes provided by the services side. Case managers generally had no further contact with service users after they completed the mandatory classes, even though they instructed users to continue to engage in job-readiness activities. Instead, as described by a manager on the business side, service users started "hanging around in the front area waiting for a job . . . and [coming] in every day to wait around to get called for a job by [the staffing coordinator]," whether or not they had been referred to the transitional work experience program by their case managers. Case managers grumbled, while staff members on the business side looked the other way.

Once service users obtained the coveted work experience positions, many stayed. Although the agency did not keep ongoing records of when service users transitioned to the work experiences and how long they remained in the positions, organizational members were aware that many service users did not transition to employment in the labor market in a timely manner, if at all. As the manager of the enterprises put it in an interview, "The [client] workers are spread out and don't see their case manager. They may end up working for us for two years!" In fact, an internal audit conducted during the study period revealed that many service users had occupied the jobs for up to ten years. Instead of a transitional work experience program, the enterprises had become a de facto sheltered workshop.

The transformation of the enterprises into a sheltered workshop model was aligned with service user preferences. A new case manager installed in the aftermath of the internal audit to increase the rate of service user transition from enterprise jobs to work in the labor market put it this way in an interview:

> Whenever a position becomes available, [service users who take the positions] feel that they have got the position and they have fulfilled their dream. They have no intention of looking for another job. Because they have found their job once they are on the [enterprise] team . . . they say the BID contractors like what they do, the supervisors like what they do, why should they transition? No matter what they were told [by the case managers], they feel that this is their position and why should they go?

CRITICAL REFLECTIVE SPACE

The gap between the professed and actual practices of Employment Services caused ongoing internal tension and conflict. The executive director, enraged by the low rate of transition to the labor market, replaced the manager of the enterprises, stating in an interview that:

> [The manager] didn't believe in his clients. He dropped the programmatic part of it—the transitional part of it—because he didn't think the clients could do it. He said he believed in the program because his daughter had been a homeless drug addict and he felt for these people. But when it came down to it he thought the best they could do was employment in [the enterprise] jobs—that they would never survive on the outside.

He also replaced the staff member who had performed the audit that had revealed that most service users stayed on the rolls for years rather than months, and fired the transitional case manager when it became clear that he was unable to transition most of the client-workers to jobs in the labor market. Yet, the firings had little impact on the practices of service providers, perhaps because the structural relations between units remained the same. Indeed, when I interviewed a staff member several years later, he said that service users still remained in the transitional work experiences for up to ten years.

Yet, the ongoing decoupling of the stated mission of Employment Services and its internal practices did more than stimulate turmoil and conflict. It also provided conceptual space for organizational members to critically reflect on the expressed needs of service users and the root causes of their problems. The professed service logic was constantly under interrogation during organizational staff meetings I attended and in my interviews with members. For example, many staff members I talked to recognized that organizational practices that aligned with user preferences were a practical response to the very real barriers that some service users faced in the labor market. Yet, they struggled to reconcile the organization's stated mission, which was to provide transitional work experience leading to employment in the labor market, with its transformed practices. The transitional case manager, for example, blamed the service users for resisting the official transitional work model and blamed staff for failing to enforce it. As he put it in an interview,

> Instead of holding [service users] accountable, we give them too much. We are nurturing them and taking care of them too much. We make excuses for them. No one says derogatory things about clients. We hold on to them and keep them here. Maybe because we think this is the only place they can get a second chance.

At the same time, he conceded that many of the client-workers had almost insurmountable employment barriers. As he told me in an interview, "All [of the long-term client-workers] have significant and multiple barriers to employment. About 127 are ex-offenders. . . . I have the rapists and murderers on my caseload . . . physical disabilities, like a prosthetic leg, or deformed body part . . . senior citizens . . . those who cannot read or write . . . mental disabilities."

Staff on the business side sometimes justified the practice of retaining client-workers in the transitional employment positions well past the three- to six-month time limit by acknowledging the structural barriers clients faced in the low-wage labor market. As the manager of the enterprises noted in a meeting, when discussing the barriers to transition, "Another problem—the Ikeas, Macys, and so forth—they don't want [to hire] anyone with a felony. By saying this they have excluded almost all of our [client] workers!" (field notes).

Discussions on potential new enterprises that would do more to enhance service users' skills dominated many meetings. Organizational members also brainstormed on new ideas such as a "transitional period" that would allow service users to ease into the workforce. In one staff meeting, for example, the manager of the enterprises mentioned a service user who had obtained a job, so he was taken off the transitional work crew. He was laid off one day later. He came to the manager, saying, "What do I do now? I can't pay my rent." As the manager noted, the situation presented a dilemma because the service user had already been replaced on the work crew. He said, "I gave the client money out of my own pocket and put him back on a crew the next week." In an oblique acknowledgment of the serious structural employment barriers faced by many service users, he argued that the agency should encourage users to obtain labor market employment but should be ready and willing to take them back when they failed (field notes).

Indeed, by all accounts, the organization was quite reluctant to enforce the three- to six-month limit on the transitional work opportunities. As service users became attached to the jobs and the security they provided, organizational members were loath to disrupt their progress by taking away their job and their income. Members feared, perhaps realistically, that withdrawing the work opportunities would push service users back into homelessness and hopelessness. Overt relations between service providers and users came to resemble a rapprochement, wherein service providers looked the other way while users retained jobs in the enterprises for as long as they needed or wanted them.

A DIALECTICAL MODEL OF SERVICE PROVISION

I find that the interactions among multiple institutional identities in WISEs lead to role ambiguity, conflict, and political struggle; yet they also provide cultural material and political opportunities for organizational change that align with service user preferences. In the case under study, the service users exploited the ambiguities in their identities and political tensions between organizational units to define themselves as workers rather than clients and, by doing so, they altered the organization's service technology. In particular, they marginalized the social service unit by avoiding it and in the process highlighted the gap between the organization's practices and its external image as an employment and transitional work program. Although the organization never abandoned its public mission, which was to help the homeless find jobs in the labor market and become self-sufficient, in practice it provided service users with the permanent sheltered employment opportunities they desired.

Yet, research suggests that many human service organizations, especially those that serve stigmatized and powerless people, routinely ignore the expressed needs and preferences of service users and are all too willing to expel, reject, or otherwise cool out service users who challenge the service logic (e.g., Gowan 2010; Lyon-Callo 2000). In his study of a homeless shelter, for example, Vincent Lyon-Callo (2000) found that staff members compelled homeless residents to locate the cause of their homelessness in personal pathologies and to accept therapy; when the residents instead blamed structural conditions such as racism or low wages, they were viewed as unwilling to help themselves and were threatened with eviction.

I argue that it was the inherent contradictions and conflicts that arose between organizational units—driven by the organization's location at the intersection of two incompatible organizational fields—that provided the political opportunity for service users to express their service preferences. The transfigured practices that resulted from these political maneuvers in turn challenged the organization's service logic, opening conceptual space for organizational members to engage in a dialectical model of service provision in which they critically reflected on the expressed needs of service users and the root causes of their problems. While the organization was not willing to integrate its actual practices into its official service model, members routinely interrogated the service logic and questioned its underlying assumptions about the causes of homelessness, poverty, and unemployment.

This ongoing dialectic also raised new moral dilemmas for the provision of human services. In particular, the organization struggled to reconcile its stated mission, which was to provide transitional work experience leading to employment in the labor market, with its transformed practices, which were to provide long-term sheltered employment to service users. The users themselves, given their multiple barriers to employment in the labor market, preferred to remain in sheltered employment at the WISE. As a result, the organization experienced uneasy tension between its formal structure and decoupled practices that periodically erupted into political conflict, as when the executive director fired the author of the audit that revealed the extent of the disjuncture.

Why, though, did the organization not seriously consider recoupling its stated mission with its internal practices—not by changing its practices but by changing its mission to align with its practices? For example, it could have built the de facto sheltered workshop model into its official array of services. Yet the executive director was highly resistant to this idea when I suggested it, and it never came up in the meetings I attended or in my interviews with other organizational members. It could be that the sheltered workshop model, if exposed, would have threatened the organization's high level of legitimacy in the homeless services field. According to the executive director, the organization attracted elite donors and large, prestigious foundation gifts not by running a sheltered workshop but by appealing to widely held beliefs that attribute poverty and homelessness to individual deficiencies such as a poor work ethic and inadequate soft skills; view personal transformation—accomplished by soft skill training and transitional work experience—as the solution; and see self-sufficiency as the desired outcome. In short, the organization had found that an organizational identity based on improving the work ethic and promoting self-sufficiency was broadly appealing and profitable in the field of homeless services. Some service users did obtain jobs while engaged in the directed job search program at Employment Services, which is the ceremony that validates the myth (Meyer and Rowan 1977), but many faced profound employment barriers that prevented them from participating in the labor market. The public identity of Employment Services in the homeless services field seemed to be a major force in pushing the organization into an ongoing and seemingly unresolvable dialectic, as the sheltered workshop template represented a tacit rebuttal to the causal model of poverty and homelessness on which it was predicated.

CONTEXT AND REFLECTION IN ACTION

As Donald Schön (1983) argues, through reflection, the service provider can bring to the surface and critique the tacit norms that inform professional judgment and guide organizational practices. If providers are to engage in a practice that is responsive to the interests, preferences, and lived experiences of service users, such reflection is critical. Reflection enables service providers, either collectively or individually, to transcend their narrow preconceptions about the service users. Using the wholeness of their experiences and understandings, they can gather information outside of their organizationally prescribed lens—including knowledge based on the lived experiences and preferences of the service users with which they interact—and incorporate such understandings into their practices. While their initial understandings of the issue at hand may be grounded in the working hypothesis provided to them by the organization, by engaging in reflection they can test this hypothesis by taking into account the experiences and responses of the service users. Using this information, they can revise their working hypothesis accordingly.

Yet, we know from street-level research that such reflection may be the exception rather than the rule—especially in human service organizations that serve stigmatized groups. Why? It is important to note that reflection does not happen in a vacuum. While service providers may be exposed to multiple and conflicting theoretical frameworks with which to guide their practices, they are more likely to incorporate the frameworks of those groups—be they organizational members or stakeholder groups—that have power over them. Service users, especially those that belong to stigmatized and oppressed groups, typically have little actual power over human service organizations that serve them. In the context of a political economy that puts service users at a political disadvantage, the organization may be more likely to ground its work in the theories of powerful stakeholders on whom they depend for resources than those of the groups they serve (Wamsley and Zald 1976). Often, these perspectives are discordant with the experiences and interests of service users.

Thus, it is not enough to say that service providers should engage in reflection. To improve the provision of services, we need to take into account the organizational and environmental context that shapes and enables practice. In this sense, context is part and parcel of practice. Reflection in practice that incorporates the lived experiences and preferences of service users is more likely when conditions of work provide political opportunities for the expression of those experiences and preferences. The experience of Employment Services demonstrates that such conditions are possible, even when serving oppressed and stigmatized groups. Institutional contradiction and conflict provided a fertile context for praxis—political action geared toward the reconstitution of social relations (Friedland and Alford 1991; Seo and Creed 2002). At Employment Services, this political conflict involved the struggle over multiple logics that were encoded in the identities of the organization and its members. Service users were able to express and advance their preferences by aligning themselves with the factions in the organization that upheld the organizational and service user identities that resonated with their interests.

The ensuing use of reflection provided the opportunity for an ongoing critique of the purpose of the organization and the most basic underlying assumptions on which its social service model was built. Eventually, these reflections became expressed in practice. At first, case managers resented service users for avoiding the client services and took exception with the business enterprises for recruiting the users before they had finished the service trajectory. Over time, however, they began to accept that many service users were unlikely or unable to transition to jobs in the labor market, despite their receipt of the organization's array of services. They became more accommodating of the wishes of service users to obtain and hold onto the jobs provided by the enterprises, and in turn their practices changed. For example, while the official service model directed the case managers to refer users to the enterprises only after the directed job search, they began instead to allow service users to "self-refer" to the enterprises without engaging in the job search. Also in violation of the official service model, over time, the case managers became less likely to pressure or encourage users to continue their job search while working in the enterprises, and in fact had little if any contact with them once they obtained the work positions (field notes).

Staff on the business enterprise side also engaged in reflection that modified their practices. They, too, came to appreciate the profound employment barriers some of the users faced in the labor market. They acquiesced to the preferences of service users who wanted to stay in the work positions well past the official three- to six-month time limit, and they always found ways to take back their past users when they failed in the labor market.

Through reflection, then, organizational members shared common interest not just with service users but also across units (see Barnes, Chapter 15, this volume). That is, service users, in exploiting the political opportunities afforded by institutional contradiction to advance their own interests, stimulated reflection in practice that created a bridge between conflicting organizational units. Reflection gave the case management and business enterprise units a common frame that was aligned with the experiences and preferences of service users.

This common frame holds the potential to provide the basis of political mobilization across units to change the official service model and practices in ways that better reflect the interests and experiences of service users. Nevertheless, while institutional contradiction at Employment Services did lead to political upheaval, ongoing dialectic, reflection, and modified practices, it has yet to substantively reshape the organization's official service model. Perhaps, as mentioned, it was less dangerous for the organization to decouple its practices from its official form than to transform its form by, for example, assuming an organizational identity as a sheltered workshop—an act that might alienate stakeholders on which it depends for resources. Admittedly, then, the potential for such a political project is hypothetical at this point in the trajectory of Employment Services.

Still, the case study suggests that struggles that give voice to typically voiceless stakeholders—especially when those stakeholders are service users who represent the raison d'etre of the organization—should be embraced as integral to the organization's service technology, because they represent an opportunity for reflection. In such a model, political destabilization provides the opportunity for service users to enter this dialogue (see Jensen and Villadsen, Chapter 11, this volume). Social workers could take a lead in exposing and reflecting on the contradictions that arise within the context of political destabilization, giving service users more room in the resulting space of ambiguities to express their preferences (see in this volume Barnes, Chapter 15; Gubrium, Chapter 1). They could also honor the choices of service users within the array of competing perspectives and practices and mobilize politically to create better alignment between official service models and service user preferences. Such alignment would enable the organization to introduce new models and frames into a broader dialogue with external stakeholders that better reflects the lived experiences and preferences of service users.

REFERENCES

Binder, A. 2007. "For Love and Money: Organizations' Creative Responses to Multiple Environmental Logics." *Theory and Society* 36(6): 547–571.

Bourdieu, P. 1989. "Social Space and Symbolic Power." *Sociological Theory* 7(1): 14–25.

Bourdieu, P., and Loic J. D. Wacquant. 1992. *An Invitation to Reflexive Sociology.* Chicago: University of Chicago Press.

Brodkin, E. Z. 1997. "Inside the Welfare Contract: Discretion and Accountability in State Welfare Administration." *Social Service Review* 71:1–33.

Desmond, M. 2014. "Relational Ethnography." *Theory and Society* 43:547–579.

Friedland, R., and R. R. Alford. 1991. "Bringing Society Back In: Symbols, Practices, and Institutional Contradictions." In *The New Institutionalism in Organizational Analysis*, edited by W. W. Powell and P. DiMaggio, 232–263. Chicago: University of Chicago Press.

Garrow, E., and Y. Hasenfeld. 2012. "Managing Conflicting Institutional Logics: Social Service vs. Market." In *Social Enterprises: An Organizational Perspective,* edited by Benjamin Gidron and Yeheskel Hasenfeld, 121–143. New York: Palgrave MacMillan.

Gowan, T. 2010. *Hobos, Hustlers, and Backsliders: Homeless in San Francisco.* Minneapolis: University of Minnesota Press.

Greenwood, R., and C. R. Hinings. 1996. "Understanding Radical Organizational Change: Bringing Together the Old and the New Institutionalism." *Academy of Management Review* 21:1022–1054.

Greenwood, R., M. Raynard, F. Kodeih, E. R. Micelotta, and M. Lounsbury. 2011. "Institutional Complexity and Organizational Responses." *Academy of Management Annals* 5(1): 317–371.

Hallett, T. 2007. "Between Deference and Distinction: Interaction Ritual Through Symbolic Power in an Educational Institution." *Social Psychology Quarterly* 70(2): 148–171.

Heimer, C A. 1999. "Competing Institutions: Law, Medicine, and Family in Neonatal Intensive Care." *Law and Society Review* 33:17–66.

Hill, K. M. 2004. "Getting Jobs and Making Progress: The Social World of a Skid Row Employment Program." PhD diss., University of California, Los Angeles.

Kraatz, M. S., and E. S. Block. 2008. "Organizational Implications of Institutional Pluralism." In *Handbook of Organizational Institutionalism,* edited by Royston Greenwood, Christine Oliver, Roy Suddaby, and Kerstin Sahlin-Andersson, 243–275. Thousand Oaks, CA: Sage.

Lin, A. C. 2000. *Reform in the Making: The Implementation of Social Policy in Prison.* Princeton, NJ: Princeton University Press.

Lipsky, M. 1980. *Street-Level Bureaucracy: Dilemmas of the Individual in Public Services.* New York: Russell Sage Foundation.

Lynn-Callo, Vincent. 2000. "Medicalizing Homelessness: The Production of Self-Blame and Self-Governing Within Homeless Shelters." *Medical Anthropology Quarterly* 14(3): 328–345.

Maynard-Moody, S., and M. C. Musheno. 2003. *Cops, Teachers, and Counselors: Stories from the Frontlines of Public Service.* Ann Arbor: University of Michigan Press.

Meyer, J., and B. Rowan. 1977. "Institutionalized Organizations: Formal Structure as Myth and Ceremony." *American Journal of Sociology* 83:340–363.

Pache, A., and F. Santos. 2010. "When Worlds Collide: The Internal Dynamics of Organizational Responses to Conflicting Institutional Demands." *Academy of Management Review* 35(3): 455–476.

Padgett, D. K. 1998. *Qualitative Methods in Social Work Research: Challenges and Rewards.* Thousand Oaks, CA: Sage.

Schön, D. A. 1983. *The Reflective Practitioner: How Professionals Think in Action.* New York: Basic.

Scott, W. R. 1995. *Institutions and Organizations.* Thousand Oaks, CA: Sage.

Seo, M., and W. E. Douglas Creed. 2002. "Institutional Contradictions, Praxis, and Institutional Change: A Dialectical Perspective." *Academy of Management Review* 27(2): 222–247.

Thornton, P. H., and W. Ocasio. 2008. "Institutional Logics." In *The Sage Handbook of Organizational Institutionalism*, edited by Royston Greenwood, Christine Oliver, Kerstin Sahlin-Andersson, and Roy Suddaby, 99–129. Thousand Oaks, CA: Sage.

Wamsley, G. L., and M. N. Zald. 1976. *The Political Economy of Public Organizations: A Critique and Approach to the Study of Public Administration.* Bloomington: Indiana University Press.

Zilber, T. B. 2002. "Institutionalization as an Interplay Between Actions, Meanings, and Actors: The Case of a Rape Crisis Center in Israel." *Academy of Management Journal* 45:234–254.

6

Between Control and Surrender in Terminal Illness

▸ GERALDINE FOLEY AND VIRPI TIMONEN

PEOPLE WITH RAPIDLY PROGRESSIVE terminal illnesses constitute specific challenges for human services given the pace of illness progression and impending death. Amyotrophic lateral sclerosis (ALS) demonstrates these challenges to the extreme. Sometimes referred to as Lou Gehrig's disease or motor neuron disease, ALS is a neurological disorder for which there currently is neither a cure nor any disease-modifying treatments that slow down the progression of the disease. Up to 70 percent of the ALS population dies within three years of symptom onset. Disease progression is unrelenting, resulting in extensive disabilities arising from paralysis of limb and respiratory muscles. Many people with ALS lose their ability to speak and eat, and some also develop cognitive impairment. Death in ALS is in most cases caused by respiratory failure (Hardiman, Van den Berg, and Kiernan 2011). Therefore, ALS poses a particularly acute challenge for understanding and improving human services provision for service users who face mounting losses of function. Adaptation in ALS is different from adaptation in chronic illnesses, which is characterized by periods of stability and movement between losses and gains. The latter process is theorized by Charmaz (1991), who encapsulates it as consisting of "good days, bad days." ALS is useful in understanding how people who have rapidly progressive terminal illnesses adapt to loss, where there are few, if any, "good days" and the "bad days" predominate.

There currently is a drive in health care research and management to design what are called "pathways" for service users, which are understood as the ideal timings and sequencings of different health care and (in the case of terminal illnesses, including ALS) palliative care interventions. They commonly are cast as intervention formulas designed to accommodate needs that arise at different disease stages (e.g., Bede et al. 2011; Bookbinder et al. 2005). Typically, these pathways rely on the assumption that a set of questions (an "instrument") can be developed that will provide a firm basis for referring individuals to the services that best meet their needs in an opportune manner. They are driven by managerial concerns with optimal scheduling and resource use, and they rely overwhelmingly on professional understandings of service user experiences (see Greener, Chapter 14, this volume). In our view, improving the human service experience of people with rapidly progressive terminal illnesses is only possible when the health care experiences of people with conditions like ALS are understood from their perspective.

In this chapter, we strive to set out that perspective and contrast it with a simplified, linear notion of disease experience, one conceived as discernible movements through time, with interventions paced in parallel to progressive needs. The chapter outlines some of our findings and theorizing regarding the everyday relational context and experience of living with terminal illness, the care preferences of ALS service users, and the ways in which the current system of human services provision is unable to fully respond to these preferences. The chapter concludes with a discussion of how human services provision can bring about meaningful outcomes for people with ALS, as well as for other people with rapidly progressing terminal conditions. We argue that this cannot happen through the design and implementation of idealized pathways but has to be brought about through deformularized encounters that place the individual's reflexive struggle between control and surrender at center stage.

CAPTURING THE SERVICE USER PERSPECTIVE

Before the study that this chapter draws on, the health care experiences of people with ALS had not been theorized. Rather, there existed a wide range of research on the cost of ALS human services provision (e.g., Van der Steen et al. 2009) and on "outcomes" of multidisciplinary care for people with ALS, with a focus on survival (e.g., Traynor et al. 2003). These studies in ALS human services did not provide insights into what aspects of human services provision matter to service users (Foley, Timonen, and

Hardiman 2012); little was known about how ALS service users' own experiences shape the human service relationship (Foley 2011). In order to address this deficit, we conducted a Grounded Theory (Corbin and Strauss 2008) study with a view toward understanding the health care experiences of people with ALS in the context of their everyday lives.

We conducted qualitative interviews with 34 people with ALS, who were sampled from the Irish ALS population-based register. Interviews with the participants in our study were unstructured, because we were keen not to preempt those domains of human services provision that might be important to them. We aimed to be as open as possible to participants' perspectives on what mattered most in their lives (Foley and Timonen 2015). In the early stages of our study, we purposively sampled participants to capture diversity in life and health care experiences. We then sampled participants based on the theory that was emerging from our analysis of those experiences.

Although data collection comprised qualitative interviews, we did not exclude service users who had already encountered problems with their speech. Neither did we seek to exclude service users with cognitive impairment. Rather, we sampled participants when they fit with our sampling criteria focused on building theory about how ALS service users engage with health and social care services. The sample comprised people with ALS with varying degrees of disability. The rapid progression of ALS is illustrated by the fact that nearly a third of the participants had died by the time we interviewed the final participant. All participants' names in this chapter are pseudonyms.

A STRIKING ILLUSTRATION

We begin by introducing a participant whose account of daily life with ALS is a particularly striking illustration of the central dynamic that ALS sets off—loss in virtually all domains of life, including the loss of control. Martin was 73 years old when interviewed, and had been diagnosed with ALS eight months before he participated in our study. He had developed symptoms of the condition ten months before his diagnosis, and he died six months after his interview. He indicated that he was experiencing unremitting and insurmountable loss in his life because of ALS. For Martin, the loss of control in all aspects of his life felt like an alien abduction:

> I read a very interesting book some years ago by Stephanie Meyer and she was talking about, it was an alien species came down to earth . . . and it took over your brain, took over your body. Well, I often think that MND [ALS] is like that. I feel like I've been taken over by a sort of an alien presence and it's, it's in my brain and I think it's like an alien that has nuclear weapons, that it can do all sorts of things to me and I'm combating it with bows and arrows. . . . So I find myself in a constant battle, day after day because this, this MND [ALS] alien that has taken over my body and that I have not too much defence against. Normally in, in a war you win some battles; I'm losing all the battles and I know for a fact I'm going to lose the war. The war, the war is lost already because MND [ALS] is going to take me anyhow, but I'm not winning any battles, because I feel that I don't have, the arms that I'm provided with in no way, can in any way defeat or even hold back this alien that is taking me over. . . . Personally I think it's, I think it's my, my own, my own body is withdrawing from my old life and I'm, I'm discarding all the things that, that I used to do, used to enjoy. I'm not doing it deliberately. My body is saying you know pull back from that and that's what's happening.

AGE AND THE FAMILY CONTEXT OF TERMINAL ILLNESS

Age, life stage, and particularly parenthood exert a central influence on resistance to and/or acceptance of ALS, and the health and social care preferences of ALS service users (Foley, Timonen, and Hardiman 2014a). In line with widespread stereotypes, participants in this research saw old age as a period of decline, resignation, and acceptance. By extension, they considered old age a more acceptable stage of life for having ALS. People who have reached a relatively high age, and have adult children, tend to be more accepting of the condition and are less inclined to seek life-sustaining interventions than younger people. People with ALS who feel deprived of the opportunity to raise their children to maturity are less accepting of ALS. Accepting death as a parent of young children was seen as particularly hard, both by people in that situation and by older and childless people with ALS.

Studies have explored how terminal illness impacts parenthood (e.g., Bell and Ristovski-Slijepcevic 2011), but we knew little about how being a parent with a terminal illness shapes how service users engage with human services. Wilson (2007) found that people with a life-limiting chronic illness (HIV) and dependent children want to live to support and protect their children. We discovered that terminally ill service users (in this case, those with ALS) also have a strong desire to "be there" for their dependent children, and they feel anxious about the effect the dying phase will have on their children. Terry, a 45-year-old father, disclosed:

> [I] just want to get them [children] across the line. . . . I've three of them, my eldest is eighteen, my youngest is, he's nearly ten, there's a bit of rearing on him left to be done . . . [but] I also know I don't want them being so young seeing me quite ill . . . so it would be peace of mind for me to think that when this thing goes so far that it'll be stopped [reference to euthanasia].

Alongside awareness of the help, care, and support that they receive, people with ALS are committed to supporting family members even when their strength and capacities are rapidly waning; many see informal flows of care and support as bidirectional (Foley, Timonen, and Hardiman 2014a). Maureen, age 62, explained how *she* provided psychological and emotional support to her family:

> I have a grandson living with me, he is twelve and his mam [mother] has a drug addiction. We have an agreement between her and me that we [Maureen and spouse] are sort of guardians [for the grandson]. . . . I have a son, he's an alcoholic and he has a condition called [congenital disorder]. . . . He [pointing to spouse] tells me that he wants to hold onto me. . . . So I need to be around for as long as I can for them.

This insight is important in light of the strong focus on the "caregiver burden" in current research and practice in the ALS field (e.g., Bruletti et al. 2015). Terminally ill service users can have family care-giving roles even if they are cared for by family.

Family members are an important conduit to formal care services and often complement or compensate for inadequate home and community human services in Ireland, as the country has a comparatively low level of formal service provision (Timonen, Doyle, and O'Dwyer 2012). Heavy reliance on family to provide care can strengthen relationships between service users and their families, but reliance on family can exacerbate conflict between service users and their families in some cases, particularly over differences in preferences for care. David shared: "I'm finding it very difficult at home. My wife doesn't seem to have any sympathy for me, empathy or whatever and we're looking at building [to make the home accessible]. . . . I'm thinking if we had [built an accessible] bedroom . . . I'll have my own little bit of independence. . . . So that's trouble now at the minute."

The associated significance of a parallel (family) care system can complement *and* complicate the human service relationship. In most cases, however, continued care at home in Ireland is only possible because of the underpinning that "complementary" family care provides. The Irish context is therefore demanding of and conducive to strong family care responsibilities, and therefore it is similar to most other health care systems, with the possible exception of those in the Nordic countries.

"NO CHOICE" BUT TO ADAPT

People with ALS feel they have "no choice" but to adapt to ALS because they have no control over ALS or the losses they encounter because of it. Adaptation in ALS is not about regaining loss, because unremitting loss, including loss of control, is fundamental to the experience of living with ALS (Foley, Timonen, and Hardiman 2014b). Neither is adaptation in ALS necessarily about accepting. Some service users accept the condition, others resist it. Some also move back and forth between acceptance and resistance. Adaptation in ALS is essentially a forced adaptation because service users have to endure losses that are beyond their control. Jennifer shared:

> It's not like one of those things where you have hope. . . . I mean it [ALS] seems to be irreversible. . . . It's been a pretty fast downward slide . . . [but] I have to deal with it. I mean I've been saying since last autumn that each week I'm just a shade weaker in some area. . . . I've had a lot of trouble getting my head around losing independence and thought it would [involve being] dressed like a child, or undressed you know. But I have to get over it.

We found that people with a rapidly progressive terminal illness such as ALS do not maintain their condition or regain in the domains of their loss because the condition (as illustrated by Martin earlier in this chapter) eradicates the prospect of a future where loss would at some point cease and allow them to regain (something of) what they had already lost. We are not suggesting here that loss in a rapidly progressive terminal illness is proportionate to the severity of the "disease." Rather, we theorize that unrelenting loss can arise from living with an illness that offers no stability or time to alleviate loss or reverse the losses that have already occurred.

The argument that psychological well-being in ALS can be regained or maintained despite illness progression (Cupp et al. 2011) is challenged by our findings. Quality of life studies in ALS had shown that people with ALS maintained psychological well-being in the face of physical decline and focused on existential domains of life to maintain well-being. In contrast, we argue that unremitting loss for people with ALS includes unremitting loss in existential domains (Foley 2014). Research participants openly mourned their multiple losses, covering *all* domains of life from health and practical to existential. This may appear particularly discouraging to health care professionals, whose raison d'être is to help service users maintain or regain what is important to them (see Eriksson and Jacobsson, Chapter 13, this volume). Loss in ALS is unremitting; normality and control are not regained in any domains of life, with the possible exception of control over human services (Foley, Timonen, and Hardiman 2014b). Hence, as care provision is virtually the only remaining area of life where ALS service users can exert control, it is particularly important to ensure that they have the highest possible degree of choice and control in relation to their human services.

EXERTING CONTROL IN HUMAN SERVICES

People with ALS exert control in human services to adapt to loss, and human services providers are potentially the primary enablers of the desire for control among people with ALS (Foley, Timonen, and Hardiman 2014b). The need to be in control of human services arises from the experience of loss (including loss of control in other domains). Being in control of human services comprises the right to either accept or decline services. Service users move at different rates in coming to terms with their loss, and they themselves judge what is amenable to them as they adapt to loss. Sally and Danielle spoke about their reluctance to use assistive devices and to accept home care services because they struggled to come to terms with losing independence:

> When the OT [occupational therapist] mentioned it [electric bed] I said "God, electric bed," oh I couldn't think about it . . . and then wheelchairs, [when] she mentioned a wheelchair I nearly died. The thought of a wheelchair, you know, and it's just that you're getting it into your head that you're losing your independence altogether. . . . I just hate it [losing independence] and I still hate the wheelchair. (Sally, age 62)

> [I]t takes a long time to get used to carers, like to have somebody come into your house and get you up in the morning and give you a shower and all that kind of stuff, it takes a lot to get used to that. (Danielle, age 45)

Having a say over the timing of services is of central importance to ALS service users because it allows them to process the life-altering impact of terminal illness.

The importance that service users attach to being in control of their care means that some might disengage from human services providers if they do not feel in control of decision making in care (see Solvang, Chapter 7, this volume). Eilish communicated what she intended to do should she encounter human services providers who did not respect her preferences for care: "Well I wouldn't go back to them. I definitely wouldn't go back to them. I'd say no I'm not coming back and that's it." However, exerting control in human services also includes the possibility to relinquish control on one's own terms. Maureen explained why she would follow through on her physician's recommendation to use noninvasive ventilation:

> [W]hen you have a pain, you say I need a pain killer. My breathing is changing but I don't want to lose control. So if you need to breathe you have to say I need that [noninvasive ventilation] to be in control.

In other words, following the recommendation of a human services provider is also a manifestation of control for some service users.

ENGAGING WITH END-OF-LIFE CARE

An especially sensitive area in human services provision is the decision making around end-of-life care. People with ALS are averse to prolonging life for the sake of increasing life span alone; in our study, most people nearing death expressed the wish to die soon. We still know too little about how people with ALS understand suffering, and what they consider appropriate in minimizing suffering. It is clear, however, that alleviation of physical distress at the end of life does not necessarily mean that service users stop suffering (Foley, Timonen, and Hardiman 2014c).

Terminally ill service users are not always informed by human services providers about end-of-life care (e.g., Bajwah et al. 2012; Wilkinson et al. 2014). We found that people with terminal illness struggle between needing reassurance about end-of-life care *and* not wanting to be fully informed about end-of-life care until they have to engage with these services. Anticipation of the dying phase can be distressing for ALS service users before they have reached the later stages of ALS. Helen, 56 years old, voiced:

> I know that near the end I'll need the hospice but I don't know anything about them [hospice]. Sometimes it'd be nice to meet them [hospice] . . . even just to say look, this is us, this is what we do . . . [but] I mean hopefully I'm a long way off the hospice. . . . I'm not inclined to jump the gun and go forward down the road too far. . . . I am not going there [planning end-of-life care] fully yet because that is something mentally very hard to deal with. . . . Right now I don't want to see myself like that [dying], imagine myself like that.

Many participants preferred to wait until they advanced in the condition before they sought end-of-life care discussions with human services, even though they spoke openly about the prospect of death and about their personal expectations of the human service relationship during the dying phase.

Life-sustaining interventions in ALS care (e.g., assisted ventilation, enteral feeding) can cause anxiety if the individual anticipates suffering as a result of the efforts to prolong life. Melanie, a 77-year-old widow who was in the end stage of ALS and who died six weeks after her interview, said:

MELANIE I mean there are days when I don't feel like living. . . . Hopefully there won't be too much future [left].

INTERVIEWER Do you have any particular feelings about life-sustaining treatment?

MELANIE Dragging it out. Well I don't see the point. . . . I think people might incorrectly believe that a life-sustaining treatment might lead to a general improvement . . . the feeling of having something [like this] dragging on and on. I don't want that.

ALS service users have anxiety about life-sustaining interventions extending their life even when they are using them or have opted for them. As discussed, some people with a life-limiting illness can have a strong desire to live on for the sake of family. However, living in a state of increased "suffering" in terminal illness is also difficult to accept. Ann, a 67-year-old retired health care professional who was severely dysarthric (losing the ability to articulate), dysphagic (having difficulty in swallowing), and in respiratory failure, had engaged with life-sustaining interventions because she felt obliged not to refuse them. She voiced concerns about the effects these interventions had on her life:

> Well I realised that life, it was out of my hands. . . . I am supposed to go the way, towards the way of preserving life . . . [but] I'm beginning to have a change. . . . I mean this [ALS] is limiting. . . . I think I'd be dead [without gastrostomy feeding and noninvasive ventilation]. . . . The RIG [gastrostomy feed] was put in before I needed it. . . . I got this [pointing to noninvasive ventilation] before I needed it . . . everything was anticipated . . . [but] the whole thing [ALS] is a nightmare, well the whole, the whole concept [of living with ALS] is a nightmare.

Terminally ill service users want to have a say over treatment decisions at the end of life (e.g., Volker and Wu 2011), and having choices over when to die is important to people with a terminal illness (e.g., Chapple, Ziebland, and McPherson 2006), including people with ALS (Cooney et al. 2012). This poses challenges for human services provision, because the system (including the rules within the system and limitations of that system) can restrict service providers in meeting service users' preferences in end-of-life care. Large-scale studies that have concluded that assisted suicide is a desirable option for some people with ALS (e.g., Ganzini et al. 1998; Maessen et al. 2014) have been conducted in countries or systems where these services are already available to service users. In Ireland, and many other countries or systems, euthanasia and/or physician-assisted suicide is not facilitated. Only a minority of participants (6 out of 34) in our study made reference to assisted suicide, which is partly a result of the unstructured nature of the interviews (i.e., the topic was not broached unless the participant raised it). However, the majority of participants in the study felt people had the "right" to sustain or end their life on their terms. Human services are in many ways un(der)prepared to accommodate these needs and preferences; therefore, they are failing to give service users the ultimate form of control—the right to decide how to live, and how and when to die.

It is important to note that, in some cases, life-sustaining interventions in terminal illness, such as assisted ventilation and enteral feeding, are also palliative in nature because they alleviate distressing symptoms. This can pose a dilemma for service users who have a preference for symptomatic care but who do not want to extend their life beyond the natural course of their condition. However, the current clinical recommendation that care of people with ALS should be palliative from the point of diagnosis (Oliver, Borasio, and Johnston 2014) is highly problematic in view of the fact that ALS service users often do not perceive their care before the dying phase as "palliative" and associate palliative care with imminent death (Foley, Timonen, and Hardiman 2014c).

SHEPHERDING AND THE SYSTEM

Most participants in our research had positive experiences in their relationship with individual health care providers. Participants felt reassured by individual health care workers as they (the participants) resigned themselves to the inevitable progression of ALS. Martin told us that he sees the health care workers as "a group of shepherds" moving him toward death:

> They've [health care workers] done as much as they can. . . . They react to whatever problems I run into and make the disease more bearable. I mean I see [neurologist] and her team as like a group of shepherds who, who are shepherding me towards you know, towards my death really. And what they're doing is there, they will insofar as they can make it more bearable for me . . . move me as gently and as bearably as possible towards when I die. And I know they'll do that with compassion and efficiency and indeed the local services [health care workers] would be, will be the same.

In contrast to the experience of individual health care providers, participants' experiences with what some referred to as the (human service) "system" were markedly negative, involving confusion and frustration with the diagnosis process, information about the condition, and about the organization of service provision. Most people with ALS in Ireland feel disconnected from the system and struggle to negotiate their way around it. As discussed, service users want to be in control of how and when they receive care, and most want to engage with human services as they approach death. However, inequity in service provision, delays, and fragmentation between different services within the system meant that participants did not always receive the care they wanted, when they wanted it. Pascal was one of many participants who felt their health care system was akin to a "grey box":

> The part that I find frustrating is like understanding what you need and where you need to get it when you want it and how long is it going to take before you get it. . . . I'm still no clearer on what I actually need to do . . . as the progression gets worse . . . not realising or not knowing where to go to get things, not realising what you are entitled to, what you need. It's quite traumatic you know . . . going to this grey box which is the HSE [public health services provider organization in Ireland].

The international research community is also part of the system in which people with terminal illnesses are processed. Researchers, in some cases, disregard the views of terminally ill service users who have cognitive impairment (e.g., Heyland et al. 2006). We found that participants in our study—which included service users with cognitive impairment—had a strong desire to participate in research and share their views about what optimal care should be. Capturing the viewpoints of ALS service users who have cognitive impairment is no less important than capturing the viewpoints of those who are cognitively intact (Foley 2015).

DEFORMULARIZING CARE PATHWAYS

Responding to what is most important for terminally ill service users is challenging for service providers because so much of what shapes how users engage with services exists outside those services. Service users' interactions with human services are intertwined with other complex interactions (in particular, family relations) that shape how they adapt to loss and engage with human services. The influence of life stage on ALS service users' approach to ALS and on their decision making in care demonstrates that the human service relationship is shaped not only by recognizable service needs but also by needs that are embedded in the lived experience and everyday context of illness (see Alm Andreassen, Chapter 2, this volume).

Our study of the experiences of the human services system for ALS service users in Ireland resonates with the challenges people face in other countries or systems in living and dealing with ALS (e.g., Hughes et al. 2005; Van Teijlingen, Friend, and Kamal 2001) and indeed with other terminal illnesses (e.g., Murray et al. 2002). Human services providers have to work very hard to bridge the gap between individuals with a terminal illness and their care systems, which are seen as confusing and alienating. An important prerequisite for evolution in human services provision is to acknowledge that care providers might not be able to improve the well-being or reverse the losses encountered by people with ALS and other rapidly progressive terminal illnesses. Nevertheless, human services have the potential to help service users cope with loss, first and foremost by allowing them to make decisions about their own care, at a time of their own choosing (see Grenier and Flood, Chapter 10, this volume).

The basic premise of the care pathways idea is challenged by our findings, which point to the importance of in-depth understanding of each individual case. We are uneasy with the idea of "instruments" that can be straightforwardly deployed to "stream" individuals toward particular interventions at "the right time." From the accounts of terminally ill service users in our study, it is evident that the person-centered, relationship-based approach serves them best by giving them the opportunity to direct their own care. It is very hard to achieve this through highly structured approaches. Our theorizing about how people with ALS engage with human services can be applied, extended, and adapted to other studies of people with terminal illnesses. ALS service users exert control over human services by deciding *when* and *how* to engage with services. Not having choices about care can diminish their control over human services. People with ALS expect to have choices about care and feel in control of their care when their preferences are accommodated. Enabling ALS service users to surrender control as they see fit also fosters control. Accommodating preferences about care reassures service users and makes ALS more bearable for them. It seems that engaging with people with ALS when *they* are ready to engage and enabling them to decide about care on their own terms is key to establishing a meaningful relationship between service user and service provider.

Pathways are detrimental to good care if they are understood and deployed as formulas for service provision that expeditiously describe, orient toward, and manage the experiences of users. The lived tension and movement between control and surrender for ALS service users contrasts with the rationalization of experience that underpins the idea of pathways. Pathways might enhance and routinize service planning and accountability, but they cannot administratively tolerate the kind of lived complexity we discovered in the lives of people with ALS. Therefore, pathways do not automatically translate into just and humane care, and indeed it is dangerous to assume that they do, especially in the case of palliative care, where the individual might not be prepared for it (because of the association with imminent death) or indeed might want to hasten death. The ALS service user experience is mediated by the continuing experiential tension between control and surrender—something that cannot be captured by the linear logic of pathways. Traditional medical research on terminal illness does not reveal this experiential tension and sometimes disregards the experiences of people with cognitive impairment who also experience this tension. At the very least, health care providers should soften the predictive stance inherent in care pathways and allow their encounters with service users to shed light on the fluid and experientially contingent course of terminal illness.

REFERENCES

Bajwah, S., J. Koffman, I. J. Higginson, J. R. Ross, A. U. Wells, S. S. Birring, and J. Riley. 2012. "'I Wish I Knew More . . .' the End-of-Life Planning and Information Needs for End-Stage Fibrotic Interstitial Lung Disease: Views of Patients, Carers and Health Professionals." *BMJ Supportive and Palliative Care* 3(1) (March): 84–90. doi:10.1136/bmjspcare-2012–000263.

Bede, P., D. Oliver, J. Stodart, L. van den Berg, Z. Simmons, D. Ó Brannagáin, G. D. Borasio, and O. Hardiman. 2011. "Palliative Care in Amyotrophic Lateral Sclerosis: A Review of Current International Guidelines and Initiatives." *Journal of Neurology, Neurosurgery and Psychiatry* 82(4) (April): 413–418. doi:10.1136/jnnp.2010.232637.

Bell, K., and S. Ristovski-Slijepcevic. 2011. "Metastatic Cancer and Mothering: Being a Mother in the Face of a Contracted Future." *Medical Anthropology* 30(6) (November): 629–649. doi:10.1080/01459740.2011.588631.

Bookbinder, M., A. E. Blank, E. Arney, D. Wollner, P. Lesage, M. McHugh, R. A. Indelicato, S. Harding, A. Barenboim, T. Mirozyev, and R. K. Portenoy. 2005. "Improving End-of-Life Care: Development and Pilot-Test of a Clinical Pathway." *Journal of Pain and Symptom Management* 29(6) (June): 529–543. doi:10.1016/j.jpainsymman.2004.05.011.

Bruletti, G., L. Comini, S. Scalvini, R. Morini, A. Luisa, M. Paneroni, and M. Vitacca. 2015. "A Two-Year Longitudinal Study on Strain and Needs in Caregivers of Advanced ALS Patients." *Amyotrophic Lateral Sclerosis and Frontotemporal Degeneration* 16(3–4) (June): 187–195. doi:10.3109/21678421.2014.974616.

Chapple, A., S. Ziebland, and A. McPherson. 2006. "What People Close to Death Say About Euthanasia and Assisted Suicide: A Qualitative Study." *Journal of Medical Ethics* 32(12) (December): 706–710. doi:10.1136/jme.2006.015883.

Charmaz, Kathy. 1991. *Good Days and Bad Days: The Self in Chronic Illness and Time.* New Brunswick, NJ: Rutgers University Press.

Cooney, G., G. Lewando Hundt, G. Goodall, and J. Weaver. 2012. "Choices and Control When You Have a Life-Shortening Illness: Researching the Views of People with Motor Neurone Disease." Oxford: Picker Institute Europe. http://www.mndassociation.org/Resources/MNDA/Life%20with%20MND/Document s/Choices%20and%20control%20FINAL.pdf. Accessed January 27, 2015.

Corbin, Jeannette, and Anselm Strauss. 2008. *Basics of Qualitative Research: Techniques and Procedures for Developing Grounded Theory*, third edition. Thousand Oaks, CA: Sage.

Cupp, J., Z. Simmons, A. Berg, S. H. Felgoise, S. M. Walsh, and H. E. Stephens. 2011. "Psychological Health in Patients with ALS Is Maintained as Physical Function Declines." *Amyotrophic Lateral Sclerosis* 12(4) (July): 290–296. doi:10.3109/17482968.2011.554555.

Foley, G. 2011. "The Complexity of Care in Amyotrophic Lateral Sclerosis." *Amyotrophic Lateral Sclerosis* 12(3) (May): 160–161. doi:10.3109/17482968.2011.554556.

Foley, G. 2014. "Loss and Wellbeing in Amyotrophic Lateral Sclerosis: Challenging the Consensus." *Amyotrophic Lateral Sclerosis and Frontotemporal Degeneration* 15(3–4) (June): 161–162. doi:10.3109/21678421.2014.896929.

Foley, G. 2015. "Cognitive and Behavioural Impairment in ALS: What Now for the ALS Patient Perspective?" *Amyotrophic Lateral Sclerosis and Frontotemporal Degeneration* 16(5–6) (September): 423–424. doi:10.3109/21678421.2015.1026830.

Foley, G., and V. Timonen. 2015. "Using Grounded Theory Method to Capture and Analyze Health Care Experiences." *Health Services Research* 50(4) (August): 1195–1210. doi: 10.1111/1475-6773.12275.

Foley, G., V. Timonen, and O. Hardiman. 2012. "Experience of Services as a Key Outcome in Amyotrophic Lateral Sclerosis (ALS) Care: The Case for a Better

Understanding of Patient Experiences." *American Journal of Hospice and Palliative Medicine* 29(5) (August): 362–367. doi:10.1177/1049909111423774.

Foley, G., V. Timonen, and O. Hardiman. 2014a. "Acceptance and Decision Making in Amyotrophic Lateral Sclerosis from a Life-Course Perspective." *Qualitative Health Research* 24(1) (January): 66–77. doi:10.1177/1049732313516545.

Foley, G., V. Timonen, and O. Hardiman. 2014b. "Exerting Control and Adapting to Loss in Amyotrophic Lateral Sclerosis." *Social Science and Medicine* 101:113–119. doi:10.1016/j.socscimed.2013.11.003.

Foley, G., V. Timonen, and O. Hardiman. 2014c. "Understanding Psycho-Social Processes Underpinning Engagement with Services in Motor Neurone Disease: A Qualitative Study." *Palliative Medicine* 28(4) (April): 318–325. doi:10.1177/0269216313512013.

Ganzini, L., W. S. Johnston, B. H. McFarland, S. W. Tolle, and M. A. Lee. 1998. "Attitudes of Patients with Amyotrophic Lateral Sclerosis and Their Care Givers Toward Assisted Suicide." *New England Journal of Medicine* 339(14) (October): 967–973. doi:10.1056/NEJM199810013391406.

Hardiman, O., L. Van den Berg, and M. Kiernan. 2011. "Clinical Diagnosis and Management of Amyotrophic Lateral Sclerosis." *Nature Reviews Neurology* 7(11) (November): 639–649. doi:10.1038/nrneurol.2011.153.

Heyland, D. K., P. Dodek, G. Rocker, D. Groll, A. Gafni, D. Pichora, S. Shortt, J. Tranmer, N. Lazar, J. Kutsogiannis, and M. Lam. 2006. "What Matters Most in End-of-Life Care: Perceptions of Seriously Ill Patients and Their Family Members." *Canadian Medical Association Journal* 174(5) (February): 627–633. doi:10.1503/cmaj.050626.

Hughes, R. A., A. Sinha, I. Higginson, K. Down, and P. N. Leigh. 2005. "Living with Motor Neurone Disease: Lives, Experiences of Services and Suggestions for Change." *Health and Social Care in the Community* 13(1) (January): 64–74. doi:10.1111/j.1365-2524.2005.00530.x.

Maessen, M., J. H. Veldink, B. D. Onwuteaka-Philipsen, H. T. Hendricks, H. J. Schelhass, H. F. Grupstra, G. van der Wal, and L. H. van den Berg. 2014. "Euthanasia and Physician-Assisted Suicide in Amyotrophic Lateral Sclerosis: A Prospective Study." *Journal of Neurology* 261(10) (October): 1894–1901. doi:10.1007/s00415-014-7424-6.

Murray, S. A., K. Boyd, M. Kendall, A. Worth, T. F. Benton, and H. Clausen. 2002. "Dying of Lung Cancer or Cardiac Failure: Prospective Qualitative Interview Study of Patients and Their Carers in the Community." *British Medical Journal* 325(7370) (October): 929–932. doi:10.1136/bmj.325.7370.929.

Oliver, David, Gian Domenico Borasio, and Wendy Johnston, eds. 2014. *Palliative Care in Amyotrophic Lateral Sclerosis: From Diagnosis to Bereavement*, third edition. Oxford: Oxford University Press.

Timonen, V., M. Doyle, and C. O'Dwyer. 2012. "Expanded, but Not Regulated: Ambiguity in Home-Care Policy in Ireland." *Health and Social Care in the Community* 20(3) (May): 310–318. doi:10.1111/j.1365–2524.2011.01048.x.

Traynor, B. J., M. Alexander, B. Corr, E. Frost, and O. Hardiman. 2003. "Effect of a Multidisciplinary Amyotrophic Lateral Sclerosis (ALS) Clinic on ALS Survival: A Population Based Study, 1996–2000." *Journal of Neurology, Neurosurgery and Psychiatry* 74(9) (September): 1258–1261. doi:10.1136/jnnp.74.9.1258.

Van der Steen, I., J. P. Van den Berg, E. Buskens, E. Lindeman, and L. H. Van den Berg. 2009. "The Costs of Amyotrophic Lateral Sclerosis, According to Type of Care." *Amyotrophic Lateral Sclerosis* 10(1) (February): 27–34. doi:10.1080/17482960802103131.

Van Teijlingen, E. R., E. Friend, and A. D. Kamal. 2001. "Service Use and Needs of People with Motor Neurone Disease and Their Carers in Scotland." *Health and Social Care in the Community* 9(6) (November): 397–403. doi:10.1046/j.1365- 2524.2001.00320.x.

Volker, D. L., and L. H. Wu. 2011. "Cancer Patients' Preferences for Control at the End of Life." *Qualitative Health Research* 21(12) (December): 1618–1631. doi:10.1177/1049732311415287.

Wilkinson, E., G. Randhawa, E. A. Brown, M. Da Silva Gane, J. Stoves, G. Warwick, T. Akhtar, R. Magee, S. Sharman, and K. Farrington. 2014. "Communication as Care at End of Life: An Emerging Issue from an Exploratory Action Research Study of Renal End-of-Life Care for Ethnic Minorities in the UK." *Journal of Renal Care* 40(S1) (September): 23–29. doi:10.1111/jorc.12084.

Wilson, S. 2007. "'When You Have Children, You're Obliged to Live': Motherhood, Chronic Illness and Biographical Disruption." *Sociology of Health and Illness* 29(4) (May): 610–626. doi:10.1111/j.1467–9566.2007.01008.x.

PART | III

Professional Work

THE CHAPTERS OF PART III take us to the professionals who provide human services to users. Here again, the focus is on everyday life, in this case everyday elements of professional "work." The quotation marks are meant to flag an insistent duality—work as a matter of applying professional skills and work as a matter of creatively adjusting those skills to the everyday contingencies of their application. Neither can adequately provide service and care on its own. Once more, we see the coexisting logics of problems and troubles come into play. Work that adequately concerns itself with users' perspectives and circumstances is imagined in terms of servicing the troubles in users' lives as well as the problems deciphered from them. That can require the deployment of strategies that apply "civil disobedience" and strive for "relational citizenship." A form of professionalism is reimagined that has as much at stake in the user-designated character and quality of experience as it has in the application of professional competence.

7

New Relations Between "Professionals" and Disabled Service Users

▸ PER KOREN SOLVANG

DISABLED SERVICE USERS HAVE LIFELONG dependent relations with health care professionals and with those professionals who provide assistance with activities of daily living. The idea of dependence has been criticized for pathologizing disability and encouraging user passivity and lack of control. This has instigated a broad range of efforts to reimagine professional work in this area by putting into place a more equitable relationship. It does not include a minority of critics who orient toward disability solely as a discrimination issue and argue that professionals keep disabled people trapped in dependency-creating relationships (see Oliver 1990). The majority of efforts focus on developing new forms of relationships between disabled people and professionals.

As Gubrium outlined in Chapter 1 of this volume, such proponents include disability scholar Dan Goodley (2011), who suggests that professionals should be working from the basic premise that disabled people can live satisfying lives with impairments, and occupational therapist Karen Hammell (2006), who frames professional rehabilitation work as a coaching enterprise in which the professional is an adviser rather than a provider of care. Hammell points to structural competence, and Bright et al. (2012) point to the goal of "being with" rather than "doing to" clients as leading the way. All of them identify with what Goodley refers to as a virgin field, even if planning and crafting services *with* users was formulated in the disability activism of the early 1980s (Zola 1972).

Focusing on professional work in disability, this chapter discusses three ways of envisioning a depathologized and less dependent relationship. The discussion is based on reviews of published studies on the topic and empirical material taken from my own fieldwork in the area. Three kinds of reimagined professionalism will be described: paid personal assistance, which adds user monetary control to the relationship; arts professionals, whose skills encourage creative, not therapeutic, engagement; and sign language communication, which equalizes the medium of exchange between professionals and users (Haualand, Solvang, and Breivik 2015).

Many attempts have been made to define professional work (see Alm Andreassen, Chapter 2, this volume). One definition is that a profession is a group of individuals with specialized skills, with a theoretical foundation for practice, and with a system of approval for qualifications (Friedson 2001). This is certainly the case for many of the professions that provide services to the disabled, such as physiotherapists, occupational therapists, and social workers. This very specific definition of a profession, however, becomes blurred when it comes to the professionals included in this chapter—personal assistants, arts instructors, and sign language interpreters. Sign language interpretation is a recognized profession, with educational programs at the university level in a few of the most developed Western countries. Arts professionals who work as theater instructors do not represent a distinct profession. They do, however, have an educational background and skills that frame them as professional art practitioners. They also are clearly differentiated from the social work professionals employed at day centers for disabled users. Finally, while the development of personal assistants is a result of an ongoing antiprofessionalism, they are seeking ways to define themselves as professionals that possibly embrace user control as defined by the Independent Living (IL) movement (see Gubrium, Chapter 1, this volume).

These new relations between professionals and disabled service users implicate user involvement and user control. These concepts—user involvement and user control—have gained a prominent position in the field of health studies and social work, particularly with respect to mental health issues. User involvement transpires in different ways. It can be framed in consumerist terms, such as being expert on one's own life, as a partner in the design of services, as research collaborators in the development of new knowledge, or even as political activists (Barnes and Cotterell 2012a). Different intellectual traditions are fueling the development of user involvement. Feminist theory provides claims that the personal is political and that all knowledge is political, the work of Paulo Freire underlines educational efforts *with* (and not for) the oppressed, and critical theory provides the concept of emancipatory knowledge. The disability movement touts a social model of disability, the need for emancipatory research, and the need to define oppression in nonpathologizing language (Cotterell and Morris 2012).

USER-CONTROLLED PERSONAL ASSISTANCE

The disability movement has given birth to the direct payment of personal assistance model, which many scholars view as a new kind of user involvement that is "the most effective means by which service users can have their say about the care and support they receive" (Barnes and Cotterell 2012b:75). The practice of hiring personal assistants whose purpose is to attend to the daily life needs of disabled people was introduced as part of the IL concept in Berkeley, California, in the 1980s. Disabled students at the university gained the opportunity to organize their daily living support needs by hiring assistants. This type of arrangement has spread to other parts of the Western world, in the United Kingdom as direct payments and in Scandinavia as user-led personal assistance. This dissemination, to some extent, has taken place by ideological export from the United States. There are, however, examples of local solutions that are seemingly unrelated to the IL concept (Askheim, Bengtsson, and Bjelke 2014).

Personal assistance and direct payments are viewed as the sine qua non or "main presupposition for user control and for freeing disabled people from their reliance on welfare professionals and unpaid carers" (Askheim 2003:227). Advocates of the direct payment strategy tend to deemphasize health and social work competence as qualifications for hiring assistants. There are, however, different personal assistant hiring models. The disabled can hire and act as employers or they can recruit assistants who are employed by a cooperative, a private care provider, or the local authority. Where IL has been implemented, the cooperative as employer seems to be the preferred model.

A large number of personal assistance and direct payment scheme studies have been carried out in the last decade. The studies have come to two main conclusions. First is that personal assistance has been a revolution for disabled people and is mainly available in the welfare states of Northern

Europe and in the United States. Second is that the professional role of assisting is underdeveloped and that the relation between the employer (the disabled) and the employee (the assistant) is potentially strained.

The Freedom Dimension

The freedom dimension of personal assistance is nicely described by the Swedish social work scholar Anna Whitaker (2012), who has conducted a life history study of parents of mentally disabled adults. Important reforms in care took place in the 1960s, 1970s, and 1980s. Curative interventions were on the rise in the 1960s. The 1970s saw social democracy reform the welfare state and young disabled people return to their families from a life in caring institutions. And the 1980s introduced the perspective of disability as a social and political construct. All of these major changes in user control pale when compared, by parents, with the introduction of personal assistance. It is said to have been nothing less than a revolution in control and equity, both where disabled persons live in the parental family home and where they live outside the parental home. Parents experience that a normal life is finally possible (see Stainton and Boyce 2004).

How can personal assistants provide this freedom? Studies have shown that disabled people do not want to employ people with a background in the health and caring professions, which resonates with IL ideology (deJong 1979; Shakespeare 2014). This is reflected in interviews I carried out in the early 1990s with a mobility disabled man who took part in one of the first experiments on direct payments in Norway. He pointed out to me that he preferred assistant candidates who were not even thinking about enrolling in educational programs in one of the health or care professions (Solvang 1994). This is because disabled people fear that health and social work professionals, or those with attitudes similar to those held by these professionals, will tend to make decisions without consulting the disabled person (Guldvik, Christensen, and Larsson 2014; Shakespeare 2014). The interviewee went on to explain that the disabled do not need a professional whose expertise is in caring. They need someone who can help them with a wide range of practical tasks. The comments show that this "new" professional role is born out of both an ideology and a concrete striving for nontherapeutic professionalism. It does nonetheless take on board a set of fairly stable skills and competencies and, as such, becomes an occupational position (see Barnes, Chapter 15, this volume).

Karen Christensen (2010) found three types of occupationalizing strategies in her cross-national study of personal assistance in Norway and the United Kingdom. The first strategy is personal and is the development of a carer biography, the assistant having been previously involved in care work, typically in their family. They form identities as carers and find this type of work rewarding. The second strategy is adopted by those who are searching for new horizons. They are typically immigrants who use the position to enter the labor market in the new country. In the United Kingdom, assistants often live in the households of the employee. The third strategy is more immediate and pragmatic. In this group, we typically find students, artists, and others with another, either imagined or real, career track ahead of them but who need money, preferably from a job that does not expect more from them than performing specific practical tasks (Christensen 2010). This approach is very much in line with the IL ideology and underlines the importance of nonprofessionalism within health and social work in the occupational role of personal assistants. These new relations between "professionals" and disabled service users form on the basis of abrogating common definitions of professionalism. The problem is located in the very idea of professionalism, which rides on a form of control tilted in favor of the professional service provider.

Emergent Challenges

A set of challenges emerges from the personal assistance model. One of these is the degree of personal involvement. Two people being alone together for long periods of time can become a friendship relationship. A friendship and a concerted professional approach must therefore be handled in a single relationship, a situation that is difficult to balance. Another challenge relates to a worker's rights. There is a danger that the likes and dislikes of the disabled employer will result in different types of discrimination in recruitment. The right to a certain level of control over the tasks an employee is to carry out may also be violated. There may also be few possibilities to develop the occupational role into a recognized career track and to achieve upward mobility by advancing skills through continuing education and by way of other systematic work competence improvements. Assistants express a wish to acquire transferable skills from the relationship (Christensen 2012). This, however, raises the question of how to educate for a profession that is founded on the sentiments or ideology of antiprofessionalism. Shakespeare (2014) suggests feminist ethics of care as a direction for working out a clearer occupational role. This highlights the interpersonal relationship that emerges, one that can be meaningful and rewarding for both sides of the care equation. Another take on this, not mentioned by Shakespeare, could be to ask whether there are established professionalisms that can work well with the needs and ambitions of disabled people and the assistants they employ.

Personal Assistance as a Caring Relationship

Claire Ungerson (1997) has presented a typology of caring relationships that is pertinent here. One of these forms of relationships is personal assistance of the kind employed by affluent households (for example, carers, housekeepers, cooks, and other "servants") or by not-so-affluent households (au pairs, for example). Personal assistants are also well known in the corporate world and more recently have also become well known in the world of celebrities. Personal assistance in the private sector has not been introduced into scholarly contributions to the field of personal assistance for disabled people. One reason for this may be that, because of physical and cognitive impairments, the dependency relations involved can resemble those of clients of caring institutions. User control and denial of the relevance of health and social work professional competence, however, does pave the way for alternative professionalisms.

The master/servant relation is one that has been referred to as a model for a new kind of professionalism (Helgøy, Ravneberg, and Solvang 2003; Christensen 2012). A servant is an occupational position in a household where the employer holds power. The relation has historical roots in subordination and poor working conditions and has little relevance in the world we live in today. The butler profession is another example of a position that can widen the discussion of the development of the personal assistant position, is also a profession with historical roots, and has comparatively high social status. There are educational programs for butlers, and there are some examples of institutional framing that provide guides of conduct. In his book on the butler, Steven M. Ferry points out that "a butler might also take on the duties of a *valet* or *personal assistant*, organizing his employer's personal and social life" (Ferry 2002:9) based on the idea that "there was a time when domestic work was an honored profession, and there is no reason it cannot again be so" (p. 7). Domestic service corporations such as City Maid have, after the introduction of the direct payment schemes recently approved by law in Norway, established subdivisions that offer personal assistance services. The development of such organizational forms, which also provide the services of butlers, housekeepers, and corporate personal assistants, suggests that there exist conduct practices and guidelines in other professional work that do not undermine the autonomy that the IL movement wants to secure and can provide personal assistants with transferable skills and career tracks.

SIGN LANGUAGE PROFESSIONALS

Deaf and hard-of-hearing people are recognized as a disability group. They make use of two sets of professional services. The first is audiologists, who provide their clients with hearing aids for a wide range of hearing losses (Olaussen 2010). The second is sign language interpreters. Deaf people's relation to sign language interpreters is not only framed by deafness being a defect that needs to be compensated for by interpretation between sign language and hearing language. Rather, using sign language interpreters can be viewed as supporting the understanding that deafness is a language minority and not a disability that needs to be compensated (Ladd 2003).

Lessons from World Congress Fieldwork

Sign language interpretation is a profession that relates to a number of user communities: deaf people, hearing people who have an interest in deaf issues, deaf interpreters, and hearing interpreters. These communities have been encouraged to work together to create the very best sign language interpreting possible (Stratiy 2005). One arena in which this is happening is the plenary sessions of the World Congresses of the Deaf, organized by the World Federation of the Deaf (WFD). Communication is at the forefront when living as deaf. Communication excellence facilitated by sign language interpreters is demonstrated when deaf people from all over the world come together at transnational arenas such as world congresses and sports festivals (Deaflympics).

Consider this example of a new professional–user relationship from the WFD congress in Montreal in 2003, where I undertook fieldwork with two social anthropologists (Haualand, Solvang, and Breivik 2015; Solvang and Haualand 2014). Only deaf interpreters worked on the stage in the plenary sessions. The hearing interpreters worked as so-called feeders, only providing translations of what was said in the oral or sign language presentations. The deaf interpreters refined the input given by this intermediate translation. Deaf interpreters are considered to have a deeper understanding of sign language nuances than hearing interpreters, which is said to raise the linguistic quality and the cultural adjustments of the interpretation carried out onstage (Boudreault 2005). One deaf participant told us she was glad to avoid "interpreter faces," a reference to what she saw as the lower visual quality of hearing interpreters. Communication is a key issue for deaf politics, and good translation to and from different languages is important in the deaf community.

Hearing people were also well catered to, the organizers providing simultaneous translation to English and French through headsets. The voicing was also an important resource for the numerous interpreters working in the many sign languages used by attendees. Not all the delegates could fluently understand the sign languages used by the three deaf interpreters in the conference hall: American Sign Language, Quebec Sign Language (local language at the conference site; usually there is only one language), and International Sign Language. International sign language was developed by frequent visitors to international arenas in the deaf world (Hiddinga and Crasborn 2011).

Professional sign language interpretation is closely linked to the culture of the deaf. The profession emerged from children of deaf adults assisting members of the deaf community. The deaf community has played an important role in enhancing the quality of this work and certifying interpreters as qualified (Cokely 2005). The professionalism of sign language interpretation has emerged from the informal helper role evolving into an advanced profession in many Western countries. The role, however, has been based on being an ally of, and working *with*, the deaf, not *for* the deaf. The deaf define themselves as a minority. This has resulted in the curricula of cultural minority courses being recommended in the further education of sign language interpreters (Janzen and Korpinski 2005). An important line of argument used when persuading a group of deaf people at a boarding school in Norway to allow an anthropologist to carry out fieldwork at the school was that a cultural minority needs anthropologists to confirm their cultural minority status (Breivik 2001). Being a cultural minority is an important frame of reference in the world of the deaf.

Sign language interpreters see themselves as allies. Their work with deaf people has the added life history dimension of a bicultural identity because many of the interpreters were born into families that practiced sign language. The WFD congresses are therefore also important to those who identify as children of deaf adults (CODAs). Many work as interpreters and attend the conferences and other major assemblies in the deaf world. In recent years, a network has been developed, and an international organization has been established based on this. The CODA issue was included, for the first time, in the official program with an evening session at the WFD congress in Montreal. About two out of three CODAs living in the United States work with deaf issues in some way, interpreting being the most frequent occupation (Preston 2001). CODAs also hold different positions with respect to deafness in their families. Some have only one deaf parent who uses sign language, while in other families the CODA is the only hearing person in their family over generations. They also differ in how they relate to the CODA identity issue. Some are attracted to CODA identity politics, finding it highly stimulating and like a homecoming. Others see it to be of little relevance. They can see the common experiences of the hearing children of deaf parents, but they do not see this as a relevant basis for forming an interest group.

Deaf people at the conferences are not only service users, coproducing communication excellence with the interpreters. By bringing other competencies into play, they also act as knowledge brokers in putting together the conference program. From a chronic illness perspective, one would expect audiologists, experts on pathologies of the ear and on how deafness is hereditary, to play an important role in the conferences. The organizers, however, hold the deaf pride position, valuing the cultural significance of sign language practice. The conference program therefore highlights language and culture, speakers being linguists, social anthropologists, and scholars in the cultural studies subdiscipline of deaf studies. This scholarly profile is also found in the parallel sessions. An off-site cultural program of deaf arts, such as pantomime and film, further promotes the minority definition of deafness by including professional competence in the fields of language, communication, and culture.

ARTS PROFESSIONALS

There are a number of ways that disabled people can relate to the arts and art professionalism. One way is that artists affiliated with disability art are disabled, use disability issues in their artwork, and find their artwork closely related to the disability movement. Disability art is a minority art practice that contributes to a common identification among those fighting for better living conditions for disabled people (Solvang 2012). A second way is through the concept of "disability aesthetics," which has developed among art historians and curators. It is a framework both for reconsidering the history of art in disability terms and for giving value to disability in the aesthetic qualities assigned to works of art (Siebers 2010). A third way disabled people relate to art is in the context of art therapy and relates to the health sciences. Its therapeutic ambitions are twofold: to give voice to suppressed feelings based on psychotherapeutic theories and to provide disabled people with a valued social practice based on social work theory (Heenan 2006; see also Miller and Kontos, Chapter 8, this volume). For example, all three play out in a well-researched case of art practice managed by art professionals for a group of mentally disabled people in the frame of the Swedish welfare state (Sauer 2004; Ineland 2004, 2005; Ineland and Sauer 2007).

Lessons from Ållateatern

The Ållateatern theater group is based in the mid-sized Swedish town of Umeå. The project is funded by the local authority. Swedish law states that adults without any opportunities for education or ordinary work have the right to daytime activation. The professionals working with the project are instructors who have been recruited based on their skills in the performing arts. Their assignment is to work as instructors with mentally disabled people who are interested in theatrical performance. Ållateatern has put on plays such as *Romeo and Juliet* and the opera *Carmen*. *Carmen* was a huge success, with critical acclaim in the press and a visit to Spain to perform the play.

The key to understanding how Ållateatern works is ambivalence. On the one hand, social services see the theater as a well-functioning center of social activation that supplements the daytime activation programs provided to the mentally disabled. To the authorities, a form of art as therapy is being provided. Ållateatern, however, is recognized in the field of culture. The theater has achieved considerable status in culture sections of the daily press for presenting artwork of high value. Reviewers pointed out that the mentally disabled actors provide an interesting take on the issue of otherness in *Carmen*, in which the relation between gypsies and the majority society is a key theme. The visible disability is aesthetically important to the theatrical performance, which is praised as an innovative version of a well-known play (Ineland and Sauer 2007).

The mentally disabled who enrolled for the project have previously experienced two different logics of care in their careers as recipients of activation. They refer to other daytime activation programs, of which they have many years of experience, as being run by "personnel" who "boss us around" and disappear into a coffee room, which the disabled cannot access. The theater project, however, is different. The project is coordinated not by personnel but by "leaders" who are present all the time, the premises are for everybody, and the disabled are even given keys (Sauer 2004:151). The art professionals point out that they have not worked on other daytime activation projects and do not know how they are run. They indicate, however, that they are committed to the established practices of theater work and that they are instructors who work together with actors to achieve a common goal, the performance of a play. They think of the theater as an arena that is well suited to people with different abilities to communicate, as the theater offers the opportunity to communicate in ways other than just by the spoken word (pp. 169–187).

COMMITMENT AND EQUALITY

What do these new relations between "professionals" and disabled service users tell us about the character of service provision for disabled people? Two keywords emerge from the research and the case material. The first is *commitment*, a strong involvement. Some personal assistants live in the households of their employers, many sign language interpreters perform a professional role based on practices going back to their early childhood, and arts professionals are dedicated to creating an artistic result that is viewed positively by the field of culture, a result that intersects with the professionals' own careers as producers of theater performances. The other keyword is *equality* in the relationship between client and professional. The mentally disabled are artistic subjects to their instructors, not clients; deaf people cooperate with sign language interpreters to achieve excellence in seamless communication; and disabled people interact with personal assistants as managers but at the same time facilitate a meaningful occupational role. Whether the relationship is leading to new opportunities for the disabled or whether it can be characterized by equality is an issue that needs to be approached with an open mind by all involved.

This chapter does not aim to develop guidelines for professionals such as occupational therapists and social work professionals. The goal rather has been to make visible the practices that can show what user involvement in services can be and what being "allied with society" implies for professionals (Goodley 2011; see Gubrium, Chapter 1, this volume). We have seen users recruiting personal assistants based on the competencies they require. Users, however, also need to involve themselves in organization building, in the development of the position of personal assistant, for example, and in the development of skills that can be transferred to other human service occupations. We have seen deaf people establishing an arena with interpreters in which excellence in communicating within and between the deaf and hearing worlds is achieved. We also have seen interpreters drawing on their biographical position in the deaf world to develop their skills as interpreters. Finally, we have seen mentally disabled people express a preference for the equality-framed mode of conduct they experience from arts professionals. We have also seen the professionals explicitly position themselves as being unfamiliar with day care practices. Their commitment as professionals, also when working with disabled clients, is therefore framed by the practice of theater work, in which the aim is to strive for a common goal.

REFERENCES

Askheim, O. P. 2003. "Personal Assistance for People with Intellectual Disabilities: Experiences and Dilemmas." *Disability and Society* 18(3): 325–339.

Askheim, O. P., H. Bengtsson, and B. R. Bjelke. 2014. "Personal Assistance in a Scandinavian Context: Similarities, Differences and Developmental Traits." *Scandinavian Journal of Disability Research* 16 (special issue 1): 3–18.

Barnes, M., and P. Cotterell. 2012a. "Introduction: From Margin to Mainstream." In *Critical Perspectives on User Involvement*, edited by M. Barnes and P. Cotterell, 1–6. Bristol: Policy.

Barnes, M., and P. Cotterell. 2012b. "User Involvement in Services." In *Critical Perspectives on User Involvement*, edited by M. Barnes and P. Cotterell, 73–78. Bristol: Policy.

Boudreault, P. 2005. "Deaf Interpreters." In *Topics in Signed Language Interpreting*, edited by T. Janzen, 323–355. Amsterdam: Benjamins.

Breivik, J. 2001. "Deaf Identities in the Making: Metaphors and Narratives in Translocal Lives." PhD diss., Department of Social Anthropology, University of Oslo.

Bright, F. A., P. Boland, S. J. Rutherford, N. M. Kayes, and K. M. McPherson. 2012. "Implementing a Client-Centred Approach in Rehabilitation: An Autoethnography." *Disability and Rehabilitation* 34(12): 997–1004.

Christensen, K. 2010. "Caring About Independent Lives." *Disability and Society* 25(2): 241–252.

Christensen, K. 2012. "Towards Sustainable Hybrid Relationships in Cash-for-Care Systems." *Disability and Society* 27(3): 399–412.

Cokely, D. 2005. "Shifting Positionality: A Critical Examination of the Turning Point in the Relationship of Interpreters and the Deaf Community." In *Sign Language Interpreting and Interpreter Education*, edited by M. Marschark, R. Peterson, and E. Winston, 3–28. Oxford: Oxford University Press.

Cotterell, P., and C. Morris. 2012. "The Capacity, Impact and Challenge of Service Users' Experiential Knowledge." In *Critical Perspectives on User Involvement*, edited by M. Barnes and P. Cotterell, 57–69. Bristol: Policy.

deJong, G. 1979. *The Movement for Independent Living: Origins, Ideology and Implications for Disability Research*. East Lansing: Michigan State University Press.

Ferry, S. M. 2002. *Butlers and Household Managers: 21st Century Professionals*. North Charleston, SC: BookSurge.

Friedson, E. 2001. *Professionalism: The Third Logic*. Cambridge: Polity.

Goodley, D. 2011. *Disability Studies: An Interdisciplinary Introduction*. London: Sage.

Guldvik, I., K. Christensen, and M. Larsson. 2014. "Towards Solidarity: Working Relations in Personal Assistance." *Scandinavian Journal of Disability Research* 16 (special issue 1): 48–61.

Hammell, K. W. 2006. *Perspectives on Disability & Rehabilitation: Contesting Assumptions; Challenging Practice*. Edinburgh: Churchill Livingstone/Elsevier.

Haualand, H., P. Solvang, and J. Breivik. 2015. "Deaf Transnational Gatherings at the Turn of the 21st Century and Some Afterthoughts." In *It's a Small World: Deaf Spaces and Encounters*, edited by M. Friedner and A. Kusters, 47–56. Washington, DC: Gallaudet University Press.

Heenan, D. 2006. "Art as Therapy: An Effective Way of Promoting Positive Mental Health?" *Disability and Society* 21(2): 179–191.

Helgøy, I., B. Ravneberg, and P. Solvang. 2003. "The Construction of Independence in Service Relations." *Disability and Society* 18(4): 471–487.

Hiddinga, A., and O. Crasborn. 2011. "Signed Languages and Globalization." *Language in Society* 40(4): 483–505.

Ineland, J. 2004. "Disability, Culture and Normative Environments." *Scandinavian Journal of Disability Research* 6(2): 131–150.

Ineland, J. 2005. "Logics and Discourses in Disability Arts in Sweden: A Neo-institutional Perspective." *Disability and Society* 20(7): 749–762.

Ineland, J., and L. Sauer. 2007. "Institutional Environments and Subcultural Belonging: Theatre and Intellectual Disabilities." *Scandinavian Journal of Disability Research* 9(1): 46–57.

Janzen, T., and D. Korpinski. 2005. "Ethics and Professionalism in Interpreting." In *Topics in Signed Language Interpreting*, edited by T. Janzen, 165–199. Amsterdam: Benjamins.

Ladd, P. 2003. *Understanding Deaf Culture: In Search of Deafhood.* Bristol: Multilingual Matters.

Olaussen, I. 2010. "Disability, Technology & Politics: The Entangled Experience of Being Hard of Hearing." PhD diss., TIK Centre for Technology, Innovation and Culture, University of Oslo.

Oliver, Michael. 1990. *The Politics of Disablement.* Critical Texts in Social Work and the Welfare State. Basingstoke: Macmillan.

Preston, P. 2001. *Mother Father Deaf: Living Between Sound and Silence.* Cambridge, MA: Harvard University Press.

Sauer, L. 2004. "Teater och utvecklingsstörning: En studie av Ållateatern" [Theatre and developmental disability: A study of Ållateatern]. PhD diss., Department of Social Work, Umeå University.

Shakespeare, Tom. 2014. *Disability Rights and Wrongs Revisited.* London: Routledge.

Siebers, T. 2010. *Disability Aesthetics.* Ann Arbor: University of Michigan Press.

Solvang, Per. 1994. "Biografi, normalitet og samfunn: En studie av handikappedes veier til utdanning og arbeid i Skandinavia" [Biography, normality and society:

A study of disabled people's roads to education and work in Scandinavia]. PhD diss., Centre for Social Research, University of Bergen.

Solvang, P. K. 2012. "From Identity Politics to Dismodernism? Changes in the Social Meaning of Disability Art." *ALTER—European Journal of Disability Research* 6(3): 178–187.

Solvang, P. K., and H. Haualand. 2014. "Accessibility and Diversity—Deaf Space in Action." *Scandinavian Journal of Disability Research* 16(1): 1–13.

Stainton, T., and S. Boyce. 2004. "'I Have Got My Life Back': Users' Experience of Direct Payments." *Disability and Society* 19(5): 443–454.

Stratiy, A. 2005. "Best Practices in Interpreting: A Deaf Community Perspective." In *Topics in Signed Language Interpreting*, edited by T. Janzen, 231–250. Amsterdam: Benjamins.

Ungerson, C. 1997. "Give Them the Money: Is Cash a Route to Empowerment?" *Social Policy and Administration* 31(1): 45–53.

Whitaker, A. 2012. "I skyggen av handikappolitikk og reformer: foreldreskap og omsorg gjennom et langt liv" [In the shadow of disability policies and reforms: Parenting and care in a lifelong perspective]. In *Livsløp med funksjonshemming* [*Life course with disability*], edited by K. Thorsen and E. J. Grassman, 217–243. Oslo: Cappelen Damm Akademisk.

Zola, I. K. 1972. "Medicine as an Institution of Social Control." *Sociological Review* 20(4): 487–504.

8

The Use of Elder-Clowning to Foster Relational Citizenship in Dementia Care

▸ KAREN-LEE MILLER AND PIA KONTOS

THE AIM OF THIS CHAPTER IS TO ROADMAP a novel relationship between service users and service providers in long-term dementia care by using elder-clown practice to illustrate how to effect a relational citizenship model.[1] We first provide an overview of the dominant discourses that concern the experiences of living with dementia and that instruct contemporary paradigms of ensuring ethical and fair treatment of individuals with dementia, including relationship-centered care, citizenship models of participation, and embodiment theory. We next review literature on the increasing use of arts-based programming in dementia care, and the specific role of elder-clowns. We then present findings from a qualitative study of elder-clowning that took place in a locked special care unit of a publicly funded residential long-term care facility for persons with moderate to severe dementia.

Our investigation found that elder-clowns enact an ethic of practice that holds profound citizenship implications for individuals with dementia. A component of elder-clown practice, what we term "relational presence" (Kontos, Miller, Mitchell, and Sterling-Twist 2015), is centered on their initiation and reception of verbal, embodied, emotional, and creative activity. We discuss the implications of relational presence for disrupting the positioning of those with dementia as passive recipients of services, and introduce our notion of relational citizenship, which we define as creating the conditions for persons with moderate to severe dementia to exercise agency and initiate engagement in relationship with others. We conclude with the wider social justice implications involved in caring for and with persons with significant dementia, discussing the role of the broader interdisciplinary health care team.

DEMENTIA AND CONTEMPORARY STEREOTYPES

Alzheimer's disease is considered the most frightening condition that faces the older population in the twenty-first century, and its diagnosis is both greatly feared and stigmatizing. Alzheimer's disease is characterized as a "monstrosity" by the lay media, with "clichéd metaphors and representations in which Alzheimer's is characteristically drawn in colorfully dramatic terms that paint vividly disturbing images" (Herskovitz 1995:152–153) such as "living death" (Matthews 2006:163) and "zombies" (Behuniak 2011:70). The source of these fears is found in much of the literature on Alzheimer's, where individuals with dementia are said to experience a steady erosion of selfhood as a consequence of the cognitive deficiencies that lie at the core of the illness (for a critique, see Kontos 2004, 2012). Thus, while Alzheimer's is usually described and analyzed in terms of the cognitive dysfunction it produces, there is also a presumed existential outcome: the loss of self with the erosion of individual agency (Kontos 2004, 2012).

These representations have serious implications for how we engage with persons diagnosed with Alzheimer's disease. Assumptions of loss of self lead to an absence of attention to human dignity, which fosters poor treatment practices such as infantilization, intimidation, stigmatization, and objectification (Kitwood 1997). Belief in the loss of agency associated with the loss of selfhood also leads to the depiction of dementia as "the sleeping beauty syndrome" (Killick and Allan 2012:65), which characterizes the person with dementia as being incapable of initiation, although it holds out some hope for a limited response following elicitation by professional and family care partners.

PARADIGMS OF DEMENTIA CARE AND TREATMENT

The classic paradigm of clinical and social care toward those with dementia has included control and containment—specifically, combinations of environmental, mechanical, and pharmacological restraints to manage challenging behaviors (Andrews 2006). The increasing disfavor of this approach because of concerns about inhumane consequences (Andrews 2006), including adverse medication effects (Katona 2001) and the harm caused by the pathologizing of distress as a dementia disease marker (Brannelly 2011; Cohen-Mansfield and Mintzer 2005), has led to alternative paradigms, including person-centered and relationship-centered care as well as the use of the arts in health care.

Person-centered dementia care (Kitwood 1997) uses the knowledge of the life biography of the individual with dementia, and their personal characteristics such as hobbies and affinities, to individualize nonpharmacological care and to understand the meaningfulness of the actions of those with dementia rather than problematizing their "behaviors" (Dupuis, Wiersma, and Loiselle 2012). The concept of personhood, which underpins this approach, has been the most influential change in dementia practice since the 1990s (Bartlett and O'Connor 2010). However, it has spawned newer paradigms intended to address important limitations, namely the decontextualization of the individual from his or her relationships with others (Nolan et al. 2002), and the ways in which issues of agency and power differentials are profoundly ignored (Bartlett and O'Connor 2010).

Relationship-centered care (Nolan et al. 2004; Adams and Gardiner 2005; see also Gubrium, Chapter 1, this volume) was developed to "fully capture the interdependencies and reciprocities that underpin caring relationships" (Nolan et al. 2002:203). It makes explicit "the centrality of relationship to good dementia care" (Edvardsson, Winblad, and Sandman 2008:213). There are two significant contributions made by this paradigm. The first is the focus on the development and maintenance of relationships between persons living with dementia, their family care partners, and professional care providers (Dupuis et al. 2014). The second is the expectation that the person with dementia will retain status as an active partner in the dementia care experience (Bartlett and O'Connor 2010). Nonetheless, the focus remains on care relationships, overlooking other relationships that individuals might have, such as those with the state and its institutions (e.g., the Ministry of Health and Long-Term Care, a provincial ministry in Canada that provides the funding for Ontario hospitals, long-term care facilities, etc.), and consequently the person with dementia continues to be positioned largely as one who needs care (Bartlett and O'Connor 2010).

Bartlett and O'Connor (2007, 2010) note that a citizenship perspective redresses some of the gaps inherent in personhood- and relationship-centered approaches. This perspective is fundamentally about the relationships individuals have with the state and its institutions over the course of their life (Bartlett and O'Connor 2010), which are rarely explicitly discussed in dementia care given the focus on relationships with family and professional care providers. However, the "rules, laws and policies of the country or jurisdiction in which a person lives" (p. 30) will inevitably influence the experiences and opportunities associated with the health and social care a person with dementia receives (Kontos, Miller, and Mitchell 2010; Reid, Ryan, and Enderby 2001). Individuals with dementia had previously been excluded from the broader service user movement, including mental health and cancer, since they were seen as antithetical to "the pro-active, rational consumer of services" (Smith et al. 2011:1466). This has changed with campaigning activities that have repositioned individuals with mild dementia as citizen-workers, yielding social and psychological benefits associated with activism, self-advocacy, and the companionship of others with similar impairments (Bartlett 2014).

Nonetheless, this classic model of citizenship, with its "emphasis on self-cognizance" (Bartlett and O'Connor 2007:108), rests on the ideal type of the fit and healthy, and thereby deepens the social devaluation of those no longer able to make recognizable contributions (Minkler and Holstein 2008), such as those with severe dementia. A proposed corrective is the passive model of social citizenship, which is concerned with "people getting what they are entitled to or have a right to expect as an equal citizen" (Bartlett and O'Connor 2010:35) without having to make a public contribution. Individuals are therefore provided with enforceable standing to complain when they are denied a treatment or service on the basis of a dementia diagnosis or other category.

Both relationship-centered care and the passive model of citizenship offer important insights into improving our understanding of the requirements of fair and equitable treatment of individuals with dementia. Yet, how this is to be accomplished in any practical sense with institutionalized and nonverbal residents remains unaddressed. Further, neither of these approaches has yet to be influenced by the emerging theoretical subfield of embodiment (Kontos and Martin 2013), which has placed the body and embodied practices at the center of dementia representations and care. In consequence, each has overlooked the importance of nonverbal communication for self-expression and interconnectedness, and the in-the-moment experiences of directing and receiving humane care within health institutions. What is needed is the fashioning of a new model of citizenship, what we term *relational citizenship*—premised on the understanding that capacities, senses, and experiences of bodies are central to the exercise of human agency and interconnectedness, and the reciprocal nature of engagement—as an entitlement at the micro-level of direct care.

In our view, elder-clowns are uniquely suited to concretize the empowerment of relational citizenship participation for those with severe dementia and can do so in a manner that incorporates the necessary care tenets of relationship-centered care and embodiment theory. Relational presence is a clown approach to the interactions between service users and service providers that offers sustained recognition of the selfhood of the individual with dementia and contextualizes social participation as the intrinsic and embodied capacities of expression and communication despite advanced dementia. In so doing, relational presence offers a novel paradigm of care that has the potential to influence the relationship between service users and service providers across the entire interdisciplinary long-term care team.

ELDER-CLOWNING

Arts-based therapies are part of a "major conceptual sea change" (Cohen 2006:7) in residential long-term care. Arts have been integrated into the new paradigms of person-centered and relational care through program-based therapeutic interventions such as music, dance, drama, and storytelling (Raglio et al. 2008; Basting 2006; Beard 2011). The most recent innovation in arts-based dementia care is the use of specialized therapeutic red-nosed clowns. Therapeutic clowns are "trained artists who use clowning to empower patients through opportunities for emotional expression, social interaction and personal control" (Blain et al. 2012:27).

Contemporary therapeutic clowning began in the 1970s in the United States (Roy 2009). Children were the first, and remain the primary, target population for most therapeutic clown programs in acute care hospital settings (Warren 2007). However, since the late 1990s, clowning has been adapted for specific use with the dementia population (Killick 2003). This adaptation is referred to as elder-clowning (Hendriks 2012; Warren and

Spitzer 2011). Elder-clowns keep their faces natural with minimal or no makeup, don a red nose, and wear clothing that harkens back to a previous era, such as colorful 1950s swing dresses (Hearts & Minds 2013; miMakkus 2013). Their intended goals are to provide social and mental stimulation, lessen social isolation, and improve feelings of well-being among long-term care residents (Gervais, Warren, and Twohig 2007).

Elder-clown interactions or plays include verbal, physical, and musical jests that incorporate fantasy, surprise, inversion, dramatic movement, physical comedy, and storytelling (Blain et al. 2012; van Troostwijk 2007). Plays additionally include "reminiscence techniques, music and song structures, and . . . bedside magic" (Warren and Spitzer 2013:xiii). To enhance their plays, elder-clowns commonly use props, such as musical instruments (Warren 2011). Clowns rely on "census information" (Gervais, Warren, and Twohig 2007:181) provided by health care staff, which includes clinical, pharmaceutical, social, and familial details (Gervais, Warren, and Twohig 2007; Warren 2009; Achcar 2007).

The vast majority of clowns often begin as professional actors with theatrical training. Actors then pursue postgraduate specialized training at clown schools such as Le Rire Medicine in France and Annie Stainer's Total Theatre School of Physical Theatre in Australia (Linge 2008). The clown curriculum usually involves instruction on the social history of clowning (e.g., the development of clown types such as commedia dell'arte or the development of contemporary organizations such as Cirque du Soleil) and the practice implications of contemporary schools of thought in clowning (e.g., LeCoq's belief that each potential clown practitioner possesses an "inner clown" that must be found through emotional or psychotherapeutic introspection). Actors-cum-clowns also receive intense instruction on skit techniques such as repetition, imitation, and exaggeration (Achcar 2007). Since 2009, the University of Haifa has offered the only academic program in medical clowning, a three-year bachelor's track in the theater department (Estrin 2012). The academicization of the profession was designed to develop an evidence base for therapeutic clown work and to legitimate clowning as a paramedical profession (Estrin 2012). To date, however, there remains no definitive universal training, or qualifying academic or practical credential, for therapeutic clowns anywhere in the world (Symons 2012). For most medical and elder-clown practitioners, the graduation requirements established by the therapeutic clown schools in which they have enrolled determine their initial or ongoing professional development training (Symons 2012).

Despite the variability in education, the fundamental goal of all clown training is to prepare the practitioner to achieve an interactional state known as "presence," which is perceived as "the ground of clowning" (de Graan 2012:61). Presence is defined as the action of being "in a sense fuller, more authentic, or more real than what we normally come across" (Davison 2008:4). Presence is said to be successfully achieved when clowns are "fully in the present moment" (de Graan 2012:69), which requires that clowns suspend their personal judgment or comparison of the unfolding moment with some past personal experience (de Graan 2012). At an individual clown practitioner level, presence is cultivated through "attentive listening" (p. 70) and extraordinary focus and sensitivity (de Graan 2012).

OUR STUDY

Our study took place from 2012 to 2014 in urban central Canada, and was a mixed-methods evaluation of a 12-week elder-clown program in a publicly funded locked special care unit for residents with dementia.

The program was delivered by four practicing elder-clowns selected using a rigorous audition process. First, casting calls for professional clowns were sent out to charitable organizations that offer clown training and elder-clown services. Two clowns were subsequently hired as the lead pair, and another two clowns were hired as backups either to work as a pair or to individually fill in for an absent member of the lead pair. Three of the four clowns had graduated from a recognized clown-training school in Canada, with a specialty in the geriatric population; the fourth clown received clown training outside of Canada. After being hired, the elder-clowns additionally received a two-day training workshop conducted by a professional elder-clown trainer to promote team building and strong duoships through a range of active and reflective creative processes, including theater games, voice and body work, role playing, and improvisation. Over the duration of the intervention, clown supervision consisted of weekly virtual support (phone calls and emails), as well as an intensive eight-hour in-person workshop with the clown trainer and research staff. The purpose of the workshop was to identify and troubleshoot study issues such as scheduling (e.g., interruptions caused by a flu outbreak), filming (e.g., capturing both the elder-clowns' and residents' responses and initiated engagement), and communication with care staff (e.g., conveying information about observed changes in pain expressions of residents).

Over the course of the study, we collected 66 hours of videotaped clown–resident interactions and 48 videotaped clown-practice reflections, and we conducted semistructured interviews with each of the four elder-clowns. In our findings presented here, clowns are identified by clown character pseudonym (Cherry, Aksom, Zazzie, Mitsy) during interactions when they are in character and by practitioner pseudonym/character pseudonym (Holly/Cherry, Camilla/Aksom, Kate/Zazzie, Ann/Mitsy) during videotaped reflections, because those were conducted when they were out of clown character.

FINDINGS

Relational presence (Kontos, Miller, Mitchell, and Stirling-Twist 2015) is an engagement practice of elder-clowns that supports the relational needs of those with moderate to severe dementia. Relational presence was achieved and experienced through a combination of processes involving affective relationality and co-constructed imagination. Drawing on examples of the affective, nonverbal, and imaginative engagements between residents and clowns, we argue that these processes support a relational model of citizenship.

Affective Relationality

Central to the training of elder-clowns is that the clown learns to become "completely attuned to the other" and is able to distinguish "with increasing subtlety between differences in how the other person relates to the world, attentively, physically, and sensorily" (Hendriks 2012:469). Much of the intersubjective communication and empathetic connection that takes place between the clown and persons with dementia is at the affect level and encompasses both joyfulness and sadness.

JOYFULNESS

In those with moderate or severe dementia, the incitement and experience of joyfulness can occur in the absence of laughter or verbal response. The intensity of positive emotion may be discerned by bright eyes, and what is known as a Duchenne smile, which is characterized by raised cheeks and mouth corners, and crow's feet around the eyes (Ekman and Davidson 1990).

In the following example, the resident nonverbally communicates her increasing state of engagement and joy. The clowns' astute perception of her responses directed them to alter the pace of their play from the lullaby they had initiated to the slapstick she clearly most enjoyed:

> Lana is sitting in an arm chair, propped up by a pillow wedged between her left side and the chair's arm rest. Her eyes are closed, and her head is fully slumped to her left shoulder. . . . Zazzie sings a quiet lullaby as she strums a few accompanying notes on her ukulele. Cherry hums in harmony as she looks at Lana, and then very gently extends her hand and touches Lana's arm. Lana responds immediately by opening her eyes. Her response is abrupt and startles both clowns, who voice an involuntary, simultaneous "Oh!" Lana smiles. At first, her smile appears as friendly but reservedly polite as she maintains strong eye contact with Cherry, who is caressing her arm. But the longer she holds the clown's gaze, the warmer and broader her smile becomes. In response to Lana's increasing engagement, Zazzie begins to stroke Cherry's cheeks and her long blonde hair, which invites Cherry into the play. Then, after carefully watching Lana's increasing engagement and facial animation, she ups the interaction to a clown pair game where she tweaks, teases and pretends to slap Cherry's face, while Cherry responds with slapstick jolts. Lana looks thoroughly amused. She briefly breaks her focus on their interaction to directly glance at Zazzie, and with eye contact signals utter enjoyment and approval of the game. Her face is now in a clear Duchenne smile.

The clowns also used music and movement/dance to play in a manner that visibly prompted joy. Residents' nonverbal but embodied expressions of joy directed further engagement by the clowns, as is aptly illustrated in the following interaction:

> Betty has clearly heard the [pending approach of the singing] clowns . . . with a broad smile, and to the beat of the music, she is moving her hands up and down, and tapping her right foot. . . . Betty focuses her gaze on Aksom, and while in keeping with the tempo of the music, she changes the rhythm of her movements so she is bobbing in double time. Aksom, in response to Betty's initiated change of rhythm, begins a slow side-to-side jive and stops just in front of Betty. With increased facial and bodily animation, Betty's

> foot tapping evolves into a stomping of her right foot, akin to a hoedown [a lively American Western country and music square or line dance], coordinated with shoulder lifts. In response, Mitsy changes the [song] phrase to "let's all stomp our feet." Aksom follows Betty's lead and mirrors her foot stomping. Betty then takes steps towards the clown while stretching her mouth with exaggerated "ohhs" and "ahhs" to the beat of the music. Aksom responds by playfully biting the air and puffing her cheeks in synchronicity with Betty's joyful facial expressions.

In both of these engagements, it is the reciprocal nature of the giving and sharing of embodied joy that is particularly salient to our analysis. Relational presence, as an engagement practice of elder-clowns, is predicated on a belief in the unique and playful expressions or offerings by those with dementia. It is the clowns' recognition and incorporation of residents' intrinsic expressiveness at the affective and nonverbal level that highlights the relational citizenship component of this form of service user engagement.

SADNESS

Contrary to the predominant belief that clowns focus on the giving of entertainment and happiness (Warren 2011; Warren and Spitzer 2013), we found that elder-clowns embrace the expression and support of sadness as a routine part of relational presence. In some cases, clowns acted as genuine and empathetic witnesses to a resident's expression of sadness. In a videotaped reflection, Ann/Mitsy recalled,

> Betty started singing a song. . . . I felt like I was watching a great performance. She would emote tremendously, like almost a sobbing cry through her song . . . that yawny note, it triggered [Betty's] tears. . . . Even though there was sadness in it, it didn't have to be negative. . . . It wasn't necessary [as part of clown practice] to take away that emotion. . . . It's not wrong to feel sadness. . . . It's not wrong to cry.

In other instances, clowns may move from simply bearing witness to a resident's sadness to affect attunement or the cosharing of an inner emotional state (Linge 2008). Kate/Zazzie explained during a videotaped reflection:

> With Ginger, there were some days where she had so much sadness in her body. . . . Just the way she was breathing, you could feel her sadness. . . . She

> expressed [her sadness] . . . in the way that she would sort of touch our hands, and touch our faces. . . . We recognized this sadness and held it in a way, allowed that sadness to be in the room. . . . We mirrored the energy with her so we felt like [we were with], or we were trying to sort of accompany her in, that state.

These examples demonstrate a shared emotional state that becomes a relational effect (Hendriks 2012) that flows from "mutual empathy," founded on "a mutual respect, maximum possible relational equality, a belief in the capacity to participate in growth-promoting relationships, and the motivation for emotional connectedness with others" (Freedberg 2007:255). The empathic responsiveness of the clowns or, more aptly, their "affective resonance" (Hartling and Littlefield, quoted in Freedberg 2007:255) forms a significant dimension of relational citizenship in the context of the interpersonal mutuality of engagement between service users and service providers.

Co-constructed Imagination

Clowns are trained to relate external stimuli such as words and objects with inner-self characteristics such as imagination, memory, and impulse (Achcar 2007). Imaginative possibility is particularly valuable in the context of dementia, where boundaries shift between time, place, and person and become more fluid and less defined (Mitchell, Dupuis, and Kontos 2013). In our study, the clowns described the importance of the relational intersection between the "imaginative reality" of their world and that of the person with dementia. Kate/Zazzie commented:

> A clown principle is the intersection of worlds. So, we bring our [clown] world, as [clown] sisters, our back story, all that kind of stuff, and our relationship into a person's space and into their world. And they have their own world happening. It's this real meshing of the two worlds that becomes the play space.

In this relational play space, elder-clowns "surrender to the participant's reality" (Symons 2012:7) and draw on the performative coherence (Hydén and Örulv 2009; Kontos and Martin 2013) of residents' storytelling to co-construct imaginative scenarios. This stands in stark contrast to the common response by care staff and family members who "try to bring someone with dementia back to 'normal' reality" (Symons 2012:7). Instead, clowns often fully embraced the imaginary as a means to counteract barriers to communication such as residents' incoherent or nonsensical speech in the presence of reminiscence or delusions. This is captured in the following videotaped observation:

> Jean says to Aksom in a reassuring tone, ". . . I'm going to call and see. You can get down, now. Right now it's too late for him. But I'll catch it." She pauses, and appears to reconsider, "And if that doesn't do it, I don't know." Aksom responds as if he is following the instructions of an older sibling, and makes to leave. He says to Jean, ". . . You catch up." Jean shakes her head sideways to signal "no," and says quietly, "I'm a breeze of an ant." Aksom asks in disbelief, "Really?" He leans heavily on the arm of the wheelchair as he coaxes, "We'll do it together. Can you do that?" Jean answers uncertainly, "I think so." . . . Jean laughs as if humoring him, "Let's see what Father has to say." Jean appears to pull an imaginary scarf from around her neck. She hands it to Aksom. Aksom queries, "Should I take it?" Then he hands the imaginary scarf back to her and says, "You take it. You have it. You are strong." Jean shakes her head and says in a rueful tone, "No, I wasn't." Aksom responds softly, "I always thought you were strong." Jean takes Aksom's hand in hers, and says in an explanatory, patient tone, "You were tired." She then adds gently, "Thanks for waiting." . . . Jean smiles kindly at Aksom, and then shifts her gaze downward. Looking into her lap, she speaks in a soft, almost inaudible torrent of words that are without coherence or recognizable sentence structure.

DISCUSSION

When examining the citizenship capacities of individuals with dementia, the key is "to consider what a person does and with what public consequence" (Lister, quoted in Bartlett and O'Connor 2010:32). However, our work with elder-clowns sheds a much different light on the relational complexity of individuals with dementia in their interactions with others. Indeed, as our findings illustrate, more advanced cognitive impairment cannot be accommodated by an exclusive focus on public and private social duties; instead, intrinsic capacities and embodied forms of engagement that persist despite even severe dementia become of paramount importance given that they constitute the primary means of engagement with the world. Thus, in order to fully support the passive citizenship entitlements of residents to long-term care, a relational citizenship model is needed that is premised on two essential values. The first is the value accorded individuals on the basis of bodily potentiality, the capacity of individuals with moderate and severe dementia to initiate as well as respond to verbal, embodied, emotive, and creative engagement. The second is the right of relationality, which captures the reciprocal nature of engagement. Embracing these values is critical to supporting the "valuing of who we are, simply *because we are*" (Minkler and Holstein 2008:203, original emphasis).

Often with only embodied self-expression and/or nonsensical speech, residents would initiate, modify, and co-construct exquisite moments of engagement with the elder-clowns. This required the use of imagination by the clowns, which has been identified as a critical source of empathetic care, particularly when premised on the communicative capacity of the body of the other (Kontos and Naglie 2007, 2009). Narrative techniques have been identified as a strategy to link subjective experience to the sociopolitical context (Baldwin 2008) within the context of an active citizenship model. However, our study demonstrated how, on the basis of empathy and relationality, the clowns eschewed distinguishing the historical accuracy of reminiscence, without losing the significance of the personal mattering of stories of self. This in turn demonstrates the significance to relational citizenship of the honoring of personal stories, independent of biographical accuracy.

Working against "the sleeping beauty syndrome" (Killick and Allan 2012:65), the clowns approached the residents with dementia as having the intention to elicit play and engagement in the clowns themselves. Thus, for clowns, it is in fact they who exist in a state of potential; their spirit of playfulness lies in wait, realized only in interaction *with* someone (Koller and Gryski 2008). In our study, the examples of nonverbal expressions of joy by residents through smiling and dancing illustrate how they directed the unfolding of the plays. We argue that this is an intrinsic capacity, and must be regarded as fundamental to how citizenship is conceptualized in the context of long-term institutionalized dementia care.

The majority of research involving clowns in health care focuses on the presence and curative potential of laughter (for a critique, see Hendriks 2012). Certainly, residents in our study experienced fun and joy when interacting with the clowns: residents' smiles, bright eyes, and laughter were not uncommon responses. Other studies have similarly found that clown interactions resulted in "dementia sufferers laughing, singing, dancing, joking, playing" (Symons 2012:4). Nonetheless, in our study, the clowns' recognition and support of residents' grief was an additional important mechanism for honoring residents' relational citizenship. The ability of clowns to bear witness to sadness, and share an inner emotional state or affect attunement, resonates powerfully with the "consumer-centricity" in care settings (Upah 2014:1).

Our emphasis on relational citizenship importantly corrects the hierarchical and unidirectional nature of most caregiving relationships in long-term institutional care and their predominant focus on the passivity of the service user. We argue that the relational presence achieved in elder-clowning offers a novel perspective with which to reimagine the relationship between service users and other care providers. Specifically, by diffusing the responsibility for enabling the creative and emotional enrichment of the health care environment, it would ensure that the residents' capacities are supported and nurtured in all aspects of institutionalized life and not exclusively through elder-clowning specifically or even arts-based programming more generally (Genoe and Dupuis 2014; Moss and O'Neill 2014). However, it is important to note that core clown competencies remain that may not be fully accessible to nursing and allied practitioners. This is evident in medical settings where, for example, physical therapists have been encouraged to employ clown techniques but in "less fantastical ways" (Upah 2014:2). Thus, clown practitioners are well positioned to provide a unique contribution to the long-term health care team; they offer a distinct cultural/aesthetic competence to which reciprocity and relationship with and by service users is fundamental. Such aesthetic enrichment supports not only good biopsychosocial care but also the more robust model of citizenship we are advocating given how aesthetics are "markers of human identity, pathways for exploration of the human condition, and key elements of personal self-expression" (Moss and O'Neill 2014:1032).

• • •

We argue for a practice engagement that begins first with mindfulness of the role of embodiment in relationship to human agency, and particularly in the case of Alzheimer's disease, as a vital source of selfhood that remains despite even severe dementia (Kontos 2004, 2012). It next recognizes the inclusion of those with dementia beyond the status of a special interest group. Yet citizenship is more than status alone; it is also a practice (Brannelly 2011). Relational citizenship as a practice uniquely addresses the tenets of engagement and care paradigms of relationship-centered care (Nolan et al. 2004; Adams and Gardiner 2005) and social justice approaches to service user inclusion (Smith et al. 2011).

New trends and directions in paradigms of treatment and care that are associated with improvements in the "image, status, role and responsibilities of people with dementia" (Bartlett and O'Connor 2010:4) are importantly occurring. Yet, much more needs to be done both in theory and in practice to reenvision individuals with dementia as more than passive care recipients. Our perspective of relational citizenship, which is predicated on the elder-clown practice of relational presence, shares some similarities to Plummer's notion of "intimate citizenship," which recognizes emerging "intimacy groups and identities" (Plummer 2003:66) and the importance of including what occurs in the private sphere among individuals as a site of citizenship claiming. Plummer (2003) has, however, neglected to include those with dementia, likely because of the troubling distinction in the citizenship discourse between "how to care for" and "how to think about, relate to and increase the capacity" of individuals (Bartlett and O'Connor 2010:14). The practice of relational presence is an important break with this distinction and heralds a new vision for the recognition of relational citizenship in individuals with dementia.

NOTE

1 This work was supported by the Canadian Institutes of Health Research Operating Grant (2012–14, MOP-114953). Pia Kontos holds a Canadian Institutes of Health Research New Investigator Award (MSH-87726).

REFERENCES

Achcar, A. 2007. "Clown Language, Performance and Children's Hospitals." In *Suffering the Slings and Arrows of Outrageous Fortune: International Perspectives on Stress, Laughter and Depression*, edited by B. Warren, 149–153. New York: Rodopi.

Adams, T., and P. Gardiner. 2005. "Communication and Interaction within Dementia Care Triads: Developing a Theory for Relationship-Centred Care." *Dementia* 4(2): 185–205.

Andrews, G. 2006. "Managing Challenging Behaviour in Dementia." *British Medical Journal* 332(7544): 741.

Baldwin, C. 2008. "Narrative(,) Citizenship and Dementia: The Personal and the Political." *Journal of Aging Studies* 22(3): 222–228.

Bartlett, R. 2014. "Citizenship in Action: The Lived Experiences of Citizens with Dementia Who Campaign for Social Change." *Disability and Society* 29(8): 1291–1304.

Bartlett, R., and D. O'Connor. 2007. "From Personhood to Citizenship: Broadening the Lens for Dementia Practice and Research." *Journal of Aging Studies* 21(2): 107–118.

Bartlett, R., and D. O'Connor. 2010. *Broadening the Dementia Debate: Towards Social Citizenship*. Bristol: Policy.

Basting, A. 2006. "Creative Storytelling and Self-Expression Among People with Dementia." In *Thinking About Dementia: Culture, Loss, and the Anthropology of Senility*, edited by A. Leibing and L. Cohen, 180–194. New Brunswick, NJ: Rutgers University Press.

Beard, R. L. 2011. "Art Therapies and Dementia Care: A Systematic Review." *Dementia* 11(5): 633–656.

Behuniak, S. M. 2011. "The Living Dead? The Construction of People with Alzheimer's Disease as Zombies." *Ageing and Society* 31(1): 70–92.

Blain, S., S. Kingsnorth, L. Stephens, and P. McKeever. 2012. "Determining the Effects of Therapeutic Clowning on Nurses in a Children's Rehabilitation Hospital." *Arts and Health* 4(1): 26–38. doi: 10.1080117533015.2011.561359.

Brannelly, T. 2011. "Sustaining Citizenship: People with Dementia and the Phenomenon of Social Death." *Nursing Ethics* 18(5): 662–671. doi: 10.1177/0969733011408049.

Cohen, G. D. 2006. "Research on Creativity and Aging: The Positive Impact of the Arts on Health and Illness." *Generations* 30(1): 7–15.

Cohen-Mansfield, J., and J. E. Mintzer. 2005. "Time for Change: The Role of Nonpharmacological Interventions in Treating Behavior Problems in Nursing Home Residents with Dementia." *Alzheimer Disease and Associated Disorders* 19(1): 37–40.

Davison, J. 2008. *The Phenomenology of Clown*. http://www.jondavison.net/images/the%20phenomenology%20of%20clown.pdf. Accessed January 13, 2015.

de Graan, R. 2012. "A Fool's View on Transformation." Master's thesis, Utrecht School of Governance, Utrecht University.

Dupuis, S., C. A. McAiney, D. Fortune, J. Ploeg, and L. D. Witt. 2014. "Theoretical Foundations Guiding Culture Change: The Work of the Partnerships in Dementia Care Alliance." *Dementia: The International Journal of Social Research and Practice*. March 31 [Epub ahead of print].

Dupuis, S., E. Wiersma, and L. Loiselle. 2012. "Pathologizing Behavior: Meanings of Behaviors in Dementia Care." *Journal of Aging Studies* 26:162–173.

Edvardsson, D., B. Winblad, and P. O. Sandman. 2008. "Person-Centred Care of People with Severe Alzheimer's Disease: Current Status and Ways Forward." *Lancet Neurology* 7(4): 362–367.

Ekman, P., and R. J. Davidson. 1990. "The Duchenne Smile: Emotional Expression and Brain Physiology II." *Journal of Personality and Social Psychology* 58(2): 342–353. doi: 0022–3514/90/$00.75.

Estrin, D. 2012. *The Healing Clowns of Haifa*. http://pri.org/stories/2012–07–30/healing-clowns-haifa. Accessed December 7, 2013.

Freedberg, S. 2007. "Re-examining Empathy: A Relational–Feminist Point of View." *Social Work* 52(3): 251–259.

Genoe, M. R., and S. L. Dupuis. 2014. "The Role of Leisure Within the Dementia Context." *Dementia* 13(1): 33–58.

Gervais, N., B. Warren, and P. Twohig. 2007. "'Nothing Seems Funny Anymore': Studying Burnout in Clown-Doctors." In *Suffering the Slings and Arrows of Outrageous Fortune: International Perspectives on Stress, Laughter and Depression*, edited by B. Warren, 175–189. New York: Rodopi.

Hearts & Minds. 2013. *The Elderflowers Programme: Watch the Elderflowers*. http://www.heartsminds.org.uk/the-elderflowers/. Accessed February 26, 2014.

Hendriks, R. 2012. "Tackling Indifference—Clowning, Dementia, and the Articulation of a Sensitive Body." *Medical Anthropology: Cross-Cultural Studies in Health and Illness* 31(6): 459–476.

Herskovitz, E. 1995. "Struggling Over Subjectivity: Debates About the 'Self' and Alzheimer's Disease." *Medical Anthropology Quarterly* 9(2): 146–164.

Hydén, L. C., and L. Örulv. 2009. "Narrative and Identity in Alzheimer's Disease: A Case Study." *Journal of Aging Studies* 23(4): 205–214.

Katona, C. L. 2001. "Psychotropics and Drug Interactions in the Elderly Patient." *International Journal of Geriatric Psychiatry* 16 (supplement 1): S86–S90.

Killick, J. 2003. "Funny and Sad and Friendly: A Drama Project in Scotland." *Journal of Dementia Care* 11(1): 24–26.

Killick, J., and K. Allan. 2012. *Playfulness and Dementia: A Practice Guide*. London: Kingsley.

Kitwood, T. 1997. *Dementia Reconsidered: The Person Comes First*. Buckingham: Open University Press.

Koller, D., and C. Gryski. 2008. "The Life Threatened Child and the Life Enhancing Clown: Towards a Model of Therapeutic Clowning." *Evidence-Based Complementary and Alternative Medicine* 5(1): 17–25. doi: 10.1093/ecam/nem033.

Kontos, P. 2004. "Ethnographic Reflections on Selfhood, Embodiment and Alzheimer's Disease." *Ageing and Society* 24:829–849.

Kontos, P. 2012. "Alzheimer Expressions or Expressions Despite Alzheimer's?: Philosophical Reflections on Selfhood and Embodiment." *Occasion: Interdisciplinary Studies in the Humanities* 4 (May 31). http://arcade.stanford.edu/sites/default/files/article_pdfs/OCCASION_v04_Kontos_053112_0.pdf.

Kontos, P., and W. Martin. 2013. "Embodiment and Dementia: Exploring Critical Narratives of Selfhood, Surveillance, and Dementia Care." *Dementia* 12(3): 288–302.

Kontos, P., K. L. Miller, and G. J. Mitchell. 2010. "Neglecting the Importance of the Decision Making and Care Regimes of Personal Support Workers: A Critique of Standardization of Care Planning Through the RAI/MDS." *The Gerontologist* 50(3): 352–362.

Kontos, P., K. L. Miller, G. J. Mitchell, and J. Stirling-Twist. 2015. "Presence Redefined: The Reciprocal Nature of Engagement Between Elder-Clowns and Persons with Dementia." *Dementia: The International Journal of Social Research and Practice*. April 23 [Epub ahead of print].

Kontos, P., and G. Naglie. 2007. "Bridging Theory and Practice: Imagination, the Body, and Person-Centred Dementia Care." *Dementia: The International Journal of Social Research and Practice* 6(4): 549–569.

Kontos, P., and G. Naglie. 2009. "Tacit Knowledge of Caring and Embodied Selfhood." *Sociology of Health and Illness* 31(5): 688–704.

Linge, L. 2008. "Hospital Clowns Working in Pairs—in Synchronized Communication with Ailing Children." *International Journal of Qualitative Studies on Health and Well-Being* 3:27–38.

Matthews, E. 2006. "Dementia and the Identity of the Person." In *Dementia: Mind, Meaning and the Person*, edited by J. C. Hughes, S. J. Louw, and S. R. Sabat, 163–177. Oxford: Oxford University Press.

miMakkus. 2013. *About miMakkus*. http://www.mimakkus.nl/?language=en. Accessed July 26, 2010.

Minkler, M., and M. B. Holstein. 2008. "From Civil Rights to . . . Civic Engagement? Concerns of Two Older Critical Gerontologists About a 'New Social Movement' and What It Portends." *Journal of Aging Studies* 22(2): 196–204.

Mitchell, G. J., S. L. Dupuis, and P. Kontos. 2013. "Dementia Discourse: From Imposed Suffering to Knowing Other-Wise." *Journal of Applied Hermeneutics.* Article 5. http://jah.journalhosting.ucalgary.ca/jah/index.php/jah/article/viewFile/41/pdf.

Moss, H., and D. O'Neill. 2014. "Aesthetic Deprivation in Clinical Settings." *The Lancet* 383(9922): 1032–1033.

Nolan, M., T. Ryan, P. Enderby, and D. Reid. 2002. "Towards a More Inclusive Vision of Dementia Care Practice." *Dementia: The International Journal of Social Research and Practice* 1(2): 193–211.

Nolan, M. R., S. Davies, J. Keady, and J. Nolan. 2004. "Beyond 'Person-Centred' Care: A New Vision for Gerontological Nursing." *International Journal of Older People Nursing* 13(3a): 45–53.

Plummer, K. 2003. *Intimate Citizenship: Private Decisions and Public Dialogues.* Seattle: University of Washington Press.

Raglio, A., G. Bellelli, D. Traficante, M. Gianotti, M. C. Ubezio, D. Villani, and M. Trabucchi. 2008. "Efficacy of Music Therapy in the Treatment of Behavioral and Psychiatric Symptoms of Dementia." *Alzheimer Disease and Associated Disorders* 22(2): 158–162.

Reid, D., T. Ryan, and P. Enderby. 2001. "What Does It Mean to Listen to People with Dementia?" *Disability and Society* 16(3): 377–392.

Roy, J. 2009. "Clowning Within Drama Therapy Group Sessions: A Case Study of a Unique Recovery Journey in a Psychiatric Hospital." Master's thesis, Department of Creative Art Therapies, Concordia University, Montreal.

Smith, M., M. Gallagher, H. Wosu, J. Stewart, V. E. Cree, S. Hunter, S. Evans, C. Montgomery, S. Holiday, and H. Wilkinson. 2011. "Engaging with Involuntary Service Users in Social Work: Findings from a Knowledge Exchange Project." *British Journal of Social Work* 42(8): 1460–1477. doi: 10.1093/bjsw/bcr162.

Symons, D. 2012. *A Study of Elder Clown Programs in Scotland, the Netherlands, USA and Canada.* Churchill Memorial Trust of Australia. http://www.churchilltrust.com.au/media/fellows/2012_Symons_David.pdf. Accessed December 30, 2014.

Upah, K. 2014. *Medical Clowning in a Physical Therapy Setting.* http://physical-therapy.advanceweb.com/Features/Articles/Medical-Clowning-in-a-Physical-Therapy-Setting.aspx. Accessed December 30, 2014.

van Troostwijk, T. D. 2007. "The Hospital Clown: A Cross Boundary Character." In *Suffering the Slings and Arrows of Outrageous Fortune: International Perspectives on Stress, Laughter and Depression*, edited by B. Warren, 137–148. New York: Rodopi.

Warren, B. 2009. "'Hi Jean!': How Clown-Doctors Help Facilitate Safe Infection-Control and Positive Health Care Practices." In *Infection Control: A Psychosocial Approach to Changing Practice*, edited by P. Elliot, 149–158. Oxon: Radcliffe.

Warren, B. 2011. "Foolish Medicine: Reflections on the Practices of Modern-Clown Doctors and Medieval Fools." *Les Cahiers de l'idiotie* 2(2): 179–195.

Warren, B., ed. 2007. *Suffering the Slings and Arrows of Outrageous Fortune: International Perspectives on Stress, Laughter and Depression*. New York: Rodopi.

Warren, B., and P. Spitzer. 2011. "Laughing to Longevity—the Work of Elder Clowns." *The Lancet* 378(9791): 562–563. doi: 10.1016/s0140–6736(11)61280–4.

Warren, B., and P. Spitzer. 2013. *Smiles Are Everywhere: Integrating Clown-Play Into Healthcare Practice*. London: Routledge.

9

Managing the Complexity of Family Contact in Child Welfare

▸ *TARJA PÖSÖ*

ULTIMATELY, DECISIONS IN HUMAN SERVICES ARE BINARY—a client either is provided services or is not. Services may include therapeutic support or may not. But this ignores the everyday practice of service provision. The processes leading to such decisions may be long and complex, and the final decision may be shadowed by uncertainty (see Järvinen, Chapter 3, this volume). Still, such decisions are made. While thinking in terms of either/or may satisfy input-output criteria, it does not tell us much, if anything at all, about *how* it is that a service is either finally provided or is not. It does not reveal the different ways either/or decisions are reached, challenging us to reimagine the service relationship in terms that recognize the complex personal experiences and institutional practices in place.

The decision of removing a child from the home and parental care and placing the child into public care is a good example of a complex but eventually binary decision. The child either is removed from the home and placed into public care or is not. But, here again, the process of making that decision is far from binary. While the place to live might change, children's relations with their family and kin remain. Memories of life before the removal are not wiped away by the decision. A break between life before and life after the removal may not even be the aim if the child welfare system intends to support parallel relations among the child, the birth parents, and the substitute caregivers while the child is in public care. The question is: what makes contacts so important but potentially complex in child welfare?

THE MORAL LANDSCAPE OF FAMILY CONTACT IN CARE

In 2011, a special booklet, *Uskomme sinuun, usko sinäkin* (We believe in you, believe in yourself as well), was published in Finland. It was aimed at children who were in care and who needed to know their associated rights. This booklet was not just a conventional publication prepared by adult professionals but a text written by so-called experts by experience, or "survivors" as they called themselves—children who were in or had been in care and who therefore had experienced what it is like. After a long series of meetings and workshops, they described in the booklet what they wanted to share with other children in care. One such message was the right to have contact with one's family and the right to withdraw from such contacts.

Under the booklet section titled "Do you lose your right to meet with your family?" survivors state that:

> When you are placed outside of your birth home, it means that the child welfare authorities have a full authority over you. The adults in your substitute home take care of your upbringing and education. You have the right to be in touch and to meet with your family and other close people. You have the opportunity to influence the decision about how often and where you want to meet your close people. The contact may be restricted if it threatens your life and development. You also have the right not to meet them. Tell about your thoughts to your social worker and caring adults. (*Uskomme sinuun, usko sinäkin* 2011:13)

The voices of the experts by experience are interwoven with not-quite-correct legal vocabulary, highlighting the inevitability of the legal dimension of child welfare. The system of authority is referred to in those situations where contacts are not welcome; the booklet encourages children in care to cooperate with social workers, who can help restrict the contacts. Although very short, this message signals a positive dependency between the children in care and the child welfare practitioners, as the practitioners have the power to influence unwelcome contacts.

This message stands in contrast with the views of a parent association called Sukupuu (Family Tree). This is a coalition of parents of children who have been taken into care, so its messages and sentiments are also those of survivors and rest on the members' own experiences. This association states its mission in the following way:

> One of the important aims of this association is to support and strengthen the contact between the child and the parents and other close ones also after the care order. This is often in the best interest of the child. Although the relation between the biological parents and child is natural, the authorities do not often respect this relation and the problems in maintaining contact are sadly common. The parents and other relatives are not always aware of their own rights and opportunities. One aim of the association is thus to share information about issues related to the care order and practical arrangements. (Sukupuu 2014)

The mission statement describes the parents' view about contact between children and parents. Contact is needed, it emphasizes, because it is both in the best interest of the child and a natural right stemming from biological ties. When emphasizing the importance of the contact, conflicting views between the parents and the authorities are raised. The moral tone of the paragraph rests on the assertion that the authorities wrongly restrict contact. The parents should be more aware of their rights to contact, and the authorities should learn to respect those rights.

Both statements take the view that contact is important, but they assign different meanings to it (see Carr, Chapter 4, this volume). Children call on the authorities to cooperate with them to restrict unwanted contacts, whereas parents criticize the authorities for restricting contacts for the wrong reasons. The contrasting messages highlight the controversial nature of contacts and the standpoints from which the vocabulary and ownership of rights are communicated. This is in accord with the conclusion of a research review that states that although contacts are often beneficial for children, they can also be unsatisfactory and even harmful (Sinclair and Jeffreys 2005). The wish to be in contact with one's family is not at all binary, such as the complication that while children generally may want to see more of their families, they also may want to see less of particular family members. According to Sinclair and Jeffreys, time and effort need to be spent on making contact a better and safer experience for all concerned. Adding to this, time and effort need to be spent on understanding how the moral complexity of the matter is managed.

Indeed, the moral landscape increases in complexity as other standpoints are taken into account (see in this volume Barnes, Chapter 15; Newman, Chapter 16). The preceding extracts demonstrate the standpoints of children and parents, but there could be other standpoints as well. Fathers' views on their right to contact could differ from those of mothers, and some members of the kinship network could insert their claim to their right to stay in contact with the child even when a parent would like to restrict that contact. If extenuating circumstances are considered, the moral landscape of contacts becomes broader than ever.

DEVELOPMENT OF FAMILY CONTACT AS AN ISSUE

In very simple terms, the development of family contact as an issue in child welfare may be summarized this way. Child welfare was initially focused on orphaned and abandoned children. Later, it began to take an interest in children who were poorly treated within their families. The latter focus is fundamentally different from the former in that now public care works with so-called dysfunctional families instead of substituting for the lack of parents and/or families as before. This development has been described in Jacques Donzelot's (1980) book *Policing of Families*. Consequently, today, child welfare deals not only with children but also with parents and increasingly with the wider kinship network. The resulting task is to assess, monitor, and change the relations between parents, families, and children, which is now the key focus of child welfare policy and practice (Gillies 2008; Ferguson 2004).

This is well recognized in Western countries, where children are taken into public care mainly as a result of problems within the family. It is the parents' right and duty to look after their children, and the accomplishment of these duties and rights is regulated by the state (Archard 2003; Gillies 2008). While some countries set a high threshold and intervene only in cases of serious neglect and abuse, others aim to intervene also in more low-risk situations, such as poor parenting (Gilbert, Parton, and Skivenes 2011). Equally well recognized is that family relations are the key target of child welfare practices and that family relations need to be supported and encouraged rather than restricted and separated, even in the case of serious family problems. If birth families fail to bring up their children, other family members or families, kin or foster families, should take over and nurture the upbringing of the child in order to provide the child with a "family home" (Gilbert, Parton, and Skivenes 2011; del Valle and Bravo 2013).

Maintaining family relations currently is envisioned from the point of view of human rights, with both the child and the parents having rights in the matter. According to the Convention on the Rights of Children (2014), not only parents but children as well have a distinctive right in family matters. As one section reads, "Parties shall respect the right of the child who is separated from one or both parents to maintain personal relations and direct contact with both parents on a regular basis, except if it is contrary to the child's best interests." The Human Rights Convention, on the other hand, states that the family as a unit should be supported by the state, which underscores the private and unique nature of family relations, and that this support entails rights that belong to every family member.

Like many other countries, the Finnish child welfare system builds on the view that children are best looked after by their birth parents (Pösö 2011). It is acknowledged, however, that parents need support in the rearing and care of minors and that the state should provide them with such support universally by way of family policy or by way of in-home services provided by the child welfare system (e.g., Eydal and Satka 2006; Pösö, Skivenes, and Hestbaeck 2014). The removal of a child from parental care should be implemented only as an intervention of last resort. In analyses of child welfare systems across countries, such an approach is called "family-service" instead of "child protection" (Gilbert, Parton, and Skivenes 2011). The Finnish legislation, the Child Welfare Act (2007:417) in particular, sets certain conditions for taking a child from parental care to public care (e.g., Pösö 2011). The important statements about care include, first, the temporary nature of care: the care order should be immediately terminated when the need for care disappears and the termination of care is in the best interests of the child. Parental rights are limited but are never terminated while the child is in care. Second, in line with the first condition, legislation underlines the importance of family reunification. Instead of separating the child from his or her parents while in care, efforts should be made to strengthen their relations to make the return of the child possible. Child welfare practitioners should plan for the parents to help them change so that reunification becomes possible. In addition, legislation encourages practitioners to support the maintenance of contact between the child and birth parents during the placement. Third, legislation states that if the contacts between the child and parents are to be restricted, there should be formal decisions made about the restrictions. Restriction is possible only when the contacts are clearly against the best interests of the child. The protocol to make and to document the decisions about the rights of the child and the parent is specified in terms of appeals and hearings. The monitoring system is also specified. This is to say that any deviations from a problem-free contact should be treated carefully, be legally correct, and also be bureaucratically transparent (Child Welfare Act 2007:417).

Reflecting the situation in most Western societies, the philosophy of the present Finnish child welfare system is summarized as "togetherness, belonging, and personhood," all of which are highly regarded qualities of human life and are connected to the family and family relations (Ribbens McCarthy 2012). According to Ribbens McCarthy, "There may be little alternative to the language of family for expressing such forms of relationality and connection." The notion of relationality is not linked to the family form itself, and it cannot be reduced to biological ties, the household, or economic arrangements. Instead, relationality has a strong emotional and existential character, suggesting that we think of individual identity in relational terms (Smart 2007). Even when the family is overshadowed by social problems threatening the integrity, health, and welfare of members, family relations and relationality play an important part in social responses to its problems. Instead of breaking up family relations, the expected response is to mend the social problems in order to support the "family" (e.g., Ribbens McCarthy, Hooper, and Gillies 2013). This rationale is clearly embedded in the present policy and practice of maintaining contact between children and parents while the child is in care, even as the child is protected from the problems and weaknesses of family life.

A STUDY OF FAMILY CONTACT

Empirical material from a study of family contact in child care practice highlights the moral complexity of the issue. The analysis is guided by the idea that contacts are not just a matter of social policy but are mediated by the circumstances of policy application. Knowledge of how contacts are experienced, avoided, dreamed about, enabled, and supervised is essential to understanding the *hows* on the ground of child welfare practice (see Gubrium, Chapter 1, this volume). The meaning and contingencies of contacts from two different standpoints are considered: from the standpoint of children who are in care and from the standpoint of practitioners and social workers, who as public authorities enable and regulate contacts so that they serve the institutional aim of supporting the child's best interests.

The data include interviews with children who are in care as well as surveys of and workshops with social workers who take care of these children. The data were collected in two Finnish municipalities in 2013 and 2014, concluding in social worker surveys and interviews with 17 children.[1] The surveys dealt with all children who were taken into care over a six-month and eight-month period of time, respectively, in two municipalities in 2013. The interviews include children from those groups whose members were seven years of age and older and who consented to being interviewed. They were given the option of choosing to be interviewed either by their own social worker (a familiar person) or the researcher (an outsider). Eight children out of 17 chose the researcher. The social workers joined the workshops with the researchers to plan the survey and to analyze the results. Altogether, 16 social workers were involved in the study as informants for the survey and/or as interviewers.

STANDPOINT: CONTACT AS LIVED EXPERIENCE

When discussing their time in care, children and young people do not talk much about their parents and family life in general. When they do talk, it is mainly about contacts. Contacts and their intensity comprise the bulk of what is said about parents and significant others. The topics of when, how often, and where one is in touch with family members are discussed at length. The focus on contacts may signal that family relations as such are a sensitive topic for interviews with children in care and are thus avoided as a topic but that maintaining contacts is something more concrete, less charged, and perfunctory, and thus easily explained. Respondents indicate that contact is very important to them (e.g., Hämäläinen 2012).

Contacts take many forms, including home visits, weekends spent at the parents' home, phone calls, and a combination of these. Very few remarks are made about the parents visiting the substitute home. However, one boy did remark that his grandfather always came to the Christmas celebration organized by the residential institution but refused to visit otherwise. Contact in the form of letter writing is not mentioned at all, although it has historically been a very important form of contact between parents and their children (Vehkalahti 2009). Some children say that they have a "phone time" on certain days during the week, suggesting that the use of the telephone is regulated.

The following extract from an interview six months after care started relates to daily phone contacts between a 14-year-old girl and her parents. The girl explains what the phone calls are about—she calls her parents to say that she loves them. This contact is repeated every evening and suggests, importantly, that contact, far from being only a matter of frequency, also references a highly emotional aspect of family life. Familial meaning sits side by side with frequency in children's contact experience.

INTERVIEWER Your parents are important to you and you keep in touch by phone almost daily, is that right?

GIRL Yeah, every day.

INTERVIEWER Both parents?

GIRL I can't go to bed if I haven't spoken with my parents. And I (have to) just say, or wish them good night. And then I've also had a habit since I was little to always tell my parents that I love them before I go to bed. If I don't say that, I can't sleep at night.

The girl being interviewed describes the phone contact as important because she has been used to expressing her love to her parents daily since early childhood. The personal meaning of this habit has not disappeared in care. Although she lives apart from her parents, the positive emotional element attached to the contact continues. In fact, very few children describe contact in a negative way. In those few that do, it is the low frequency that is underscored—the lack of contact is mentioned as a welcome situation while being in care. Lack of contact is, for example, a good way to keep distant from the parents when the child is not on "good terms" with them, as one teenage girl put it. Being in care made it possible for her to stay away from her parents. Another example of the significance of fewer contacts comes from a boy who qualifies his feeling that he enjoys his contacts with his father during the weekends although his father often gets drunk. If the father turns out to be very drunk and difficult, the boy explains that he has other relatives he can visit during the weekend. The contact itself is still important to him and is not destroyed by his father's behavior.

While home visits may be said to be regular and routine, this is not simply a matter, say, of visiting every second weekend with the parents, every second weekend in the substitute home, and the like. Unexpected contingencies enter the matter, such as a parent's work schedule. Routine and contingency work together in practice, which simple tallies of frequency fail to convey (see Gubrium, Chapter 1, this volume). The following extract from an interview with a 15-year-old boy suggests that while the child regularly commutes between his parental homes and the substitute home, their social relations exist in parallel.

INTERVIEWER How often do you meet your parents?
BOY Three times a month. Sometimes more often.
INTERVIEWER Do you visit home then sometimes during the week as well?
BOY I have, we go there sometimes to talk during the week.
INTERVIEWER So it is with your family worker.
BOY Yes.
INTERVIEWER If that happens on a weekday, can you then still go home at the weekend?
BOY Mm.
INTERVIEWER So it goes like this: you first visit your mother, and then you visit your father, and then you go again to your mother. Is that it, is that the rhythm?
BOY Yes, but it depends how it suits my father. He has quite a lot of work.
INTERVIEWER So you always find the times out and you know beforehand where you go. Is it like one week before the visit?
BOY I normally ask about it.
INTERVIEWER Do you think that you meet your parents often enough?
BOY Of course, hm, it's always too little, it's not ever enough.

For some children, routine translates into continuously updating a visitation plan. For example, one of the girls interviewed stated that she regularly visits her birth mother, her grandmother, and her birth father, all of whom live in different homes and have individual schedules of their own. Making matters even more complex, the mother tends to regularly lose her apartment and thus moves around a lot, which makes contact planning into a field of visitation. The girl describes this routine as taking the form of "a state of the art" rather than as a predictable array of contacts in a particular time period. She indeed keeps in touch with her parents and grandparents, but the places they live and their schedules crystallize in terms of a state of the art.

Restrictions on contact also are part of children's lived experiences in care. These can be associated with long-forgotten reasons for the restrictions. Some children mention in passing that contact restrictions apply to only one parent, for example. When asked to explain, they state that they do not recall the reasons for the restriction. This poses an interesting dilemma. According to legislation, the children are to be informed about the restriction of contact and the reasons for it, but the reasons are not recalled in the interviews. It is possible that the formalities of informing the child about the restriction of contact are not comprehended by the child in a way that the child can convey in an interview. The dilemma is that while legislation requires it, it is based on an overdrawn sense of agency in children, a matter that raises issues of equal rights and citizenship.

STANDPOINT: CONTACT IN SERVICE PRACTICE

For social workers, contacts between the child and the parent(s) entail a great deal of monitoring and decision making. While the social workers were mandated by law and policy to make professional decisions in matters of contact, decisions were continually contingent on ongoing developments in the matter. This was evident in workshop conversations between the social workers of the two municipalities and the researchers of the study.

Much of the decision making centered on the need to document contacts numerically in terms of frequency per time period. For example, a specific contact schedule needed to be formulated: how often per week, for example. At the same time, the policy imperative that the intensity of the contact schedule should meet the needs of the child entered the mix. Oddly enough, what constituted the needs of the child might be an outcome, not so much a determinant, of frequency.

Needs were assessed in meetings between the child, the social worker, the parents, and the foster parents and residential staff. Contact decisions were recorded in the child's care order, which was shared with all parties to ensure that everyone was aware of the order and their related rights in the matter. The start of the care order was commonly regarded as a period of "settling down," so contact at this point was often less frequent than it otherwise might be. Spending a weekend with the parent every second week was not unusual.

As the child's parents might not live together, the order also needed to be adjusted so that every parent/parental home was included in the contact schedule. The location of the contact was one of the tasks for the practitioners also to work out, because of the multiple families of children and sometimes because of the poor state of the homes of some parents. The child's trips to the parents needed to be organized and financially arranged as well. And it was important that contacts suited the needs and preferences of the substitute home and its household schedule. If the parent was willing to visit the child in the substitute home, similar financial and timetable adjustments had to be made.

The following social worker's comments demonstrate the complexity of organizing the contacts between the child and parent from the point of view of the social worker, which required balancing institutional and familial contingencies. In this case, the divorced parents do not cooperate with each other, and they request an equal number of contacts with the child. The meeting schedule is thus shadowed by disagreements between the parents.

> The child's contact with her parents has needed attention several times. Biological parents who are divorced are not capable of cooperating with each other and both insist on having an equal number of contacts with the child. Child welfare is however concerned about these contacts and also about where they could be carried out.

In the next extract from a survey questionnaire, the social worker writes about contacts held in the grandparents' home because of the unstable life of the birth mother. There is no "maternal home" in which the child can meet her mother, and therefore the grandparents' house is decided to be the contact venue. Although the mother's life situation is unstable, the relevance of maintaining contact is not contested. At the same time, it is noted that the child's foster parents need some psychosocial support and supervision, as the contact tends to cause some confusion for them. Hence, contrary to child welfare system understandings, the need for the child welfare system to provide psychosocial support to families might not effectively be restricted to the child and the parent.

> The child's contact with the biological mother. It was decided in the client plan meeting that due to her unstable living situation that the mother would meet the child only at her parents, that is, at the grandparents of the child. Supervision needs to be organised for the foster family.

Decisions in matters of contact are further complicated by surprise developments on the home front. This makes care planning anything but a linear process in practice, as is indicated in the following extract from the survey questionnaire of a social worker. As the father in the case now has a prison sentence abroad, related contacts will be difficult to organize, and this disappoints the child. The child's disappointment, not the arrangements of the contacts, seems to be a key point in this extract.

> A client plan meeting which was held in the home of the father and his partner. The plan was that the child's visits would be infrequent and supported at the father's home. The child liked this plan but soon after the meeting the father was sentenced to prison for a quite long period of time. Did not speak anything about his sentence in the meeting, he serves the sentence in another country, therefore it is really difficult to maintain the contact and this is a deep disappointment to the child.

It is evident in the data that the child's emotional well-being during and after the contacts is an important factor in contact planning. The child's emotional state after the contact—a weekend spent at the parental home, for example—is normally a focus of attention. The foster parents or the staff in residential institutions report about it to the social workers. If the reports are worrisome, they take that into account when planning future contacts. On this front, the future is a matter not of timing but of interactional developments that take place along the way and the monitoring that entails, which work against a linear sense of the matter, additionally complicating the idea of planning.

Conflicting views ending up in complaints add to the mix. The social workers mentioned parents in particular in regard to complaints about the nature and intensity of contacts. In some cases, the complaints of the parent ended in formal administrative appeals. In the following extract from the social worker survey, the appeal has been made in a situation in which the contact between the child and parent had been restricted.

> The termination of care which was planned in cooperation with the parents was stopped because of the parents' substance abuse in September 2013. Therefore a lot of work has been done to plan and to make the contacts possible. The mother has made a complaint about the contract restriction order. We have given our arguments to the administrative court.

INSTITUTIONALIZED CONTACT AND NEW RIGHTS

The phrase "normalizing the troubles in family" has been used to describe policies and therapeutic practices in which family troubles become part of the institutional system of practice (Ribbens McCarthy, Hooper, and Gillies 2013). This stands in contrast to approaches that pathologize family problems, which aim to change or even to abolish the problems. In the child welfare system, the aims of working with the child in care fall somewhere in between. On the one hand, the family's troubles are seen to be serious enough that the child has to be separated from his or her parents, thus pathologizing family troubles. On the other hand, normal family relations are seen to be so important that family contact outweighs the separation of the child from those troubles (see Gubrium, Chapter 1, this volume).

In the context of child welfare, the balance between treating the problems in family relations as normal, pathological, or both leads to a formalization of those relations. This refers to the schedules, plans, meetings, and documented decisions that maintaining contacts requires from the institutions, practitioners, children, and parents. For children, contact is transformed into the routine service and care that rests on the contracts agreed on by practitioners and parents. The contacts are not normal in the sense that they would take place spontaneously or intimately. A child needs to have permission to call his or her parents, and the parents' whereabouts must be known to the child welfare agency so that the child's visit can be arranged. The aftermath of contact is scrutinized, documented, and shared by practitioners. If family relations in general are considered personal, when in care these relations are turned into formal agreements, assessments, and whatever privacy and intimacy is involved is thereby monitored and documented. Institutionalized contact becomes the new normal.

As such, maintaining children's contact with families becomes as much an occupational task for practitioners working in the child welfare system as it is a matter of child and family rights. Institutionalized contact is mediated by the formal element of contact management, which requires time and effort by substitute carers, social workers, and eventually, in cases of appeals against decisions for contact restrictions, judges in the administrative courts, possibly including legal representation. The occupational task is carried out under the aegis of transparency and accountability. Decisions made need to be extensively recorded and justified, and need to be able to withstand any criticism from stakeholders and any monitoring by managers. This is why documentation and related client-information systems play such an important role in child contact. Psychosocial supervisors, educators, and therapists may be involved directly or indirectly in this practice as well. Some children's homes actually teach the parents how to behave with their children (Laakso 2012). Indeed, in some situations, maintaining contacts requires a variety of staff for enablement. There may even be some therapists included in maintaining the contact, as some children are in need of therapy in order to make them resilient enough to meet an abusive parent (Forsberg and Pösö 2008).

The formal and occupational elements of maintaining contacts are needed to support the protection of everyone's rights to family contact. The trouble is that, under the circumstances, this view of rights ultimately requires applying the binary standard that something is or is not a right (King 2004). The view is individualistic insofar as the logic deploys something like the idea that rights have particular owners. Jim Ife (2001) argues that the individualistic view of rights is rarely practical in social service, as the working messiness of issues, people's relations, and their standpoints and related stakes in the matter are almost always palpable. A broader view of rights recognizes rights' relational contours, the enduringly unfinished business of rights embedded in the practice of service provision.

Seen from this perspective, contact between children and their parents is bound to be continually unfinished business. Children, parents, and practitioners are positioned in constantly changing roles, shifting the boundaries of what administratively divides them. Children may claim the ownership of their rights, but they also may be the target of someone else's rights—simply because contact, as with all of everyday life, is about a relationship. Service practitioners may have the right to provide contact, but they also have the right to restrict it. Shifting coalitions between those actors add to the social dynamics of rights largely unrecognized by social policy.

Equally importantly, although the child welfare system aims to manage the complexity of contact and related rights while the child is in care, the system cannot capture and master its experiential turns. Children will always find ways to stay in touch with close and important people, family or not. Parents present or absent will have an impact on children, because family is so strongly rooted in our culture as a way of being related to others. The system cannot manage the imagination, dreams, and memories of children or their parents. All such things remain outside of the purview of systems of human management and accountability.

Standpoints on the horizon will add to the mix. When the condition of the child welfare system in Finland was thoroughly reviewed in 2013, the review group recommended that, in the future, child welfare should include advice given by experts by experience (*Toimiva lastensuojelu* 2013). Local authorities are being asked to establish groups of experts by experience to guide child welfare decisions locally. The voices and sentiments of survivors and Sukupuu mentioned at the start of this chapter will have a say in decision making. Such input into decision making will mean an unsettling of the existing divisions between service providers and service users by incorporating another standpoint into the process. It is unlikely that a univocality of rights regarding child welfare will be reached, as there is good reason to believe that new complexities will transpire (see Newman, Chapter 16, this volume).

NOTE

1 The majority of children taken into care in the two municipalities studied were teenagers: 22 children out of the 37 were 13 years of age or older. Three children were six or younger. At the moment of the first data collection, 19 children lived in a residential institution, 15 in foster homes or professional family homes, and 2 elsewhere. One care order had already been terminated during the first six months.

REFERENCES

Archard, David. 2003. *Children, Family and the State.* Aldershot: Ashgate.

Child Welfare Act. 417/2007. (unofficial translation). www.finlex.fi. Acccessed 10/20/14.

The Convention on the Rights of Children. http://www.ohchr.org/EN/Professional Interest/Pages/CRC.aspx. Accessed October 20, 2014.

del Valle, J., and A. Bravo. 2013. "Current Trends, Figures and Challenges in Out of Home Child Care: An International Comparative Analysis." *Psychosocial Intervention* 22:251–257.

Donzelot, J. 1980. *Policing of Families*. London: Hutchinson.

Eydal, G., and M. Satka. 2006. "Social Work and Nordic Welfare Policies for Children—Present Challenges in the Light of the Past." *European Journal of Social Work* 9:305–322. doi:10.1080/13691450600828358.

Ferguson, H. 2004. *Protecting Children in Time: Child Abuse, Child Protection, and the Consequences of Modernity*. Basingstoke: Palgrave Macmillan.

Forsberg, H.e, and T. Pösö. 2008. "Ambiguous Position of the Child in Supervised Meetings." *Child and Family Social Work* 13:52–60.

Gilbert, N., N. Parton, and M. Skivenes, eds. 2011. *Child Protection Systems: International Trends and Orientations*. New York: Oxford University Press.

Gillies, V. 2008. "Perspectives on Parenting Responsibility: Contextualizing Values and Practices." *Journal of Law and Society* 35:95–112.

Hämäläinen, K. 2012. *Perhehoitoon sijoitettujen lasten antamat merkitykset kodilleen ja perhesuhteilleen* [*Meanings Given by Foster Children to Their Home and Family Relations*]. Jyväskylä: Jyväskylän yliopisto.

Ife, J. 2001. *Human Rights for Social Work: Towards Rights-Based Practice*. Cambridge: Cambridge University Press.

King, M. 2004. "The Child, Childhood and Children's Rights Within Sociology." *King's Law Journal* 15:273–300.

Laakso, R. 2012. "Lastensuojelun laitostyön arki ja ammatillisuus" [The everyday life of residential work and professionalism]. In *Lasten erityishuolto ja—opetus Suomessa* [*Special Care and Teaching of Children*], edited by Markku Jahnukainen, 127–153. Helsinki: Lastensuojelun Keskusliitto.

Pösö, T. 2011. "Combatting Child Abuse in Finland: From Family to Child-Centered Orientation." In *Child Protection Systems: International Trends and Orientations*, edited by Neil Gilbert, Nigel Parton, and Marit Skivenes, 112–130. New York: Oxford University Press.

Pösö, T., Marit Skivenes, and Anne-Dorthe Hestbaeck. 2014. "Child Protection Systems Within the Danish, Finnish and Norwegian Welfare States—Time for a Child-centric Approach?" *European Journal of Social Work* 17:475–490. doi:10.1080/13691457.2013.829802.

Ribbens McCarthy, J. 2012. "The Powerful Relational Language of 'Family': Togetherness, Belonging and Personhood." *Sociological Review* 60:68–90.

Ribbens McCarthy, J., Carol-Ann Hooper, and Val Gillies. 2013. *Family Troubles? Exploring Changes and Challenges in the Family Lives of Children and Young People.* Bristol: Policy.

Sinclair, I., and T. Jeffreys. 2005. *Fostering Now: Messages from Research.* London: Kingsley.

Smart, C. 2007. *Personal Life: New Directions in Sociological Thinking.* Cambridge: Polity.

Sukupuu. 2014. http://www.sukupuu.fi/toiminta-ajatus/. Accessed October 5, 2014.

Toimiva lastensuojelu [*Functioning Child Welfare*]. 2013. Report 19. Helsinki: Ministry of Social Welfare and Health.

Uskomme sinuun, usko sinäkin. 2011. http://www.lskl.fi/files/1274/Usus_nuorten_kasikirja_nettiin.pdf. Accessed 10/10/14.

Vehkalahti, K. 2009. *Constructing Reformatory Identity: Girls' Reform School Education in Finland, 1893–1923.* Bern: Peter Lang.

10

Risk, Trust, and the Complex Sentiments of Enacting Care

▸ *AMANDA GRENIER AND CRISTI FLOOD*

THE NOTION OF RISK IS OFTEN TAKEN for granted in policies and institutional practices of care. Dominant approaches to risk in North American care settings include the measurement of risk according to "objective" standardized assessments that are heavily influenced by biomedical interpretations, judgments about safety and security, and deeply entrenched ideas about compliance that operate in the management of older people's needs. Yet, detailed attention to the enactment of care across health care and social care practices reveals that relationships and interactions about risk are subjective, imbued with complications and emotion. Risk operates in a practice context that is characterized by client desires for autonomy and agency; takes place (or is ideally meant to take place) in intimate settings such as the home; and is dependent on care providers, who through their everyday interactions are acutely reminded of power relationships in society and their own families. As a result, encounters between care providers and service users include an inherent tension between the larger sociocultural interpretations of risk and those that operate in practice and inform lived experience.

This chapter problematizes "risk" in the context of care. It explores how care is enacted in relation to risk, and it outlines the contradictions experienced by care providers and older people as service users. First, we review key understandings and approaches to risk. This includes how social risks are considered to have increased as a condition of modernity, the standardization of risk in North American care practices, how dominant ideas about risk shape care relations with older people, and the overriding focus on the minimization of risk that occurs in care practice. Second, reaching across health care and social care settings with older people in home care and shelter settings, we demonstrate how risk is relational and depends on context, location(s), and subjective experiences. Here, illustrations from home care with "frail older clients" and shelter work with older homeless people are used as contrasting cases. Third, we move into a discussion of the complexities of enacting care and outline the tensions that exist between risk, agency, and trust. Finally, we end with a call to reconsider seemingly straightforward policy and practice notions such as risk and devote renewed attention to the development of care practices that are capable of containing the contradictions of risk. This includes, for example, a turn toward trust and relational practices as a means to counter risk-centered practice.

UNDERSTANDINGS OF AND APPROACHES TO RISK

The concept of risk is central to the ideas and practices that operate in health care and social care practices in North America and Canada. In care, the concept and measurement of risk is primarily associated with the shift to case management that began in the United States in the 1980s (see Kane 2000) and came to replace frameworks based on "rights" and/or "needs" in countries such as Canada, the United Kingdom, and Australia (see Means, Richards, and Smith 2003). Such practices reflect the dominance of biomedical interpretations of older people's needs, a neoliberal political agenda, and the accompanying managerialism of care in Canada. In neoliberalism, government spending is reduced, and care is increasingly situated in the private economy—a context that is referred to as the "mixed economy of care" (Aronson and Neysmith 1997; Armstrong and Armstrong 2001; Bourgeault et al. 2001; Duncan and Reutter 2006). At the level of practice, it is health care and social care professionals who are charged with the responsibility of rationing public services through standardized assessments.[1] Risk—and risk assessment—are thus central to eligibility for programs, service delivery, and the "management of care" for older people. Eligibility tends to be assessed through standardized assessments that are heavily influenced by medical interpretations of need—most often articulated as functional impairment, "frailty," or falling (see Grenier 2007; Katz 2015). The corresponding services offered to those deemed eligible continue the neoliberal rationale structured according to individual interpretations and principles of minimizing risk.

Social Risks and the Risk Society

Macro-level analysis outside the domain of care practice has focused on the increase in risk, safety, and risk discourse as a phenomenon unique to modern society (Giddens 1990; Beck 1992). In theorizing risk, Beck (1992) outlines how technological advances in modernity have presented society with increased risk and have in turn generated macro-level responses intended to minimize risk and increase predictability. For example, Beck (1992) outlines how the invention and resulting dependence on nuclear energy created a new risk of disaster that initiated a social response organized around calculating and managing the potential of nuclear catastrophe. Beck's theory of the risk society also outlines how risk is both shared and distributed unequally. For example, while the risk of the nuclear disaster is shared or generalized, particular types of risk are unequally distributed across and between societies (i.e., the poor living closer to sites of threats or waste; e.g., garbage dumps). Understandings of risk as generalized and unequal are particularly relevant to the consideration of older people's experiences, where aging can be understood as both a universal phenomenon and an accumulation of a life course of inequalities. The "risk society" therefore provides another means to understand how approaches to care have become organized around responses to and the avoidance of risk, and from there a critique of the inequalities that underpin individualized care practices.

Although there is debate as to whether the actual level of risk faced by individuals and societies has increased,[2] there is agreement that modernity is marked by an increased *focus* on risk (Giddens 1990, 1991; Adams 1995), that the preindustrial trusting tradition has been replaced by an emphasis on risk and trust as fundamentally conflicting features of modernity (Giddens 1990), and that the discursive constructions of risk are highly political (Giddens 1990; Beck 1992; Green 1997; Lupton 1999). Scholarship on risk has focused, for example, on the control of risk, which can be seen through risk management as a means to predict and mitigate risk to avoid accidents (Green 1997). Likewise, researchers have outlined the turn to insurance-based schemes of protection[3] and the individualization of risk, as opposed to shared systems of social protection (Laliberte Rudman and Durdle 2008; Funk, Stajduhar, and Purkis 2011).[4] Care practices can be considered as sites where the movement to risk in systems and services is acutely apparent.

The Standardization of Risk in Care Practices

Care practices that respond to risk as rational, predictable, and controllable reflect this increased focus on and attempt to mitigate risk. Although "risk" in care practice is often taken for granted as a concept that can be measured and avoided, the exclusive focus on predicting and responding to risk at the expense of other types of interventions is problematic. With the shifting focus of control—or perhaps the sense of losing control in modern conditions—practices have become organized as attempts to gain control over risky situations. In care practice, the concept of risk is "signified and storied through biomedically influenced evaluations of uncertainty and related experiences" (Russell and Babrow 2011:239). In care, risk becomes a "reality" that can be measured, standardized, controlled, and thus prevented through individual behavior or intervention. Once risk is assessed, services are organized around prevention and the minimization of risk. Older people are expected to change their activities, and professionals are expected to encourage, control, and/or police their compliance. Beck's (1992) thinking allows us to understand that standardized, individualized responses to risk are deeply entrenched in neoliberalism and the rationing of public services in national and local contexts (Adams 1995; Tansey and O'Riordan 1999; Tulloch and Lupton 2003), as well as part of a larger political and global response to the perils of modern society.

Many authors have criticized the acceptance of an objective and standard notion of assessing risk, and the subsequent individualized interventions organized around minimizing risk. In particular, approaches to risk are considered to impede understandings of the complexities of the body and the social world (Skolbekken 1995). Research has called for a move toward complex conceptualizations of risk that better reflect the realities and service needs of older people (Skolbekken 1995; Wenger 1997; Tansey and O'Riordan 1999; McLaughlin 2008).[5] Such critiques have drawn attention to the prevalence of deficit model assessment tools (see Petersen and Lupton 1996; Wenger 1997) and suggested biographical, or at a minimum biographically informed, approaches to risk assessment (Webb 2006; Grenier 2007). Suggestions have also been made for interventions that would more accurately capture the dynamic processes of care, including trust, and decision making between reasonable and unreasonable risks (Skolbekken 1995; Tansey and O'Riordan 1999). The inclusion of voices and experiences of older people in care systems is also considered as a way to bridge gaps, increase quality of service, decrease stereotypical views of older people, and increase service users' quality of life (Gubrium 1991; Wenger 1997; Zinn 2005; see also Miller and Kontos, Chapter 8, this volume). Yet, what is often overlooked in the debate between professional systems and lay interpretations is the mutual dependence and coconstruction that occurs between macro-structures and individual experiences. It is the interplay between the larger social and cultural response and the practices in health and social care that reveals the problems of dichotomous interpretations of risk and trust, and the dominance of individualized risk-based interventions.

The Framing of Identities and the Individualization of Risk

Public policies, discourses, and macro-level influences, such as those organized around objective and individualized understandings of risk, are considered to play a role in shaping older adults' experiences and, by extension, their identities (see Hendricks 2004). In his explanation of the reflexive shaping of self-identity as a modern project, Giddens (1991) posits that a macro-level emphasis on risk shapes, and is shaped by, individuals' self-identities. With regard to aging, Hendricks (2004) has highlighted that risk-based policies are contingent on the qualifying, stereotyping, and classifying of older adults and their experiences. Risk discourses in practice, for example, have simultaneously depicted older people labeled "at risk" as powerless, vulnerable, and dangerous (Webb 2006; Grenier 2007; McLaughlin 2008), overlooking how social locations, such as ethnicity, sexual orientation, gender, nationality, and geographic location, can influence conceptions of risk (Tulloch and Lupton 2003). Such practices also create anxieties and fears among older people, which can result in older people constantly evaluating risks, engaging in risk avoidance, and experiencing reduced community mobility (Lupton 1999; Laliberte Rudman and Durdle 2008).

At the same time, practices aimed at preventing and minimizing risk at the individual level can perversely increase anxieties and risks for older people and their caregivers (see Adams 1995; Richards 2000). Older people may, for example, doubt their abilities and become fearful of their bodies and their actions. This may result in the creation of further decline, marginalization, or otherness (e.g., older people reducing their participation in life) (Lupton 1999; Tulloch and Lupton 2003; Hendricks 2004). On the other hand, older people may also enact their agency and/or resistance to overcome the restrictions that are imposed on them. To prove their independence or abilities, they may engage in activities that they would not otherwise have done. This idea that risk can be controlled at the individual level (i.e., individualization of risk) is thus both a sociocultural frame and a practice that can result in decisions that reduce older people's participation for fear of being unable to manage risk (Lupton 1999; Laliberte Rudman and Durdle 2008). As such, risk-based practices can perversely prevent older people from fully experiencing health, regardless of their actual health status (Pickard 2009), and make older adults feel as though they are dependent and fundamentally unsuccessful at aging (Laliberte Rudman et al. 2010).

Contradictions of Care and the Minimization of Risk

Models of practice that are organized to minimize risk present a number of contradictions for service providers and older people alike. Interventions are organized around discourses of risk minimization. However, care services for older people are undoubtedly dominated by an apocalyptic discourse of costs associated with "greying societies" (see Gee and Gutman 2000), neoliberal restructuring of health and social care systems (see Armstrong and Armstrong 2001; Bourgeault et al. 2001; Grenier and Bidgoli 2015), and enacted through processes of risk assessment and insurance-based models that are intended to control the costs of care (see Kane 2000; Baines 2004; Grenier 2007; Neysmith 2009). Whereas the Canada Health Act provides universal coverage for medical needs (often within medical or institutional settings), the social needs of older people and people with disabilities that take place "at home" and "in the community" are provided within what is most commonly referred to as a "social" or "mixed" economy of care (see Armstrong and Armstrong 2001; Grenier and Guberman 2009).

This means that care is either provided by informal caregivers, through minimal services rationed by means of strict eligibility criteria, or purchased from the private market. Thus, the organization of practices, despite being led by and organized around discourses of risk, can, at the practice level, structure problems of access that lead to increased risk. Older people who do not qualify for services or are not willing to accept the labels applied to them, for example, may be required to purchase services from the private market—which may not only place them at greater risk as a result of not seeking care but also demonstrate the contradictions between stated intent and realities of practice.

The minimization of risk is contradictory as a discursive frame, and, unfortunately, service providers also experience its implications in their practice. At a base level, organizational policies that emphasize clients' choices to live "at risk" seem closely aligned with older people's concerns for autonomy (Ceci and Purkis 2009). Yet, when considered within a broader analysis of risk, such measures are less about preserving older adults' agency and more about decreasing government and organizational responsibility for the provision of care, which is typical of neoliberal frameworks (Ceci and Purkis 2009). Care providers, then, face ethical dilemmas in trying to mediate professional standards of minimizing risk—and, by extension, minimizing costs—and encouraging client participation and independence (Jakobsen and Sørlie 2010; see also Newman, Chapter 16, this volume). This unresolved tension can lead to workers feeling devalued, frustrated, and overwhelmed with the dilemmas that exist between organizational policies and care that they believe would increase service users' quality of life (Cabin 2007, 2008; Vik and Eide 2012; Grenier and Bidgoli 2015; see also Solvang, Chapter 7, this volume). Feeling unable to successfully negotiate between contradictory discourses, practices, demands of providing care, professional values, and their own consciences (Juthberg et al. 2008; see also Jensen and Villadsen, Chapter 11, this volume), many care workers suffer from burnout (Glasberg, Eriksson, and Norberg 2007; Juthberg et al. 2008).

Similarly, the contradictory nature of the minimization of risk as a philosophy of practice has deleterious effects on service users' experience of care. Aimed at reducing costs, risk-based interventions may challenge older people's autonomy—something that older people strive to maintain while simultaneously weighing the risks of doing so (Laliberte Rudman et al.

2010). Consequently, service users who insist on maintaining their autonomy or independence can come to be seen as refusing care, despite the fact that their refusal is often rooted in a belief that the available care options are inadequate (Grenier 2007; Ceci and Purkis 2009). Thus, while the creation of standardized assessments of objective criteria may *seemingly* cut costs at the level of administration (see Cabin 2007, 2008), managing care through the minimization of service users' risk (Tanner 1998; Webb 2006) has negatively impacted both service providers' and service users' experiences of care (e.g., Lymbery 1998; Ballinger and Payne 2002; Webb 2006; Cabin 2007, 2008; McLaughlin 2008; Delp et al. 2010; Jakobsen and Sørlie 2010; Glasdam et al. 2013).

Safety and litigation may also play into how decisions about risk and care are implemented. The value of autonomy and agency may come into direct conflict with the agency and professional requirements of caregivers to avoid fault and/or litigation. In a context where assessments of risk could later be tied to a failure to act, and thus result in the threat of litigation, "risky behaviors" are not well tolerated. Despite organizational claims that service users can choose to live at risk, and notwithstanding older people's desire to maintain autonomy, individual professionals do not place a high value on clients' independence when client safety is construed as being low and client risk is construed as being high (MacCourt and Tuokko 2010). Such restrictions could thus be experienced by workers as imposing limitations that are not in the clients' best interests, and by older people as decisions being made for them and not by them (see Foley and Timonen, Chapter 6, this volume). The contradictions experienced by service users and professionals while receiving and/or enacting care demonstrate the extent to which policies and practices based on standardized, objective assessments and individualized practices of minimizing risks can actually constrain service and meaningful care interactions.

THE COMPLEX SENTIMENTS OF CARE ENCOUNTERS

While the literature makes a convincing case for introducing a critical reading of risk into care practice, it tells us less about the relativity of risk, and about how different contexts, positions, and trajectories that inform experience can create complex care encounters. Further, the other side of the balance—trust—is often lost in the critique; this is especially the case when attention focused on the macro-level economic or neoliberal context is disconnected from the practice or relational and personal levels of care. As mentioned, the emphasis that was once placed on trust and trusting tradition is now being replaced by an emphasis on reducing the risks associated with high modernity, resulting in an increased difficulty in cultivating trust (Giddens 1991; Seligman 1997; Sztompka 1999). Despite this erosion of trust in others, there are "foundations of trust" that can encourage an individual actor, such as a service user or service provider, to trust—or distrust (Sztompka 1999). Relationships enacted through a variety of micro-, meso-, and macro-level interactions can promote trust and trustworthiness between individuals, in society, and in culture more broadly (Sztompka 1999). When considered complementary rather than in competition, fostering trust and the encouragement of a "culture of trust" can shape individual and relational experiences in care contexts (Sztompka 1999). In this regard, policies that promote trust and counter risk through relational models of practice can profoundly affect interpersonal and intrapersonal experiences of trust and distrust, and, by extension, shape interactions and sentiments. Furthermore, policies that promote trust offer alternatives to the deleterious effects of risk management while being no less effective at controlling the essentially uncontrollable uncertainties of modernity.

Thus, our intent is to move the consideration of risk into the relatively uncharted territory of trust and the variable sentiments of enacting care. Moreover, we aim to demonstrate that risk is not only a product of neoliberalism but also a response to the conditions of modern society that is too often taken for granted as the only approach in the context of care. Drawing on interviews with service providers enacting care and older people experiencing care, we highlight the thorny emotions that seep into seemingly objective care practices, and the subsequent contradictions that exist for older people and service providers alike. The illustrations of home care and shelter work practices that follow problematize risk-based assessments and practices as currently enacted in North American and Canadian contexts of care. As such, these examples inform our reconsideration of risk, prompting us to consider models of practice that counter risk-based models of care, and can promote trust between service users and service providers, as well as society more broadly.

Illustration A: Older People "At Risk" in Home Care Services

Much of the critical work in the field of care for older people takes place in relation to home care rather than institutional settings (e.g., long-term care) and is dominated by discourses and discussions of risk and fall prevention.[6] Yet, risks and rewards experienced in care vary according to role and structured location. Risks for workers are related to their position (e.g., professional or paraprofessional), visible minority status (i.e., the racialized labor force of immigrant or nonstatus workers), level of education, and job security, with those having lower levels of education having more physically demanding jobs with lower pay (see Neysmith and MacAdam 1999). Such differences are extremely important in assessing the unequal distribution of risk, and the types of experiences that workers bring into the care encounter (e.g., experiences of colonization, racism, discrimination, and so forth). The shared values about care—whether they are personal or professional—and desire for change, however, are also a source of conflict in care practices (Neysmith and MacAdam 1999; Grenier and Bidgoli 2015). The desire for change that tends to underpin the vocational call of workers and sustain their involvement in a difficult context of work can be experienced as a source of conflict. Practices organized around minimizing risk create tensions between what care providers believe they are meant to do and what they can do within the confines of practice (Grenier and Wong 2010).

Care workers also bring personal trajectories, relationships with their families and kin, and fears and anxieties into care. The needs of the older person and their styles of interaction are understood through their interpretive lens—often as it aligns or conflicts with their past experiences (i.e., personal experience and practice knowledge).[7] The care encounter may vividly trigger sentiments of past successes or failures, and it may surface in their expectations for their work and relationships with clients. If the tension between risk and trust is essential to the care encounter, then the level of trust and the possibility of communication between the care providers and service user are key. Consider the following example from earlier work of the first author:

> Joyce, a young social worker, is discovered, crying quietly to herself in the corner of an empty staff room. Asked what is the matter, Joyce eventually starts to talk about George, an 81 year old former sergeant in a famous Scot-

> tish infantry regiment who is popular on the ward as an eccentric leg-puller and an indulged comic turn. Why is the social worker upset? He reminds her of her grandfather who was, in her words, "a right bastard." He abused his wife, Joyce's grandmother, as well as her mother and he "ruled the roost." The social worker began to cry again because she felt that she must like all her clients. . . . "Why can't I like him like everyone else in the ward seems to?" (Grenier and Leonard 2006)

But personal trajectories and constraints in the care setting may hinder and/or facilitate the communication and personal connections that are the foundation for trust. Relationships between service providers and service users are at the heart of any intervention, yet infrequent are the discussions of how personal trajectories and life course experiences may impact these encounters. In decisions about risk, service providers grapple with their own historical relationships with family members, their history with "clients," their judgment of the person's ability in connection with their "objective" assessments (e.g., denial), their professional values and desires, and their professional responsibilities. The following question is often found at the base of their interventions: can they trust that Mrs. X will listen to their advice and thus will remain safe? Such decisions rely on trust between care provider and recipient but also place enormous responsibility on the shoulders of the workers. And, of course, if Mrs. X does not "listen" (i.e., to be read as comply), workers not only have the personal implications of "poor judgment" but the failure as a professional and the risks that this failure may entail on a professional level (e.g., questions about their competence, legal action, etc.).

Service users bring similar contradictions, family experiences, and anxieties into care. Differing in nature from the risks of organizational pressures experienced by care providers, older people's constraints relate primarily to maintaining dignity and autonomy in the face of decline. The risk of whether their autonomy will be maintained is balanced in many ways with their "right" to stay at home, thus escaping—or perhaps delaying—institutionalization as long as possible. In this context, however, older people come to the encounter in a less powerful position, with encounters shaped in part by whether they will be permitted to continue their activities, autonomy, and independence (i.e., they worry about dependence and becoming a burden). Any interaction is thus a representation both of larger sociocultural interpretations of their decline and the risks that they embody—to the care system and themselves. Interactions also carry the weight of relationships and performances enacted with service providers, friends, and family. What the objective measures fail to capture, therefore, is how older people feel about their "abilities" and how this informs their decision making with regard to risk.

The clash between practices of minimizing risk and the desire for autonomy is witnessed in unintended or undesired outcomes of interventions. This includes, for example, how older people may internalize risk discourse in ways that may be harmful to their well-being. Workers give accounts of how they prevented movements and falls by using obstructions and obstacles that can actually increase risk-taking behaviors (Richards 2000). For example, in one team meeting, "workers discussed practices . . . whereby the furniture from the hospital room was placed at the bedside to prevent Mrs. K from getting up. . . . Mrs. K then proceeded to climb over the bedrails and the furniture [used as a] means to restrict her movement" (Grenier team meeting notes 2009). Interventions therefore result in older people being sanctioned to remain in one room or one level of their house in order to mitigate the risk of falling. Yet, in doing so, they risk isolation and exclusion within their homes (see Laliberte Rudman and Durdle 2008). Alice's example speaks to this restriction and the decisions she makes to continue her daily activities and mitigate risk. You will notice that although she realizes the risk, she continues the activity, but in a different way (she brings her phone):

> Well, they suggested, practically forbid me . . . instilled upon me—not to go down to the basement because it's very dangerous if I fell. Of course I know that . . . [and later . . .]. If you fall in the basement you could lay there for a while and no one would know. I generally take my portable phone. (Alice) (Grenier and Guberman 2009)

It is here that insights from people living with disabilities can be useful in pointing to the risks that one can take on a regular basis—and that adapting to such changes may require time and a supportive process for older people who are new to experiences of impairment. It is here also that the lived experiences of uncertainty conflict directly with the sociocultural emphasis on certainty, control, and prediction that are articulated through practices based on minimizing risk. Aging—and the acquisition of impairment in late life—brings an inherent uncertainty that can be neither predicted nor controlled (Grenier 2012). The care encounter is thus replete with a number of contradictory influences, including trajectories of need, healthy or strained family relations, dynamic changes to the user's body and needs over time, the dilemmas that these changes represent, and the emotions that seep into the seemingly objective processes of care practice. Practices that attempt to standardize, objectivize, and control risks can thus create an unrealistic and contradictory site of practice where emotion, trust, and relationships are concerned.

Illustration B: Shelter Work with Older People Who Are Homeless

A contrast in thinking about the relativity of risk and the implications for care encounters can be found in the example of work with older people who are homeless. In the case of older homelessness, the practice-based interventions are not focused around risk-based discourses and practices such as those in home care. Instead, they focus on basic needs such as food and housing, human rights/dignity, and safety/stability. While the differences between the settings are quite substantial, and thus relevant for problematizing risk in practice, it is important to remember that the historical developments and realities of the work differ significantly. Shelter work belongs in the realm of community-based practice rather than professionalized practice (e.g., as accredited by professional associations such as nursing, social work, and occupational therapy). This results in there being less of a shared professional value base, in addition to less competitive and/or territorial domains of practice. Consequently, although shelter work does tend to be routinized around meal times, shower and bed times, and safety guidelines, most do not use standardized assessment procedures in their practices. Similarly, interventions are framed not around risk but around helping people who are homeless to gain stability and support. As shelters are only beginning to see older people, this type of work represents a new area of practice within the shelter system that is likely to develop over time, especially where demographic change and interactions with the broader health care and social care systems are concerned.

Consideration of the case of shelter work with older people who are homeless reveals that both the existing "objective" frame for understanding risk and the idea of minimizing risk are context dependent and could be reconsidered as a primary frame for practice. At the broadest level, homelessness in late life represents the unequal distribution of risks as well as how structural and personal trajectories may intersect to create homelessness, both in the present and on into late life. Risks that are seen at the site of older homelessness cannot merely be understood as individualized phenomena but must also be considered within the context of major social issues such as poverty, a lack of affordable housing, violence (e.g., women's homelessness), health inequities (e.g., mental health), colonization (in the case of Aboriginal peoples), family breakdown, and trauma. Shelter users bring these histories and trajectories into the care encounter, perhaps expecting marginalization, a breakdown of trust, and the continuation of unmet needs.

The trajectories of homelessness among older people call into question the individualization of risk as well as the assumption that risk can be predicted and controlled. Interviews with older people echoed the message, "I simply don't know how this happened to me. I don't know how I ended up on the streets at my age." Here, the time frame of older homelessness is relevant: risks that would normally be framed as "potential" in home care practice have already taken place in the case of homelessness among older people. The situation of the older homeless person thus presents us with a failure of systems and strategies in modern society. While homelessness is often misleadingly interpreted as a choice about the freedom to live outside of the establishment, in its realities, homelessness of older people represents a situation out of control—a narrative that is expressed both by the older person and by the professional. Few acceptable options are available to older homeless people, who become caught between care systems (many of which require a home, as in the case of "home care"), emergency shelters, and decent, affordable, and safe housing. The risks for older people who are homeless are of safety, injury, or illness, a continued life on the streets, and/or death on the streets (see McDonald, Dergal, and Cleghorn 2007; Grenier et al. In Press). Their well-being is seriously compromised by their condition of being homeless. At the same time, their stories illustrate the ways in which individual responses to risk must be understood in relation to larger global and national issues that occur at the intersections of housing, income support, care, and age.

It was not surprising that work with older people who were homeless significantly altered the care dynamic. Unexpected, however, was that staff, accustomed to working with homeless people, were deeply affected by the presence of older people in the shelter. Workers resoundingly replied that "homelessness in late life shouldn't happen." To express their dismay, discussions of their own grandparents came up. One worker said, "You are not meant to be in here at this age. . . . I think of my grandfather." Following this, workers expressed the constraints they experienced in the context of the system. One says, "What can I do? I have no place to send these women. . . . I can't have her living in an unsafe housing block." As with home care workers, their personal values conflicted with the options available. Their reflections demonstrate that their trust in systems and social responses has for some reason broken down. Yet, while the risks that resulted in homelessness and the risks to health and well-being were apparent, their discourse did not turn to discourses of "risk," the prevention of risk, or restriction/control. Instead, they framed their discussions and interventions around trust, humanity, rights, and personhood as the necessary foundations for care relations. Workers highlighted the need to trust and communicate directly with people who were homeless in order to understand their needs. Admittedly, in care settings, it seems that discourses such as personhood or rights seem to surface more where older people are considered to have less—or where these rights are severely constrained (e.g., dementia, homelessness, etc.). At the base for older people, however, is the need to know that they will be "cared for," that they can trust the services, that the care they receive will meet their basic needs, and that their histories and well-being will be taken into account.

THE COMPLEXITIES OF RISK

A careful consideration of care encounters reveals the inherent tensions and contradictions within risk-based discourse and practice. While it is possible that the differences between the discourses used in home care settings and those used in shelter work can be explained by different historical trends in care, shelter workers' use of a discourse based on trust calls into question the predominance of a standardized risk discourse and individual risk-based models of practice in home care and other health and social care settings. Risk discourses and practice are, at the same time, a feature of modern society, a response to shared and unequal conditions in society, and a means by which to ration and distribute services in a scarcity model.

Although there is a tendency to view risk within health and social care as a powerful social practice that is enacted by professionals as part of a system, the various interpretations and contextual locations of risk draw attention to a more complex reading.

Professionals and service users both come to the care encounter with conflicting interpretations of the tension between control and freedom that "care" represents—tensions that are enacted in a system that can (and does) constrain decisions and available options. Care providers and service users also enter care relationships that are shaped by structural contexts, including the way that their needs are framed (whether this is as "risk" or stability/support). Yet, entrenched in neoliberalism, post-welfare society, and late modernity, the dominance of individualized risk and risk-based practices can overlook the trajectories that led to the need for care, as well as the complex dynamics and emotions that take place in care encounters. Nowhere is the failure to respond more acute than in the case of homelessness in late life.

The complex sentiments of enacting care are thus articulated in the tensions between the control and/or management of risk and the notions of freedom and trust that characterize interactions and relationships in health and social care. Thinking through the various contexts of risk, balanced with personal trajectories and the sentiments of care, provides an approach to understand the inherent tensions of care practices. Such thinking allows us to extract what takes place at the micro-level as an enactment of sociocultural discourses of risk, and reflections of larger macro- or political structures that shape and sustain risk. Specifically, the variations between contexts of risk allow us to more carefully consider the underlying unequal distributions of the "risk-society," the differences that exist between sites of practice, and the ways in which particular trajectories can produce varying relationships to risk. As such, the differences between home care and homeless shelters draw attention to the relativity and changeability of risk, as well as the fallibility of fixed and objective notions of preventing risk relative to location and setting. Focus on risk as it is enacted through care practices can therefore provide insight into the complex sociocultural interpretations and interpersonal dynamics and exchanges that inform and influence care.

The contradictions that exist within and between practice sites draw attention to the need for practices that encourage trust as a central feature of care practice. Social responses, including those of care, have become unbalanced in their attention to risk over trust. We need a new critical model of care practice that promotes trust and allows for the complicated relationships that are inherent in the practices of risk management. To achieve such a model, care work needs to be understood beyond an individualized risk-based model of intervention, and service providers must be able to trust that they can improve service users' lives while simultaneously maintaining their own personal and professional values. In this regard, trust needs to take place on the part of professionals (e.g., that the risk they take with regard to their clients will be permitted and supported) and on behalf of the service users (e.g., so that the risks taken can allow for contexts of care and well-being). One suggested model to achieve a better balance between risk and trust is through a relational care practice.

Relational models that better balance risk and trust offer an alternative to risk-based approaches to care. In relational practices, service providers and service users draw on existing social relationships and networks to achieve therapeutic outcomes (Tosone 2004; Ornstein and Ganzer 2005; Folgheraiter 2007). This includes using the therapeutic relationship and dynamic exchange to prompt larger changes within service users' relationships with and constructed meanings of themselves, other individuals, community systems, and larger sociocultural institutions (Tosone 2004; Ornstein and Ganzer 2005). Relational practices operate on the principle of inherent interconnectedness and relationality by acknowledging the extent to which one's emotions and sentiments are affected by seemingly abstract, distant social institutions, as well as one's understandings and meanings of these social institutions (Tosone 2004; Ornstein and Ganzer 2005). Relational practices thus acknowledge service users' emotions, as well as the complex factors and relationships that shape these emotions, rather than encouraging a denial or suppression of emotion (Ornstein and Ganzer 2005; Morrison 2007). As such, the emphasis on relationality shifts the focus from an individual-level intervention into a reconstruction of the interpretations of micro-, meso-, and macro-level social relationships. In doing so, the therapeutic relationship represents a space within which to foster trust with the service provider as well as in broader social relationships, interactions, and institutions (Ornstein and Ganzer 2005). Such modes of practice have been suggested as being capable of containing the tensions of the increasing neoliberal, managerial, and, by extension, shifting context of care enactment (Butler and Drakeford 2005; Ornstein and Ganzer 2005; Morrison 2007).

Illustrations from the context of shelter work with older people demonstrate the possibility of reframing risk as a need for care and stability. The realities of homelessness in late life create a moment for pause about risk and how we understand and respond to it. Shelter work illuminates the socially embedded features of risk, and the timing of risk as the accumulation of experience rather than as a fixed event. This provides an important contrast to risk in home care practice. The interactions between staff and shelter users (albeit limited in the therapeutic sense) demonstrate that a shift in discourse and practice is not only possible but also essential to creating change in the lives and experiences of older people. Extending the lessons from this illustration, we suggest that sentiments that call for the importance of relationships could form the base for care practices that rebalance and promote trust in care encounters, and as such thwart the contradictions that are embedded in the dominance of risk-based care practices.[8] In this way, illustrations from care practices such as those discussed here disprove and destabilize standardized objective notions of risk through their situation-dependent interpretations of risk and risk-based discourse. They broaden understandings of risk beyond the individual-level intervention and, in doing so, call for a practice that subverts the minimization of risk through practice relationships of trust and relational practice.

In conclusion, we argue that in order to reimagine the relationship between care providers and service users, the seemingly straightforward interpretation of risk that operates in policy and practice, shapes service providers' work, and affects older people's experiences of care needs to be reconsidered. Objectivity and the minimization of risk as enacted in care practice is misleading—disguising the complex interconnections of structural, relational, and emotional dynamics that are involved in the assessment and response to risk. The focus on objective measures of risk that take place on the body overlook the populations that "end up" in public care or in shelters. Although the degree of need varies from home care to shelters, in both cases it is older people with high care needs who have limited financial resources (or insurance), and small social networks of care kin, that require care. While an insistence on broad-level change may be difficult to achieve, the work of care providers needs to be situated in the larger contexts within which they care (i.e., social and cultural emphasis on rationality and control, the uneven distribution of risks, neoliberalization of care, etc.), and risk-based responses need to be adjusted accordingly. Furthermore, there must be an increased awareness of the risk society, the unequal conditions that result in the need for care in late life, the contradictions workers face in practice, and both the suggestions to advocate for broad-based change and the solutions of training and support.

We need a new critical model of practice that allows for the conflicts and tensions inherent in care practices that are organized around risk. A binary opposition between powerful practices and subjective experiences is at times implied in the professional versus lay experience debate on risk. Yet, moving forward requires a model of risk that is premised on contextual and shifting notions of risk, integrates the value of risk taking, and promotes the establishment of trust that would lend itself to risk taking as part of the care process. Service providers need to trust that they can make changes and improve people's lives in ways that match their personal and professional values. Older people receiving care need to be able to rely on care—they need to believe and trust that someone will care for them. They also need to know that their life experience and decision making that is rooted in their histories and relationships will be acknowledged and respected. Whereas unequal risks and unmet needs experienced across the life course are best illustrated in the case of older homelessness, the need to foster well-being beyond physical risk is most evident in the case of home care practice. While these contrasting cases are differentially situated with regard to risk, they underscore the need to develop trust and relational care practices capable of containing the contradictions between risk and trust. It is only through a foundation of trust and acknowledgment of the position of the other that service providers and service users can address the ways in which they rely on each other for support and to have their needs met.

NOTES

1 While there is variation across the Canadian provinces, public home care services tend to provide limited forms of support (e.g., rehabilitation equipment, functional devices, and/or a bath) to those deemed eligible, up to a maximum level of support (many programs max out around 12 to 14 hours per week).

2 Giddens (1990, 1991) disagrees with Beck's (1992) claim that modernity is marked by increased risks. Instead, Giddens, like Adams (1995), argues that modernity is marked by an increased *focus* on risk, despite the fact that the actual level of risk with which individuals and societies are faced has not increased.

3 The political nature of constructing risk is exemplified by post-welfare changes characterized by a movement from share risks to individualized insurance-based schemes. Such changes make it an individual responsibility to purchase insurance policies, annuities, and pensions, resulting in better protections to persons who can minimize their risks through the purchase of these market-based schemes (see Means, Richards, and Smith 2003; Funk, Stajduhar, and Purkis 2011).

4 This process through which risk has become increasingly viewed as an individual's responsibility rather than the government's has been referred to as "responsibilization" (Funk, Stajduhar, and Purkis 2011).

5 The issue of technology is also key here. The increased emphasis on risk is intimately tied to the development of technology (Skolbekken 1995; Russell and Babrow 2011), creating a dependence and faith in technology that has resulted in changed perceptions of the locus of control (Skolbekken 1995). Areas of life over which humans were previously thought to have little control are now being viewed as something that humans can, in fact, control through advancing technologies (Skolbekken 1995; Russell and Babrow 2011). This shift in the locus of control over health issues has been exacerbated by the dominance of risk management through health promotion, epidemiology, probability statistics, and computer technology (Skolbekken 1995; Petersen and Lupton 1996), and necessarily shapes care practices and experiences of care (Skolbekken 1995; Webb 2006).

6 There is a significant body of literature on the risks of home care practice, and some on the rewards. We thus focus less on home care practice in this chapter, outlining only the key strands of thinking.

7 Such discussions, while outside the scope of this chapter, often take place with regard to the phenomenon of transference and countertransference as a fundamental power relation in social work practice (see Ornstein and Ganzer 2005; Grenier and Leonard 2006).

8 A word of caution is important here. Our research demonstrates that a shift in shelter work has taken place. Shelter work at our research site was once characterized by disciplinary modes of practice (i.e., physically large workers responsible for "control and regulation"). However, this context is undergoing a shift toward a more therapeutic context, which can be understood in relation to changing sociocultural ideas and policies that view shelters as points of contact for housing, rather than only emergency services. The "age relation" component, however, may also give a very different reading than work with younger groups. The question is thus perhaps overstated by workers in this regard. I would suggest that older people may represent the location where practices must be different from usual shelter practices—that is, they must be gentler and more relational (important reflections on these social and cultural constructs in their own right).

REFERENCES

Adams, John. 1995. *Risk*. London: University College London Press.

Armstrong, Pat, and Hugh Armstrong. 2001. "Women, Privatization, and Health Reform: The Ontario Case." In *Exposing Privatization: Women and Health Care Reform in Canada*, edited by Pat Armstrong, Carol Amaratunga, Jocelyne Bernier, Karen Grant, Ann Pederson, and Kay Williams, 163–216. Aurora: Garamond.

Aronson, Jane, and Sheila M. Neysmith. 1997. "The Retreat of the State and Long-Term Care Provision: Implications for Frail Elderly People, Unpaid Family Carers and Paid Home Care Workers." *Studies in Political Economy* 53:37–66.

Baines, Donna. 2004. "Caring for Nothing: Work Organization and Unwaged Labour in Social Services." *Work, Employment and Society* 18(2): 267–295.

Ballinger, Claire, and Sheila Payne. 2002. "The Construction of the Risk of Falling Among and By Older People." *Ageing and Society* 22(3): 305.

Beck, Ulrich. 1992. *Risk Society*. Beverly Hills, CA: Sage.

Bourgeault, Ivy Lynn, Pat Armstrong, Hugh Armstrong, Jacqueline Choiniere, Joel Lexchin, Eric Mykhalovskiy, Suzanne Peters, and Jerry White. 2001. "Everyday Experiences of Implicit Rationing: Comparing the Voices of Nurses in California and British Columbia." *Sociology of Health and Illness* 23(5): 633–653.

Butler, Ian, and Mark Drakeford. 2005. "Trusting in Social Work." *British Journal of Social Work* 35(5): 639–653.

Cabin, William D. 2007. "The Phantoms of Homecare: Homecare Nurses' Care Decisions for Medicare Home Health Alzheimer's Disease Patients." *Home Health Care Management and Practice* 19(3): 174–183.

Cabin, William D. 2008. "Revaluing Social Work in Homecare: Lessons from Innovators, Rebels, and Hospice." *Home Health Care Management Practice* 20:265–272.

Ceci, Christine, and Mary Ellen Purkis. 2009. "Bridging Gaps in Risk Discourse: Homecare Case Management and Client Choices." *Sociology of Health and Illness* 31(2): 201–214.

Delp, Linda, Steven P. Wallace, Jeanne Geiger-Brown, and Charles Muntaner. 2010. "Job Stress and Job Satisfaction: Home Care Workers in a Consumer-Directed Model of Care." *Health Services Research* 45(4): 922–940.

Duncan, Susan, and Linda Reutter. 2006. "A Critical Policy Analysis of an Emerging Agenda for Home Care in One Canadian Province." *Health and Social Care in the Community* 14(3): 242–253.

Folgheraiter, Fabio. 2007. "Relational Social Work: Principles and Practices." *Social Policy and Society* 6(2): 265–274.

Funk, Laura M., Kelli I. Stajduhar, and Mary Ellen Purkis. 2011. "An Exploration of Empowerment Discourse Within Home-Care Nurses' Accounts of Practice." *Nursing Inquiry* 18(1): 66–76.

Gee, Ellen, and Gloria Gutman. 2000. *The Overselling of Population Ageing: Apocalyptic Demography, Intergenerational Challenges, and Social Policy.* Toronto: Oxford University Press.

Giddens, Anthony. 1990. *The Consequences of Modernity.* Oxford: Polity.

Giddens, Anthony. 1991. *Modernity and Self-Identity: Self and Society in the Late-Modern Age.* Cambridge: Polity.

Glasberg, Ann Louise, Sture Eriksson, and Astrid Norberg. 2007. "Burnout and 'Stress of Conscience' Among Healthcare Personnel." *Journal of Advanced Nursing* 57(4): 392–403.

Glasdam, Stinne, Nina Henriksen, Lone Kjær, and Jeanette Praestegaard. 2013. "Client Involvement in Home Care Practice: A Relational Sociological Perspective." *Nursing Inquiry* 20(4): 329–340.

Green, Judith. 1997. *Risk and Misfortune: The Social Construction of Accidents.* London: University College London Press.

Grenier, Amanda. 2007. "Constructions of Frailty in the English Language, Care Practice and the Lived Experience." *Ageing and Society* 27(3): 425–445.

Grenier, Amanda. 2012. *Transitions and the Lifecourse: Contested Models of "Growing Old."* Bristol: Policy.

Grenier, Amanda, Rachel Barken, Tamara Sussman, David Rothwell, and Valerie Bourgeois-Guerin. In Press. "Homelessness and Aging in Canada: Setting a Research Agenda for Evidence-Based Policy and Practice." *Canadian Journal on Aging* 35(1).

Grenier, Amanda, and Elham Bidgoli. 2015. "The Emotional Consequences of Organisational Change." *Canadian Social Work Review* 35(1–2): 181–200.

Grenier, Amanda, and Nancy Guberman. 2009. "Creating and Sustaining Disadvantage: The Relevance of a Social Exclusion Framework." *Health and Social Care in the Community* 17(2): 116–124.

Grenier, Amanda, and Peter Leonard. 2006. "Interpersonal Acts Within Organisational Practices: Power and Resistance Within Public Health and Social Care for Older Persons." In *Foucault and Ageing*, edited by Jason L. Powell and Azrini Wahidin, 101–113. New York: Nova Science.

Grenier, Amanda, and Trudy Wong. 2010. "The Process of Health and Social Service Reform in Quebec as Experienced on the Frontline." *Canadian Social Work Review* 27(1): 41–61.

Gubrium, Jaber F. 1991. *The Mosaic of Care: Frail Elderly and Their Families in the Real World*. New York: Springer.

Hendricks, Jon. 2004. "Public Policies and Old Age Identity." *Journal of Aging Studies* 18:245–260.

Jakobsen, Rita, and Venke Sørlie. 2010. "Dignity of Older People in a Nursing Home: Narratives of Care Providers." *Nursing Ethics* 17(3): 289–300.

Juthberg, Christina, Sture Eriksson, Astrid Norberg, and Karin Sundin. 2008. "Stress of Conscience and Perceptions of Conscience in Relation to Burnout Among Care-Providers in Older People." *Journal of Clinical Nursing* 17(14): 1897–1906.

Kane, Rosalie. 2000. "Long-Term Case Management for Older Adults." In *Assessing Older Persons: Measures, Meaning, and Practical Applications*, edited by Robert L. Kane and Rosalie A. Kane, 438–457. New York: Oxford University Press.

Katz, Stephen. 2015. "Ageing, Risk and the Falling Body." In *Handbook of Cultural Gerontology*, edited by Wendy Martin and Julia Twigg, 165–172. London: Routledge.

Laliberte Rudman, Debbie, Suzanne Huot, Lisa Klinger, Beverly D. Leipert, and Marlee M. Spafford. 2010. "Struggling to Maintain Occupation While Dealing with Risk: The Experiences of Older Adults with Low Vision." *OTJR: Occupation, Participation and Health* 30(2): 87–96.

Laliberte Rudman, Deborah, and Michelle Durdle. 2008. "Living with Fear: The Lived Experience of Community Mobility for Older Adults with Low Vision." *Journal of Physical Activity and Aging* 17:106–122.

Lupton, Deborah. 1999. *Risk*. London: Routledge.

Lymbery, Mark. 1998. "Care Management and Professional Autonomy: The Impact of Community Care Legislation on Social Work with Older People." *British Journal of Social Work* 28(6): 863–878.

MacCourt, Penny, and Holly Tuokko. 2010. "Marginal Competence, Risk Assessment, and Care Decisions: A Comparison of Values of Health Care Professionals and Older Adults." *Canadian Journal on Aging* 29(2): 173–183.

McDonald, Lynn, Julie Dergal, and Laura Cleghorn. 2007. "Living on the Margins: Older Homeless Adults in Toronto." *Journal of Gerontological Social Work* 49(1–2): 19–46.

McLaughlin, Kenneth. 2008. *Social Work, Politics and Society: From Radicalism to Orthodoxy*. Bristol: Policy.

Means, Robin, Sally Richards, and Randall Smith. 2003. *Community Care: Policy and Practice*, third edition. Basingstoke: Palgrave Macmillan.

Morrison, Tony. 2007. "Emotional Intelligence, Emotion and Social Work: Context, Characteristics, Complications and Contribution." *British Journal of Social Work* 37(2): 245–263.

Neysmith, Sheila M. 2009. "Closing the Gap Between Health Policy and the Home-Care Needs of Tomorrow's Elderly." *Canadian Journal of Community Mental Health* 8(2): 141–150.

Neysmith, Sheila, and Margaret MacAdam. 1999. "Controversial Concepts." In *Critical Issues*, edited by Sheila Neysmith, 1–26. New York: Columbia University Press.

Ornstein, Eric D., and Carol Ganzer. 2005. "Relational Social Work: A Model for the Future." *Families in Society* 86(4): 565–572.

Petersen, Alan, and Deborah Lupton. 1996. *The New Public Health: Health and Self in the Age of Risk*. London: Sage.

Pickard, Susan. 2009. "Governing Old Age: The 'Case Managed' Older Person." *Sociology* 43(1): 67–84.

Richards, Sally. 2000. "Bridging the Divide: Elders and the Assessment Processes." *Journal of the British Association of Social Workers* 30(1): 37–49.

Russell, Laura D., and Austin S. Babrow. 2011. "Risk in the Making: Narrative, Problematic Integration, and the Social Construction of Risk." *Communication Theory* 21(3): 239–260.

Seligman, Adams. 1997. *The Problem of Trust*. Princeton, NJ: Princeton University Press.

Skolbekken, John-Arne. 1995. "The Risk Epidemic in Medical Journals." *Social Science and Medicine* 40(3): 291–305.

Sztompka, Piotr. 1999. *Trust: A Sociological Theory*. Cambridge: Cambridge University Press.

Tanner, Denise. 1998. "The Jeopardy of Risk." *Practice* 10(1): 15–28.

Tansey, James, and Tim O'Riordan. 1999. "Cultural Theory and Risk: A Review." *Health, Risk and Society* 1:71–90.

Tosone, Carol. 2004. "Relational Social Work: Honoring the Tradition." *Smith College Studies in Social Work* 74(3): 475–487.

Tulloch, John, and Deborah Lupton. 2003. *Risk and Everyday Life*. London: Sage.

Vik, Kjersti, and Arne H. Eide. 2012. "The Exhausting Dilemmas Faced by Home-Care Service Providers When Enhancing Participation Among Older Adults Receiving Homecare." *Scandinavian Journal of Caring Sciences* 26(3): 528–536.

Webb, Stephen A. 2006. *Social Work in a Risk Society: Social and Political Perspectives*. Basingstoke: Palgrave Macmillan.

Wenger, G. Claire. 1997. "Social Networks and the Prediction of Elderly People at Risk." *Aging and Mental Health* 1(4): 311–320.

Zinn, Jens O. 2005. "The Biographical Approach: A Better Way to Understand Behaviour in Health and Illness." *Health, Risk and Society* 7(1): 1–9.

11

"Civil Disobedience" and Conflicting Rationalities in Elderly Care

▸ SIGNE MIE JENSEN AND KASPAR VILLADSEN

DURING THE LAST TWO DECADES, welfare services have undergone reforms aimed at increasing their quality, efficiency, and transparency with respect to costs and outcomes. In the Danish context, these reforms took their inspiration from New Public Management (NPM) and the idea that the traditional core welfare services should be opened to inspection based on evaluation criteria not integral to the character of traditional care services. Along with employees in other social services fields, professionals working in the elderly care sector also have been exposed to increasingly critical mass media scrutiny, resulting in a fear of becoming the subject of scandals over poor care or employee slacking.

This chapter focuses on the challenges confronting lower-level managers and frontline workers in residential elderly care. In order to obtain a better understanding of these challenges, detailed observations were undertaken over a period of seven months in the residential care service of the Danish municipality of Tønder. During that time, a project for improving management and facilitating organizational innovation was carried out. The project, led by an external consultant, offered a window for uncovering the different rationalities that the professionals need to balance in their daily practices.

A key finding was the existence of conflicting rationalities—in brief, the mixed logics of legality, care, and economics that employees felt placed paradoxical demands on their ability to provide professional care to their elderly clients (see Gubrium, Chapter 1, this volume). To cope with these conflicting demands, what care workers called "civil disobedience" had become a popular doctrine to designate activities guided by professional judgment—care and service—rather than by administrative regulations and standardized service protocols. This chapter describes how managers and care workers attempted to navigate the inherent ambiguities of contemporary welfare provision (see in this volume Garrow, Chapter 5; Järvinen, Chapter 3). It argues that principles and new solutions developed on "the front line" and "on the floor" may provide a resource for innovation, and that welfare managers need to consider ways of supporting the kinds of creativity and "disobedience" that yield such solutions. The findings are of relevance beyond the context of residential elderly care and could resonate in other areas of current welfare provision now being targeted by NPM-style reforms.

THE PRESSURE OF CONFLICTING RATIONALITIES

Those who manage care professionals have conventionally exercised leadership by invoking professional codes of care. However, they are increasingly required to keep abreast of their organization's financial status; thus, they must also manage through economic rationality while ensuring that they meet various statutory regulations for treating their clients.

This situation of conflicting demands has been described as "cross-pressures." Focusing on the front line of welfare, Michael Lipsky's (2010) thesis on cross-pressure begins from the premise that employees of welfare institutions seek to treat people as unique individuals with specific needs. However, the structure of their work organization prevents them from doing just that, because the logic of case management, by which individuals are assessed and placed into categories of eligibility, requires that professionals prioritize resources and categorize clients to fit them into the welfare system's regulations and service offers. Niels Andersen (2003:35–36) uses the term "organizational polyphony" to describe the coexistence of conflicting demands and situations of fundamental indeterminability between diverse rationalities. This polyphony has allegedly intensified in the public sector as a result of the reforms of the past two decades, both in Denmark and in other Western welfare states (Pedersen 2008:9).

Scholars of welfare reform have described how the quest for getting "more welfare for less money" has given rise to numerous technologies aimed at ensuring greater (financial) efficiency and accountability in the processes of welfare production. Novel technologies have been put in place that enhance surveillance, evaluation, and documentation in order to allow more evaluative comparisons between service-providing units and to place more budgetary responsibility on the frontline managers (Pedersen 2008:29). Yet, along with these increasing controls, we have witnessed parallel reforms aimed at decentralizing responsibility, deregulating certain bureaucratic activities, and facilitating a higher level of self-management in the frontline units of welfare provision.

This objective of decentralization reflects a recognition that the kind of professional knowledge necessary for ensuring a high level of service quality is principally generated "on the floor" in welfare institutions. One of the key purposes of decentralization was indeed to "liberate the creativity and professional potentials of the frontline employee" (Majgaard 2009:267). A commonplace assumption was that, before the reforms, frontline managers had been bound to the rigid borders of professionalism and legal requirements, and that they were faced with demands for decoding, negotiating, and reconciling various sets of values (Pedersen and Hatley 2008:327).

At first glance, this development would appear to be an increase in autonomy for the local units of service provision. However, the enhanced local autonomy was coupled to greater responsibility for documenting and controlling how this new responsibility was practiced. Hence, it has been argued that the paradigm of self-management was in fact a form of reregulation rather than deregulation (Majgaard 2009:267; Pedersen 2008:339). This duality of delegation and responsibilization has created contradictions between self-management and control, as well as between centralized and decentralized administration. It has been argued that these contradictions now constitute an integral and ubiquitous part of the frontline managers' working conditions (Majgaard 2009:283; Thygesen 2009:8).

The point of this short account of current developments in public welfare services is to support the thesis of the increasingly conflicting demands placed on frontline managers in welfare institutions (Pedersen 2008:29–31; Jensen 2009). These demands are exacerbated by recent welfare reforms (NPM) in terms of the emphasis on greater cross-disciplinarity, economic efficiency, and service delivery according to legal regulations and user satisfaction, all of which has been accompanied by increasing mass media attention. We do not argue that this polyphony of demands is something entirely novel, but rather that we are witnessing an intensification of long-standing contradictions in modern welfare provision.

More than ever, frontline professionals such as the residential care workers and their managers in Tønder, for example, locally confront the challenge of having to communicate and conduct their work in relation to the heterogeneous rationalities of care, economy, and law. As a result, they must often try to shape decisions in what is a somewhat indeterminate space, a grey zone lying between conflicting demands (Jensen 2009:16). The situation is not unique to the provision of home care services. Hence, Majgaard described cross-pressures in child and youth services, where the rationalities of economy, law, and professionalism collide, with the resulting pressure on harried managers (Majgaard 2009:278). Similarly, Villadsen (2011) investigated the challenges that arise when diverse organizations involved in reintegration work with homeless people adhere to conflicting evaluation criteria.

THE TØNDER STUDY

The Tønder study was carried out at the same time as a project for management development and improved work quality was under way in the residential elderly services of the municipality. Performing field observations during the time of this project was a great opportunity, since issues of key relevance to our research problem were continuously placed at the center of discussions between employees and managers. The consultant who organized the project took a semistructured approach by encouraging the participants to actively shape the discussions and activities. In order to help the participants articulate issues of concern related to work practices, the consultant highlighted three themes for debate: quality and efficiency, well-being and pleasures of work, and creativity and innovation. What kinds of work practices yield quality and efficiency? And what prevents it? These were the key issues brought up in the three discussion themes that spurred managers and employees to discuss their work and that gave the consultant material to work with. Prioritization in terms of making choices on how to spend time and resources in home visits also became a central theme during the project. The process included a series of workshops, supervision at individual care centers, interviews with representatives from the care administration, local managers, and working environment representatives, department meetings, and joint seminars.

One of the authors, Signe Mie Jensen, was an observer at 12 activities, making up about half of the activities in the innovation project, which included four of the six local centers of Tønder's residential elderly care. Thus, our approach took shape as structured fieldwork, with the qualification that it was structured by the consultant and not by the researcher (Kristiansen and Krogstrup 1999:47–48). This gave us the opportunity to act exclusively as participant observers, and hence we did not mediate or guide the debates. In all cases, observations were carried out after receiving informed consent from our informants. When it was not possible for the authors to participate in these meetings, the consultant reported to the authors by telephone and in writing.

We supplemented our observations with documentation of the management development project, including the municipality's brochure titled *Quality Standards for Personal Care and Practical Assistance* (Tønder Kommunes Social-og Sundhedsforvaltning 2011); descriptions of the various protocols and procedures used to determine which care services an elderly person should receive; and a letter of information about the development project, sent to middle managers.

We pursued the following principles when registering and analyzing the communication that unfolded at the meetings in the residential service centers. First, we started from what was actually communicated by the participants, the viewpoints and shared meaning that emerged, and refrained from immediately explaining communication with reference to external factors, underlying structures, or subjective (unarticulated) motives. In this regard, we followed David Silverman and Jaber Gubrium's (1994) insistence on beginning with the locally constructed discourse before moving to possible explanatory factors. This is not to say that there are no external influences that play a constitutive part in institutionalized everyday communication but rather that our focus was on investigating how such influences were articulated in specific contexts and hence shaped by the local and institutional cultures (Gubrium and Holstein 1999:530). Second, we wished to pay attention to how particular institutional norms, values, and categories are routinely articulated by those concerned, allowing for their capacity to modify, twist, and develop these institutional imperatives (p. 524).

Third, we recognized speakers as active in enacting and developing discursive categories over time (p. 526).

Our analysis draws broadly from Niklas Luhmann's systems theory, which helps to highlight communication patterns, paradoxes, and contradictions. In this context, systems theory serves as an alternative, or at least a relatively rarely utilized approach, in the English-speaking research tradition on welfare issues. Luhmann's systems theory has already been applied to social work in Germany (Baecker 1994; Bommes and Scherr 2000) and in the Scandinavian context (Villadsen 2007; Moe 1998). While systems theory may not immediately speak to ethnographic particulars by way of its status as perhaps "the last grand social theory," we believe that it offers an empirically sensitive orientation for analyzing communication practices. In this regard, we concur with the argument that systems theory can produce theoretically guided modes of observing patterns of institutionalized everyday communication (Gibson, Gregory, and Robinson 2005; Villadsen 2011). The approach affords a multifaceted framework for understanding communication in modern organizations, including welfare services faced by divergent rationalities and complex demands.

In particular, Luhmann's concept of observation provides a helpful tool for analyzing localized discourses. For Luhmann (1993:485), observation is an operation that cleaves the world into two parts by indicating something within the framework of a distinction. This observation creates one positively marked inner side and an unmarked reflective side: for example, lawful/unlawful, healthy/unhealthy, learning/nonlearning, and so on. The theory rests on the premise that one cannot observe or communicate about anything without indicating one side of a distinction (Luhmann 1993). Such distinctions are not set in stone but should be conceived of as temporary ways of observing the world that for a period of time obtain stability and instill certain expectations as to how communication may continue (Villadsen 2007:3). Notably, the idea that communication relies on the drawing of distinctions implies no theory of underlying structure but requires a detailed empirical description of recursive patterns in organized communication, as we will illustrate in the following empirical material.

The leading goal of the analysis is not simply to identify the appearance of a specific distinction but rather to carefully describe the types of communication and logics that unfold when a particular distinction is drawn on and sets expectations for subsequent communication. A fundamental advantage of approaching communication as the drawing of distinctions is that this analysis makes it very clear what is assigned a positive value in the statements under scrutiny. Once a statement has indicated, for instance, legality in communication, concerns of pedagogical, economic, or aesthetic nature become secondary issues by consequence (Villadsen 2011). In the analysis to follow, we witness instances where what is positively indicated by speakers at the expense of other latent possibilities certainly does make a significant difference.

KEY POINTS OF FRUSTRATION

Increasing complexity in the management of welfare organizations helps explain key points of frustration and resolution found in our empirical material.

Legitimate Illegality

In an exemplary meeting, a manager from the Tønder municipality's Department of Nursing and Care noted that some residential care workers and managers used the term "civil disobedience" to underscore their "professionalism" in dealing with clients. The term "professionalism" was used as an equivalent to "the use of common sense." The notion entailed being creative and using one's informed judgment according to the professional competency that social and care workers obtain through their education and training. Accordingly, "professionalism" was used as a descriptor for the correct form of care, and pursuing it rather than the proverbial rules and regulations had become the civil disobedience doctrine. It should be noted here that, in the Danish context, the term "citizen" is often used for service recipients when professionals wish to emphasize the recipient's formal position and rights in regard to welfare provision (see Miller and Kontos, Chapter 8, this volume). At a workshop involving employees, managers, and administrators, one employee referred to the need to have more influence based on personal evaluations of the citizen's situation.

During an interview, a frontline manager similarly articulated the connection between professionalism and exercising civil disobedience. In the following excerpt from her comments, note how she expresses a certain pride in employees taking responsibility even when it happens at the border of regulations:

> I feel good about my employees being a little disobedient. For example if they take their work vehicle to go buy a liter of milk [for the elderly person whom they are caring for]. They should be allowed to think for themselves and to use their professional competences. However, I like to know when they do so, so that I can back them up if someone phones me to say that they have seen a home helper out buying groceries while wearing their uniform. If I can give reasons for why we do what we do, then nobody can come after us.

A large proportion of the health and social workers who participated in the project did not feel that the legal requirements and other written rules on how to perform services in home help and care were conducive to providing proper care. The care workers and some of their managers who have the same training in care work saw the rules, legal requirements, and other coded demands as foreign to the values of their profession. They responded to this frustration with practical and discursive inventiveness.

The perspective of systems theory prompted us to be sensitive to how the care workers discursively parsed illegality into, respectively, "legitimate illegality" and "actual illegality." Linked to this parsing process, the term "civil disobedience" was used to refer to "the correct kind of care." This is the care provided when the worker acts according to his or her professional judgment regarding what the citizen needs, which coincidentally might be perceived as being contrary to the rules.

A working environment representative applied the same notion of "illegality" at another interview when discussing the assessment protocols used to determine the types of services and duration of visits for which the client is eligible, which were called "packages." The representative explained how the workers felt that they sometimes had to take minutes from one client and use them to care for another person deemed to be in greater need of care and help:

> The stupid thing about the [assessment] packages is that there is a jump from 32 to 120 minutes, which forces us to play Robin Hood and take a little time here and there.

Relatedly, at the start of the project, one worker lamented:

> I feel limited by all the rules. For example, I am not even allowed to help the citizen go to the bakery [to buy bread] instead of cleaning.

And, at a workshop on the theme of quality, the antithesis between professionalism and legally defined tasks was expressed by way of a concern for the person assigned both to managing the care routine and to assessing the needs of the citizens:

> The case worker is stuck between a rock and a hard place. Should you stay within the limits of the package or should you be loyal toward your professional values?

At first glance, it seems paradoxical that the legal requirements intended to safeguard proper conditions for the citizens receiving assistance are viewed by the caregivers as the antithesis of the very care they were to ensure. The consequence of this paradox is that conflicts constantly arose because of the tension between the conceptions of proper care and legality.

During interviews and in the meetings, however, the managers and care workers made distinctions that transformed the conventional, clear-cut differentiation between care and legality. The result was communicative inventions in which professionalism figured as the correct definition of care but was constructed as being "legitimately" opposed to legality.

Sverre Moe's (1998:46–61) analysis of the function system of care provides for a partial explanation of this conflict between professionalism and legality. Moe applied systems theory to the care system, arguing that inherent to the care system's self-description is that only the care system and its professionals have the discretionary competence to determine the need for help. In the case of Tønder, however, the political system has mobilized the medium of law in an attempt to determine clients' needs and control welfare services. Arguably, this coupling has prepared the ground for the health workers' and social workers' invention of the notion of care as (legitimate) civil disobedience. In principle, the employees acknowledge the legitimacy of judicially specified care services, but they do not recognize it as guaranteeing adequate quality. Quality care, they explain, can be provided only through the exercise of their professional competencies. Their complaints related to juridical regulation center on the loss of professional discretion, as priority decisions about how much and which kinds of care are to be given each service user are moved out of the hands of the individual care worker.

Cost Restrictions, Professional Care, and Scandal

The increasing emphasis on judicial regulation is not the sole factor generating increased complexity and the care workers' perception that their profession is under threat. As a result of the frontline managers' greater responsibility for fulfilling budgetary demands, the presence of economically coded communication has become more pronounced on the front line of service provision. Because communication shaped in the economic code instills a rationality of scarcity and prioritization, it is not surprising that the residential care workers in Tønder drew a direct line between more cost restrictions and less time for what they view as proper care. This view was clearly expressed by a local trade union representative during a supervisor meeting:

> We lack time with the citizen. We don't feel that we get things done properly, because we only have 15 minutes to do them.

During a workshop, a care worker explained:

> There isn't any time for the weakest clients. There is no time for care. We dare not ask how the citizen is doing, because we do not have time to deal with it if the citizen starts to cry.

During the entire project, the perception of the tight financial situation was omnipresent. When asked at a workshop what concerned the managers most, a frontline manager replied:

> Finances. Everything is determined by the economy. It's hard making ends meet.

At another workshop, a manager said:

> It [the work and services] is not determined by needs. It's determined by the economic conditions.

Managers and employees alike related that there used to be more room for the care aspects of their work. Before the NPM reforms, they asserted, considerations at the front line had been dominated by the care rationale. A working environment representative explained:

> We used to have more time. Now that there is less time, there is much more focus on doing the stuff we have to do in time. . . . Today our work is dominated by routines, rules and habits.

During a workshop on quality and efficiency, well-being and pleasure in work, and creativity and innovation, a care worker referred to the new rules on documenting the use of materials:

> It used to be so that if we needed any extra materials, we could just ask for them if we gave a proper explanation for why we needed them.

This quotation is emblematic of how the employees tend to refer to a past when "things were better." But it also exemplifies how the workers' sentiments of distrust articulate the irony of recent NPM reforms that aim to regain public trust by introducing a distrust-based control mechanism (Van de Walle 2011:309). In the following, we will explore how this distrust was articulated at the residential care centers of Tønder and why, with the intensification of complexity, distrust of their organizational surroundings had become pronounced among the frontline workers.

Conventionally, such rules and demands originate from the central political and administrative authorities, but because of the decentralized administrative structure, their implementation often falls on local managers. This means that it is not easy to grasp whether new requirements derive from the managers or from external actors, which results in employees' distrust toward managers, who might actually be quite sympathetic to care workers' civil disobedience. The following quotations from supervision workshops illustrate a shared feeling of lack of trust. At one of the workshops, an employee said:

> There is a lack of trust. One needs to specify everything in detail and know all the right words to achieve the right resources.

During an interview, a working environment representative similarly expressed the feeling of a lack of trust:

> There is a lack of trust. We do not want to do less; in fact we would like to do more. If this wasn't the case, we wouldn't be in this job.

Apart from emphasizing the contradictory demands that financial and efficiency requirements place on residential care work, a pronounced fear of mass media scandal was repeatedly expressed at the meetings. In the past decade, Danish media have reported numerous instances of mistreatment in nursing homes and of care workers allegedly running private errands during working hours (Kristensen 2010:15). None of these stories implicated the municipality of Tønder, but the Tønder care workers were nonetheless very much aware of the public scrutiny of their work. For example, during an interview, a frontline manager told the story of a care worker who had purchased a chocolate bar while refueling his service car. A couple of young men saw this and drew the conclusion that the care worker was buying sweets during work hours. They followed him, yelled at him, and even threw rocks at his car. This happened not long after a scandal had appeared in the news about poor residential care in Copenhagen, far away from Tønder. Still, the manager stressed that such episodes were rare but were nevertheless present in the minds of the employees. In a different conversation, another frontline manager mentioned that employees are very careful to avoid, or to document, anything that might arouse the suspicious gaze of journalists looking for scandal. The fear of scandals and the stories sustaining them is an example of how events in the external environment can become significant components in local discourse, flagging the systemic linkages of conflicting rationalities.

STRATEGIES FOR MANAGING CONFLICTING RATIONALITIES

Consider the strategies care workers deploy for managing conflicting rationalities.

Strict Rule Adherence

One of the strategies consisted of care workers' rigid adherence to rules and regulations. From early on in the project, we observed numerous accounts indicating a marked "overinterpretation" or overly strict interpretation of the regulatory demands. Our data suggest that the care workers' overemphasis on rules and regulations was associated with the intensification of contradictory rationalities at the front line. This overemphasis, in turn, prompted managers and employees to use the term "civil disobedience" to legitimate actions in accordance with their professional standards, even if they contravened formal procedures.

The overly strict interpretation of rules took different shapes. Sometimes the workers did not dare act unless the services they performed were explicitly described in the set of rules, regulations, protocols, checklists, and the like. In other situations, their actions were based on misconceptions or "myths" about rules that in fact did not exist or, conversely, a habitus that was not founded on written rules.

Employees repeatedly articulated "we are limited by rules" and similar pronouncements. They felt as if their professional competencies were distrusted by the environment around them and, as a result, they were anxious about not complying completely with the rules. In the past two decades, their work practices had been subjected to increasing scrutiny through ever more detailed requirements for documentation and more detailed regulations, all of which was perceived by the frontline professionals as a manifestation of distrust (Hildebrandt 2013). This has been a general issue in the Danish public sector, which led the Ministry of Domestic Affairs to initiate "trust-reform" for the public sector in 2013 (Møller 2013).

As noted, myths play a significant role in this. To illustrate, a Tønder employee had become convinced that she was not allowed to boil an egg for a person in her care. Asked why she would think that, she explained that she assumed so because the care professionals no longer cooked for the elderly. Instead, meals were delivered by an outside catering company and were only to be prepared by the care worker, not cooked. The employee reasoned that since the care workers were no longer to cook warm meals, they were not allowed to use any cooking utensils either, not even a pan for boiling an egg.

During some of the workshops early in the project, which included employees as well as managers, we took note of numerous statements of this kind, such as "We are not allowed to" or, emphatically, "But we are not allowed!" These statements left managers and administration representatives dumbfounded, leading some to wonder: "But it doesn't say anywhere that you cannot do that." Addressing this issue in an interview, a working environment representative recounted how she had asked a care worker in a teaching mode, "Why do you say you are not allowed to do that? Because you are!"

It was said by some that the workplace was virtually haunted by such myths. The management development project revealed the existence of these myths to the central managers, who were quite surprised. The frontline managers, however, were somewhat aware of the myths but were taken aback by the suggested widespread overly strict interpretation of rules. According to one manager:

> People have a hard time understanding that they ARE allowed to do something which is not spelled out on a piece of paper.

Another said:

> People call and ask about things they could easily work out themselves.

There were many remarkable myths of overly strict rule adherence allegedly based on imaginary rules and regulations. For example, many frontline employees perceived it as paramount to always make their client's bed in the morning. The morning shift is the busiest of all the shifts during the day, and it would be beneficial for employees working this shift if they could leave less urgent tasks for those working the afternoon or evening shifts. This relates to the conflicting belief that allowing the bed to get cold before making it reduces the risk of dust mites. Nevertheless, the care workers insisted on making the bed in the morning. We found that fear of scandal had increased the perseverance of the legally coded communication. One care worker cautioned, "What would the relatives and next of kin think of us if they came to visit and saw that the bed was not made?" Another care worker said:

> The employees find it hard to let things go that [are] not even essential because they fear that the neighbor may visit. . . . The relatives focus on whatever might be missing.

For some employees, strictly abiding by the rules—including mythical ones—was a virtual shield against the possible scandal. The rationale for this, according to one worker, was, "If I do everything on the checklist, no one can come after me." This mentality, of course, was a great hindrance to innovation and dynamic development of the relationship between service provider and client. According to the care professionals, the result of the proliferation of documentation requirements and indeed other assumed rules was a workday dominated by strict adherence to routine. Oddly enough, routines diminish the space of professional judgment, which in turn impairs the experience of quality of the work performed on the part of the provider as well as the receiver. The aforementioned notion of civil disobedience was the counterstrategy and symbolic opposite of strict rule adherence. At a more advanced stage of the innovation project, a central manager said:

> We need to challenge the rules. How else are we to figure out whether we need to change them?

Overcaring

A second strategy for managing perceived work dilemmas consisted in "overcaring" for service users. This implies that the care workers would be so preoccupied with complying with all requirements and needs for care that they risked placing their users in a passive or "clienticized" role. The risk of providing "overcare" has been posited as a general challenge of residential care (Mandag Morgen, Aarhus Kommune 2013:12). Tønder employees reported that the fear of not fulfilling the statutory regulations led to situations where they helped the elderly with tasks they could have managed by themselves. A union representative gave this example:

> I was assisting a citizen who had just had a bath. Automatically, I helped him put on his shirt. He dryly commented that he could do that himself.

Another employee described how the assistance she and her colleagues offered impaired the service user's own initiative:

> Once I asked a citizen, "What would you like for breakfast?" His reply was, "Why, your colleague has written it in the blue book."

Accepting Contradictions

A third strategy was to accept the perceived contradictions and dilemmas as an integral and enduring component in residential care work (see in this volume Garrow, Chapter 5; Carr, Chapter 4; Grenier and Flood, Chapter 10). In notable cases, this led to creative and innovative approaches to the dilemmas instead of hoping for, or demanding, their ultimate resolution. Taking contradictions as virtually coming with the territory, one employee said at a workshop that she felt that:

> The rigid requirements made professional creativity necessary in order to make the daily working practices manageable.

In regard to innovation, the organizational development project had somewhat of a snowball effect. The project created a communicative space in which it was acceptable to talk about which factors made management and employees satisfied or dissatisfied, what would be nice to change, and so on. The extensive articulation of the care workers' tasks provided a break from those very tasks. It allowed for sharing experiences from the floor, which had not yet been a part of the common communication between staff members. The sharing paved the way for a relegitimation of professionalism and professional judgment.

For example, at a workshop about prioritizing, the care workers were asked to divide their tasks into "must-do tasks" and "nice-to-do tasks." In the discussion of where to place the tasks, ideas generated by the care workers in conjunction with their clients were shared. New ideas on how to improve the daily care process also arose from these discussions. In this framework, professional creativity was used to navigate issues *within* the reality of the conflicting demands. Consider a few examples on this front. Early on in the project, a union representative said:

> It's the small, visible things which matter to the relatives, and this is on the minds of the care workers. They [the relatives] don't see all the other important work, we do.

Later, during a workshop about prioritization, a care worker suggested that a note could be put on the dishpans in the homes of the elderly citizens, saying, "Dishes will be done once a day." This would calm the day shift, making room for them to do their work without the feeling of racing against time:

> We have to be better at leaving some tasks for the evening shift. But we try to do everything during the day shift. The dishes for example, so the relatives don't see them, if they visit.

During one workshop, several ideas were presented by frontline managers and by union and working environment representatives suggesting that sometimes a new perspective on the care receiver was a good thing. A related issue was that sometimes care workers start to feel "ownership" over certain service users. It makes it more difficult to make schedules when the manager knows that they will have dissatisfied employees, because "someone else got Mrs. Hansen." Counteracting employees' feelings of ownership, it was suggested, would make it easier to plan or replan schedules, especially on days where a lot of employees call in sick.

In the workshop, it was noted that the care professionals would be more challenged and could better develop their professionalism if they were exposed to new service users instead of staying with the same ones for years. A different example of this exposure to novelty was when a manager let a care worker who had day shifts only try an evening shift. The worker really enjoyed that experience, it was said. The day and evening shifts are very different from one another since they involve different tasks. But because of the lack of knowledge sharing up until the point of the innovation project, the managers had not further expanded on this possible innovation.

Related to the issue pertaining to care workers who work with the same service users for extended periods of time is that they can become blind to the citizens' abilities to take care of themselves. This risk of overcare was expressed recurrently. At the prioritizing workshop, a care worker succinctly stated this risk of excessive care:

> I can't help but to think back on when we were on strike, suddenly a lot of the elderly could take care of themselves for a while.

In this light, letting other care workers bring a new perspective on a citizen can be a good thing. The idea was expressed at the workshop that every now and then the frontline managers should accompany their employees to witness the employees' everyday routines, which could help bring new perspectives on particular cases and uncover their employees' everyday innovation.

From a systems theory perspective, the key to formulating an innovative management strategy is to focus on the paradoxes observable in communication; for example, concerning "the right kind of care." Systems theory suggests that paradoxes resulting from conflicting rationalities cannot simply be put aside or eliminated. Instead, they are drivers integral to the communication process (Majgaard 2009). This means that rather than seeking to eliminate the tensions between the professionals and novel management technologies, the challenge of the frontline manager is to explore how paradoxes and conflicting rationalities can be brought on board to breed innovation dynamics within the system. The assumption is that paradoxes can be made productive if it is acknowledged that they constitute a fundamental condition under which organizations function.

• • •

In this chapter, we have explored how conflicting rationalities and related working demands are managed by lower-level managers and employees on the front line of welfare services. The institutional context in which these contradictions and creative responses were articulated was made up of multiple components, including demands derived from NPM reforms, legal and economic requirements, and fear of mass media scandals. In our study, we did not attempt to grasp the external factors in their "objective" or material reality, since we approached them merely as they emerged and were articulated in the locally produced discourse at the residential care centers. Our study presented varied responses to the external demands, which were perceived as contradictory.

Employees practiced a multipronged strategy of working strictly by the formal rules and regulations but nevertheless insisting on providing care and inventing solutions rooted in their professional values. These contradictory practices can be viewed as a response to particular working conditions at residential care providers, where they served to expand the maneuvering space at the front line without violating administrative policies, legal stipulations, and budgets. Most of the frontline managers were aware of the "civil disobedience" doctrine, and some even condoned it. Understandably, then, the frontline managers largely expressed support for this response by which employees dealt with the conflicting demands in their daily routines. Recent NPM reforms of welfare services have advanced solutions to issues of transparency and efficiency derived from management theories and sectors outside of the welfare professions, such as systematic measurement, contracts, and performance-based resource allocation. However, there is little solid evidence that such reforms generate higher public trust (Van de Walle 2011:314). The reliance on "evidence-based knowledge" and hard, measurable data risks neglecting "soft" data in terms of employees' opinions and solutions developed informally "on the ground": "Too often we are seduced by deceptive metrics and false polarities that would have us believe that only structural studies based on 'hard' data can provide satisfactory explanations of social phenomena which lead to successful policy interventions" (Silverman and Gubrium 1994:194). This study points at the potential for shifting this emphasis.

REFERENCES

Andersen, Niels Å. 2000. "Politisk Administration." In *Diskursteorien på arbejde*, edited by T. B. Dyrberg, A. D. Hansen, and J. Torfing, 71–103. Frederiksberg: Samfundslitteratur.

Andersen, Niels Å. 2003. "Polyphonic Organisations." In *Autopoietic Organization Theory: Drawing on Niklas Luhmann's Social Systems Perspective*, edited by T. Bakken and T. Herness, 151–182. Oslo: Copenhagen Business School Press.

Baecker, Dirck. 1994. "Soziale Hilfe als Funktionssystem der Gesellschaft" [Social Help as Functional System of Society]. *Zeitschrift für Soziologie* 23:93–110.

Bommes, Michael, and Albert Scherr. 2000. *Soziologie der Sozialen Arbeit* [The sociology of social work]. Weinheim: Juventa.

Gibson, Barry, Jane Gregory, and Peter G. Robinson. 2005. "The Intersection Between Systems Theory and Grounded Theory: The Emergence of the Grounded Observer. *Qualitative Sociology Review* 2:3–21.

Gubrium, Jaber F., and James A. Holstein. 1999. "The Nursing Home as a Discursive Anchor Point for the Ageing Body." *Ageing and Society* 19(5):519–538.

Hildebrandt, Steen. 2013. "Efter New Public Management." MM Blog 14.05, Mandag Morgens hjemmeside. https://www.mm.dk/blog/efter-new-public-management.

Jensen, Annette. 2009. "Udfordring: Velfærdsledelse skal praktiseres." In FOA–Fag og Arbejde, CBS–Copenhagen Business School, UCC–University College Capital, KL–Kommunernes Landsforening: *Velfærdsledelse. 6 indlæg om offentlig ledelse*, 16–20. Copenhagen: FOAs trykkeri.

Kristensen, Dennis. 2010. "Velfærdslederen i fokus." In FOA–Fag og Arbejde, CBS–Copenhagen Business School, UCC–University College Capital, KL–Kommunernes Landsforening: *Værdfærdsledelse—det handler om praksis. Syv indlæg om offentlig ledelse*, 5–8. Copenhagen: FOAs trykkeri.

Kristiansen, Søren, and Hanne Kathrine Krogstrup. 1999. *Observationsmetoden og dens former, i Deltagende observation—introduktion til en forskningsmetodik*. Copenhagen: Hans Reitzels Forlag.

Lipsky, Michael. 2010. *Street-Level Bureaucracy: Dilemmas of the Individual in Public Services*. New York: Russell Sage Foundation.

Luhmann, Niklas. 1993. "Observing Re-entries." *Graduate Faculty Philosophy Journal* 16(2): 485–498.

Majgaard, Klaus. 2009. "Slip paradokserne løs!" *Økonomistyring and Informatik* 32(4): 261–302.

Mandag Morgen, Aarhus Kommune. 2013. *Kærlig Kommune—fremtidens sundhed og omsorg, i Aarhus* [The caring municipality: The future of health and care in Aarhus]. Copenhagen: Mandag Morgen, Aarhus Kommune.

Moe, Sverre. 1998. *Den moderne hjelpens sociologi: Velferd i systemteoretisk perspektiv*. Oslo: Apeiros Forlag.

Møller, Bjarke. 2013. "Den vigtige tillidsreform." Mandag Morgens website. https://www.mm.dk/vigtige-tillidsreform.

Pedersen, Dorthe. 2008. "Strukturreformens styringspolitik: En overskridende dynamik." In *Genopfindelsen af den offentlige sektor—ledelsesudfordringer i reformernes tegn*, edited by D. Pedersen, C. Greve, and H. Højlund, 23–49. Copenhagen: Børsens Forlag.

Pedersen, Dorthe, and Jean Hatley. 2008. "The Changing Context of Public Leadership and Management: Implications for Roles and Dynamic." *International Journal of Public Sector Management* 21(4): 327–339.

Silverman, David, and Jaber F. Gubrium. 1994. "Competing Strategies for Analysing the Contexts of Social Interaction." *Sociological Inquiry* 64(2): 179–198.

Thygesen, Niels Thyge. 2009. "Udfordring—når man skal udvikle teori om velfærdsledelse." In FOA–Fag og Arbejde, CBS–Copenhagen Business School, UCC–University College Capital, KL–Kommunernes Landsforening: *Velfærdsledelse. 6 indlæg om offentlig ledelse*, 8–10. Copenhagen: FOAs trykkeri.

Tønder Kommunes Social-og Sundhedsforvaltning. 2011. *Kvalitetsstandarder for personlig pleje og praktisk hjælp*. Tønder Kommune website. http://www.swiflet.com/tk/aeogh/30/1/. Accessed February 17, 2014.

Van de Walle, Steven. 2011. "NPM: Restoring the Public Trust Through Creating Distrust?" In *The Ashgate Research Companion to New Public Management*, edited by Tom Christensen and Per Lægreid, 309–321. Farnham: Ashgate.

Villadsen, Kaspar. 2007. "'Polyphonic' Welfare: Luhmann's Systems Theory Applied to Modern Social Work." *International Journal of Social Welfare* 1(17): 65–73.

Villadsen, Kaspar. 2011. "Ambiguous Citizenship: 'Modern' and 'Postmodern' Welfare at the Margins." *Distinktion: Scandinavian Journal of Social Theory* 12(3): 309–329.

PART | IV

Reimagined Service Relationships

THE CONCLUDING CHAPTERS THAT COMPRISE PART IV consider instances of reimagination. Their point of departure is that in the contingent world of everyday life, fixed borders and roles are illusory. Interactional roads are always two-way streets, and identity detours are to be expected along the way. Alternative routes that blur service roles and missions are possible, yet these routes, too, come into conflict with lingering structures of interaction. The first two chapters in this part present concrete examples of service relationships that cross the professional–nonprofessional divide that Weber and Kafka put into place a century ago and that still typifies models of service delivery and administration. The last three chapters discuss ways of reconceptualizing the roles of service providers in more dynamic and reflexive terms. Service roles, for instance, are viewed as context pertinent rather than administratively fixed. Terminology continues to be telling, with "border work," "crossing borders," "tension and balance," "stewardship," and "negotiated power" leading the way.

12

Mental Health Self-Knowledge

CROSSING BORDERS WITH RECOVERY COLLEGES AND TOJISHA KENKYU

▸ *TOM SHAKESPEARE AND RACHAEL COLLINS*

HISTORICALLY, APPROACHES TO MENTAL HEALTH have been strongly polarized. In contrast to the dominant medical model within psychiatry, antipsychiatry perspectives have been very vigorously adopted within the mental health service user field, as evidenced by the positions of organizations such as the World Network of Users and Survivors of Psychiatry. However, the late twentieth century saw the growth of user involvement initiatives, both as a reaction to the limitations of the medical model and as a reflection of the shift toward a human rights ethos.

In this chapter, we will discuss two recent mental health service developments that seek to bridge the gap between the psychiatry and user perspectives, namely Recovery Colleges (Britain) and Tojisha Kenkyu (Japan). Each is based on a changed conception of the roles of professionals and service users. The chapter will show some of the similarities and differences between the two activities and discuss the potential of this new thinking both for overcoming the service divide and for improving the lives of people with mental illness.

Because of the exploratory nature of the research, we have adopted the case study method (Denzin 2006; Crowe 2011). First, this chapter draws on an extensive literature review of service user involvements in mental health, particularly published material and grey literature relating to Tojisha Kenkyu and Recovery Colleges. Second, it draws on a visit made by the lead author to Japan in April 2013 to attend a workshop on Tojisha Kenkyu, and on a workshop held at the University of East Anglia in September 2014, funded by the Great Britain Sasakawa Foundation, at which both

Tojisha Kenkyu and Recovery College participants presented and discussed their activities. Third, it draws on discussions with peer tutors and mental health workers involved in Tojisha Kenkyu and Norfolk and Suffolk Recovery College.

BACKGROUND

In England until the eighteenth century, the approach toward individuals with mental illness focused on control rather than treatment, with such individuals being confined to "Madhouses" (Rush 2004). One of the earliest examples of service user involvement is the "Petition of the Poor Distracted Folk of Bedlam" in the 1620s, though perhaps the most notable early user group was the Alleged Lunatics' Friend Society created by John Perceval in 1845 (Rush 2004; Wallcraft and Bryant 2003). In the postwar period, the consolidation of the "medical model" of health confirmed professionals as the experts and required service users merely to comply (Rush 2004). This was often experienced in terms of forced confinement, depersonalization, and objectification (Crossley and Crossley 2001).

The work of R. D. Laing and the Anti-Psychiatry Movement in the 1960s opened spaces for new thinking about mental illness and made it easier for the general public to listen to people with mental illness. One consequence was the emergence of the leading mental health advocacy and support organizations of today, such as Rethink (originally the National Schizophrenia Fellowship, founded in 1972) and MIND (originally National Association for Mental Health but changed its name in 1972) (Wallcraft and Bryant 2003).

In the early 1970s, service users reemerged as "survivors" through the growth of organizations such as Campaign Against Psychiatric Oppression and the British Network for Alternatives to Psychiatry (Crossley and Crossley 2001; Tait and Lester 2005). Groups such as Survivors Speak Out, UK Advocacy Network (UKAN), and the Hearing Voices Network began to use the term "survivor" to promote a positive image of individuals who had survived the mental health services (Crossley and Crossley 2001; Tait and Lester 2005) and to build a collective identity (Crossley and Crossley 2001). Such service user groups campaigned on a range of issues, such as improving conditions of services, closing large long-stay psychiatric hospitals, and giving users greater autonomy (Wallcraft and Bryant 2003). During the 1980s, Britain saw an increase in mental health service protests, with more user groups developing, including forums, movements, patient councils, and self-help and advocacy groups (Wallcraft and Bryant 2003). It is estimated that the service user movement in the United Kingdom has grown from 15 groups in the mid-1980s to over 700 today (Thornicroft and Tansella 2005). This growing survivor voice challenged the voice of authority, namely the medical model of psychiatry and the health system as a whole (Crossley and Crossley 2001): instead of "mental illness," the term "mental distress" is often used to signal this changed perspective.

The survivor and the recovery movements in mental health have coincided with wider developments within health policy. During the 1980s and 1990s, free-market ideas about challenging paternalism and monopolistic provision coincided with grassroots perspectives about user empowerment and self-help. Milestones such as the 1990 NHS and Community Care Act, the Patients' Charter (Department of Health 1991), and later the 2001 Health and Social Care Act shifted thinking about service user involvement and promoted the idea of patients as consumers or service users, not passive recipients of care (Crossley and Crossley 2001; Rush 2004). For example, it has become accepted that the National Health Service (NHS) should engage service users in the planning and evaluation of services and provide opportunities for treatment decision making (Wallcraft and Bryant 2003; Tait and Lester 2005). In the 2001 report "The Expert Patient: A New Approach to Chronic Disease Management for the 21st Century," the Department of Health recommended the introduction of self-management led by service users to all areas of the NHS by 2007 (Department of Health 2001). More recently, the Department of Health white paper "Equity and Excellence: Liberating the NHS" (Department of Health 2010) highlighted the importance of "shared decision-making" between service users and professionals (El Enany, Currie, and Lockett 2013). In 2011, service user involvement as an aid to recovery was promoted in the Department of Health's "No Health Without Mental Health" (El Enany, Currie, and Lockett 2013). However, it is not necessarily straightforward to transfer self-management approaches from physical health to mental health (Davidson 2005).

The notion of recovery emerges from the way in which the mental health survivor movement has developed its own "therapeutic language of healing and recovery" (Crossley and Crossley 2001:10; Slade et al. 2014). In contrast to clinical recovery—absence of symptoms—personal recovery is about taking control over one's life, having a satisfying and meaningful life, and participating in the community (Slade et al. 2014). The recovery philosophy is about focusing on strengths, rather than problems, and restoring hope. Often, the stigma and discrimination that people with mental illness face can be as big a difficulty as the illness itself. Rather than symptom control, people are looking for acceptance. The outcome of a recovery process should be that individuals with continuing mental health issues feel empowered to live better lives (Repper and Perkins 2013:12; Shepherd et al. 2008).

It has been argued that the development of service user initiatives has been influenced by prevailing political and social climates and that the promotion of user involvement in the industrialized world has coincided with the crisis in the funding of health care (Lomas 1997; Rush 2004; Slade et al. 2014). For example, in the United Kingdom, the current emphasis on recovery and self-help may partly be a response to the closure of psychiatric hospitals and outpatient services as part of the Coalition and Conservative governments' austerity program of funding cuts (e.g., Dooher and Rye 2013). Yet, services have to be available for times of personal crisis in someone's life, even if the individual is managing their mental health better through the recovery philosophy.

Mental health policy and practice in Japan offers a considerable contrast to that in the United Kingdom (Taplin and Lawman 2012). In Japan, mental health services remain dominated by institutional provision, with more than 80 percent of Japan's psychiatric hospitals being privately run, and with treatment being based on high-dose polypharmacy (Ito 2012). This has proven a disincentive to progress toward community-based care. From 1974 onward, there were attempts to encourage outpatient treatment by reforming reimbursement policies, but these did not lead to significant reductions in inpatient beds. For example, in 2010, there were 27 inpatient beds per 10,000 population, compared to just under 8 per 10,000 in the United States and just under 6 per 10,000 in the United Kingdom (2004 figures, quoted in Ando and Thornicroft 2012). Often, day care centers were adapted from inpatient wards on the same hospital site.

A turning point in mental health policies came with the Utsunomiya Hospital scandal (1983), when human rights abuses and deaths were revealed to have occurred at a private mental hospital. This led to a new emphasis on the protection of the human rights of mental patients. Mental health service user groups started in Japan in the late 1980s (e.g., Osaka) and early 1990s (e.g., Tokyo). These were mainly top-down initiatives, reflecting a governmental desire to keep up with current best practices in mental health, and the groups were more successful in some areas than in others (Lawman 2012).

The year 2004 saw another landmark, when a service user joined a government committee of the Ministry of Health, Labour and Welfare for the first time. That same year, the government announced the intention of shifting from institutional to community care, with the goal of reducing the number of inpatients with schizophrenia from 215,000 in 1996 to 124,000 in 2026 (Lawman 2012:44). In 2007, the Japanese government signed the Convention on the Rights of Persons with Disabilities, which in theory commits the country to promoting community living and inclusion. In 2011, the government Mental Health White Paper promoted the recovery model, discussing the value of peer support models and how this approach could boost the confidence of service users. Despite these positive signs, Sandra Lawman's recent review concluded that, "The user movement in Japan is fragile and needs further nurturing" (Lawman 2012:111).

Since 1990, consumer participation in mental health has been a global trend, seen not just in the United Kingdom but also in Australia (Lammers and Happell 2003; McCann et al. 2008) and the United States (Davidson et al. 2006) and other high-income settings. In 2011, the World Psychiatric Association (WPA) stated a key goal for best practices when working with service users and carers is to promote the meaningful involvement of users in the planning and implementation of services and the development of person-centered care (Wallcraft et al. 2011). The benefits of self-help and social support outside the service context, and of hearing user perspectives on their conditions within the service context, have long been acknowledged (Wallcraft and Bryant 2003; Tait and Lester 2005; Faulkner and Kalathil 2012). However, research finds that user involvement is more likely to be on the model of consultation rather than partnership (Rutter et al. 2004). Moreover, while there may be support among professionals for service users' involvement in the planning and management of services, there seems to be less support for service user involvement in care and treatment (McCann et al. 2008; Soffe, Read, and Frude 2004). It may be that professionals are reluctant to concede their specialist expertise and the status that comes with it. Recovery principles around user involvement in care can also come up against professional anxieties around risk avoidance, and the danger of tragic outcomes in mental health (Davidson et al. 2006; Schwartz et al. 2013; Tickle, Brown, and Hayward 2014; see also Grenier and Flood, Chapter 10, this volume).

RECOVERY COLLEGES

The Recovery College approach uses education to support the recovery and social inclusion of people with mental health issues. Recovery Colleges began at Boston University in 1984, and they are now being developed in Italy, Ireland, and the United Kingdom (Slade et al. 2014). In February 2011, the Department of Health commissioned Sainsbury's Centre for Mental Health and the NHS Confederation's Mental Health Network to pilot the Implementing Recovery through Organisational Change (IMROC) program across 29 UK NHS sites. One of these sites was Norfolk and Suffolk. Aspects of the Recovery Project include Recovery College (coproduced education and training), Peer Supporter Workers, Staff Journeys (including discovering "Hidden Talents," the label for staff who have experienced mental distress), and Life beyond Illness (partnerships, positive stories, and finding opportunities).

As part of the IMROC program, Recovery College seeks to adopt an educational and coaching model rather than a therapeutic frame. A curriculum of recovery-focused workshops and courses is offered, whereby staff and peer tutors can help people make sense of what has happened, find meaning, and become expert in managing their own lives. Coproduction is key to the Recovery College approach: the educational activities are developed by professionals and users, working together, and are delivered by dyads of staff and peer tutors; "co-produced, co-delivered, co-received" is the slogan.

Characteristic of the recovery movement is that peer support workers—people with lived experience of mental distress—become part of the staff team (Gillard et al. 2013; Slade et al. 2014). When this is done effectively and not simply as a tokenistic response, it has the potential to transform mental health care relationships. The extensive evidence base for the benefits of peer support workers includes RCTs in Australia, the Netherlands, the United Kingdom, and the United States. The use of peer support workers helps both clinical outcomes and subjective outcomes, and the benefits of peer support workers are equivalent to those of professionals in similar roles (Repper and Carter 2011; Slade et al. 2014).

Thus, the recovery movement has implications for the relationship of the professional to the service user (see Greener, Chapter 14, this volume). Because most professionals do not have personal experience of profound mental illness, their insights are necessarily limited. Also, professional practice may enforce clear boundaries that prevent personal disclosure. Therefore, service users may turn to other people who have faced the same challenges, called experts by experience, rather than turning only to professionals:

> The critical thing is that, as mental health workers, we acknowledge and respect these differences, accept our own limitations, and recognize the wisdom endowed by first-hand experience. People can gain a great deal of support, information and hope—a vision of the possible—from those who have faced similar challenges. (Repper and Perkins 2013:13)

A staff tutor from the Norfolk and Suffolk site talked about moving beyond "us and them":

> working in partnership, recognising assets rather than traditional relationships where the professional knows best.

The emphasis of Recovery Colleges appears distinct from that of previous activities emphasizing the role of service users in researching service or social barriers in the community (Beresford 2000). Evidence from other settings suggests that, for example, promoting the capacity of people with schizophrenia to have insight into their condition may be of therapeutic benefit (van der Meer et al. 2013). In this changed approach, mutual aid is very important, together with a change in the power and role of professionals:

> Recovery is not a professional intervention, like medication or therapy, and mental health workers do not hold the key. (Repper and Perkins 2013:47)

A peer tutor said, "I wanted to give something back to the Trust, because these lovely people had been listening to my problems for so long." This individual talked about the danger of her diagnosis becoming her identity. She felt it was too easy to take on the patient role, which she described as an excuse for disengaging, to wait for others to cure her: "In the blink of an eye, I became a delinquent child." The same service user expressed the view that too little had traditionally been expected of people with mental illness, and that people could take more responsibility for themselves. She also criticized the "them and us phenomenon" she had encountered as a user of mental health services. For example, she had encountered facilities where there were separate staff toilets. She reflected, "As far as I know, mental illness can't be caught by using the same toilets." In contrast, for her, "Recovery College can help break down boundaries."

A staff tutor active in the Norfolk and Suffolk Recovery College talked about how, in her previous professional work as a modern matron, she had been told to maintain borders between the staff and service users:

> I graduated after 4 years of training providing me with theories and methods and depressing opinions about life-long disability and low expectation. But also with an expectation that I will offer only clinical advice, that I should remain boundaried and never to admit any personal lived experience—I think the expectation was that I wouldn't have any. . . . I should present myself as the perfect, healthy, expert nurse!

For example, she had been told off for sitting on the floor with patients. She had always felt uncomfortable about her own power as a professional. Despite her training as a psychiatric nurse, often she had not felt like an expert when confronted with the distress and disorder of service users' lives. In a traditional psychiatry setting, she felt care was not individualized, and there had been low expectations for the patient. She also disclosed her own lived experience of mental health issues. In contrast to her previous work, the Recovery College was inspirational for her. She talked about the benefits of working alongside peer tutors, and the partnership that had been created between professionals and service users, which she described as "magical interactions." She concluded by saying, "It's what I came into the profession for."

A key aspect of the Recovery College approach is that it recognizes that professionals themselves will possibly have experienced mental distress. For example, the Norfolk and Suffolk Recovery College has what they call a "Hidden Talents Group," mentioned earlier, where staff can discuss their own experiences of mental health issues. This openness potentially helps diminish the divide between professional expertise and the patient or service user, who traditionally is considered lacking in expertise. If both the professional and the service user have lived experience of mental distress, and if both are considered to have relevant expertise, that opens up new and more equal ways of working. The service user may have additional confidence in the professional because they have shared similar difficulties.

But there are also some dangers here. One is about the authentic voice. Professional experiences of distress are unlikely to be of the gravity or complexity of the conditions with which service users are presenting. It could be dangerous if the professional felt empowered to speak for service users rather than recognizing the importance of their voice and experiences. This requires a sensitivity and respect on the part of the professional. One service user said: "It's about how you use your lived experience in your everyday work. . . . It's not a pissing competition."

A second problem is about the focus of the professional encounter, which should always be about the needs of the service user. One professional said: "You don't want to overwhelm the person you're working with, with your own difficulties and problems." At best, the lived experiences of the professional can help build rapport, and possibly also encourage the service user to think that recovery is possible and that they, too, may be able to resume expert roles. However, the service user might lack confidence in the professional if the latter disclosed that they had experienced difficulties themselves.

> It is not the case that professionals lack expertise; rather that they do not have a monopoly on wisdom. The real challenge we face as practitioners involves placing this expertise at the disposal of those with mental health problems rather than making decisions for them. (Repper and Perkins, 2013:187)

TOJISHA KENKYU

Urakawa is a small town in Hokkaido, the most northerly island in the Japanese archipelago, home to approximately 14,000 people. Bethel House began in 1978, with four former mental hospital residents with schizophrenia, who began to live in the community, supported by two other people and a social worker, Ikuyoshi Mukaiyachi. Given the context of Japanese mental health policy, this was a very rare initiative, and few thought it could succeed. The group sought livelihood activities, such as gathering seaweed for sale, and subsequently opened a shop. From the outset, the group communicated with other residents of the town, particularly through paradoxical slogans such as: "Welcome! Prejudice and discrimination. We never criticize you"; "Meeting is more important than eating"; and "Your vulnerability is connected to fellowship, fellowship connects with strength."

Over time, the project grew and consolidated. Now there are 150 members of Bethel House, mainly people living with schizophrenia. There are 11 group homes, a factory, a farm, and two shops. People say that what they like most about living in Urakawa is fellowship:

> If we seek it, we can find rich and wealthy human relationships and fellowships inside [the] local community. Human relationships in the local area such as Urakawa have the power to care for patients suffering from mental disorders and the power to both develop and empower both patients and medical staff. (Imamura 2012:81)

People living with profound mental illness are able to be supported, and to support each other, through working together, group self-help meetings, role playing, creative work, and social activities. Urakawa hospital chief psychiatrist Toshiaki Kawamura says: "When we work together, we can face our problems, face our realities." As a service user commented, "Bethel is a place to study yourself."

The project members have made books and DVDs to communicate with others about their daily lives, and they also give lectures about their experiences. Through these various public activities, people with mental health issues campaign for greater acceptance, not by denying difficulties or vulnerabilities but by demonstrating that they have come to terms with them. For example, one of the most famous activities of the Bethel community is the Annual Delusion and Hallucination Festival each year. In this televised event, people with psychosis who have the most excellent delusion or auditory hallucination get a prize:

> What is an excellent delusion? It can be serious or strange but this is not the best part of this festival. Whether their symptoms have associations with their friends in the local community is important for them. (Imamura 2012:81)

The Urakawa approach is based on the recovery principle, which does not mean cure or remission of symptoms but rather that "patients come and live their daily lives with other citizens as citizens." Key features of the model are that service users take a leading role in their own treatment and that, conversely, health and social care staff make themselves vulnerable. In other words, a formerly hierarchical and differentiated relationship is equalized to a large degree. As Toshiaki Kawamura has said:

> It's no good if people feel better because they think we did something for them. It's no good if they think that I cured them. We're always noting that people who think "we cured them" always relapse. On the other hand, people get better the Bethel way because of everyone's help. (quoted in Nakamura 2007)

While mental health professionals support self-help group discussions and activities, service users also take a role as facilitators and take paid roles in the organization. For example, Kohei Yamane is both a Bethel member (service user) and the IT manager for the community.

Tojisha Kenkyu started in Urakawa Bethel House in February 2001 among service users, supported by social workers. The Japanese phrase "Tojisha Kenkyu" (study by tojisha [service users] themselves) refers to a unique activity of mental health service users in which they study their symptoms and everyday worries with their peers and social workers. Tojisha Kenkyu shifts mental health outside the therapeutic frame and relocates it into the research frame.

The self-study that is involved in Tojisha Kenkyu can be based on an individual or a group of individuals experiencing similar difficulties. According to Mukaiyachi (quoted in Ishihara 2015), there are five steps to the process:

1. Externalize the problem—as opposed to introspection, problems are brought out into the open. For example, a problem might be auditory hallucinations.
2. Give a name (*jiko byomei*) to the problem, such as "schizophrenia thought broadcasting type" or "allergy to humans and addiction to evaluation by others."
3. Elucidate the problem or symptoms through pictures or role playing.
4. Devise a way of helping the individual, and rehearse the technique.
5. Evaluate the research process, and highlight the good and bad aspects of it, to learn lessons for other people and future research.

Tojisha Kenkyu has now spread beyond people affected by schizophrenia to include people with other mental health conditions, addictions, developmental disorders, cerebral palsy, and other afflictions.

Tojisha Kenkyu is thus a form of mutual aid, in which peers work with a person to understand the mental health symptoms and devise ways of living more successfully with the condition or modifying their attitudes toward their problems. The philosophy does not reject the insights of psychiatry—for example, diagnostic labels—but adapts these concepts for personal use, finding innovative strategies for self-help or peer support. As Ishihara writes, "Professionals are authorities on medical diagnosis and medical treatment, but not on difficulty and the troubles accompanying medical diseases" (Ishihara 2015).

Yet service users are not quite experts either. The motto of the Japanese disability movement (Tojisha Undo) is "we know what we need; we decide what service should be provided," which parallels the global disability rights motto, "nothing about us without us." However, Tojisha Kenkyu assumes that service users do not know themselves well and need to study themselves. As Ishihara (2015) notes, "the *kenkyu*-attitude could make patients capable of addressing their own problems." Thus, the theme of Tojisha Kenkyu is that "We don't know ourselves well. We ask ourselves who we are, what we will do, together with peers" (Kumagaya 2013, quoted by Ishihara 2015).

In Tojisha Kenkyu, service users are exploring their experiences, and connecting to peers, supported by professionals. The British audience who heard about the Japanese approach thought it more radical—one commented that it had the spirit of "punk rock"—compared to the British Recovery College approach, which operated within the context and confines of the National Health Service, although there is a sense in which the recovery movement could be seen as a new social movement, straddling both the NHS and the community (Smith-Merry and Sturdy 2013). Conversely, while the Urakawa community and the other Tojisha Kenkyu groups are islands of progressive practice amid the very traditional Japanese mental health services, there are also signs that the psychiatry profession in Japan is beginning to learn from and be influenced by these innovations (Ishihara 2015).

IMPLICATIONS FOR THE HUMAN SERVICE RELATIONSHIP

Generally speaking, mental health conditions entail disruption to autonomy. A person with manic depression, schizophrenia, or another form of profound mental illness may have their capacity to make decisions questioned or removed. They may be subject to involuntary confinement or compulsory treatment. For this reason, mental health user movements have emphasized regaining control. Second, mental health conditions have been viewed as person-defining, as incurable and incapacitating. Therefore, it has been vital within the recovery model to emphasize hope and the potential for people with mental illness to lead a good and productive life, albeit with intermittent episodes of mental ill health.

Whereas Tojisha Kenkyu relocates from a therapeutic to a research frame of reference, Recovery Colleges adopt an educational frame of reference. In both cases, the more hierarchical and medicalized relationship between professional and patient is reformed into a more equalized staff tutor/peer tutor model. This relies on a twofold movement: emphasizing the vulnerability of the professional and valuing the strengths of the service user. While these initiatives may both appear very positive, it is important also to consider some challenges.

Some service users will not want greater involvement in their own treatment or recovery process (Lammers and Happell 2003; McCann et al. 2008; Tebeanu and Macarie 2013). Because of either their socialization or their basic attitude toward their illness, they will expect and desire a mental health professional who can take charge, treat them as a patient, and help them emerge recovered. They may not want to take responsibility for their own care or to participate in user groups. For example, one London study found that those participating in user involvement activities were not typical of the wider patient group (Rutter et al. 2004). It has been suggested that people who are more educated and empowered to begin with are more likely to want to participate in recovery activities. Correspondingly, people with more severe symptoms may be less likely to participate and take control of their recovery (Lammers and Happell 2003).

The peer support role is a complex one. The consumer/advocate may find that he or she has "crossed over to the other side" when operating as part of a professional staff team and may now have to act professionally or have boundaries. There may be a lack of role clarity. Adequate training and supervision is vital (Kemp and Henderson 2012). Conversely, staff may have concerns about confidentiality of other service users, or about the mental health needs of the peer support workers themselves. It can be very demanding to be a peer support worker, and some people who express initial enthusiasm may drop out (Gillard et al. 2013). There are tensions both for staff and for peer support workers.

Mental health user movements have sometimes been keen to devalue professional knowledge and to establish equality between the expert and the service user. However, while a more equal and participative relationship is preferable when developing mental health policies, this is not necessarily always desirable within mental health treatment. From the professional point of view, the notion of professionals disclosing their own vulnerabilities could also be questioned. Arguably, personal experience is not relevant to treatment, and to make it central undermines the professional expertise of the mental health professional, as if to say that their training and research background are less relevant than any symptoms they may have personally experienced. The therapeutic stance depends on having a structured relationship, with clear boundaries. There may be a need to maintain the differentiation in status and expertise between the patient and their therapist; for example, psychodynamic psychotherapy depends on the transference between client and therapist. From the point of view of the service user or patient, they may not want to hear about the mental health conditions that their therapist has personally experienced. Some patients may be very anxious about boundary violations and value a strong framework.

Even within recovery and self-help activities, professionals retain an important role. The availability of professional support can be reassuring to peers running self-help groups, particularly when the illness of key individuals means that the self-help process is in danger of collapse; backup when needed is essential (Lammers and Happell 2003). The recovery movement is not a rejection of psychiatry, medication, or even inpatient care. Having service users and professionals working together is usually the preferred and most beneficial model. For example, self-management approaches might involve a service user and a professional working together to develop a crisis plan for when things go wrong with the user's mental health. This suggests the professional role as "companion or fellow traveller rather than as expert" (Davidson 2005:32). Equally, research has found that dialogue between consumers and providers, where both sides can acknowledge and tell stories of vulnerabilities, can lead to greater understanding and transformation (Schwartz et al. 2013).

Recovery could be seen as simply a fashion in mental health care (Pilgrim, 2009; Tickle, Brown, and Hayward 2014), adopted in a superficial or limited way, with no deep understanding or genuine commitment from professionals (see Eriksson and Jacobsson, Chapter 13, this volume). There is also a danger of tokenism, if and when the recovery or Tojisha Kenkyu models become more widely adopted (El Enany, Currie, and Lockett 2013; Tait and Lester 2005). If a directive arrives from the top, it may be that some minimal participation of service users is adopted, to satisfy the new trend, but genuine participation is not achieved (Lammers and Happell 2003; Soffe, Read, and Frude 2004). Mental health experts may continue to believe that service users do not have anything meaningful to contribute (Slade et al. 2014; Shepherd, Shorthouse, and Gask 2014; see also Järvinen, Chapter 3, this volume). This may be the case particularly when service users are included as members of management and planning structures, where a sole user voice is outnumbered by professional and policymaker expertise (Rutter et al. 2004).

Professionals may hold supportive views but practice in more traditional ways (Summers 2003; Soffe, Read, and Frude 2004). They may be pessimistic or defensive with regard to service user involvement (Shepherd, Shorthouse, and Gask 2014). It may be difficult to express negative views, given the general consensus regarding the value of service user involvement. While the majority of respondents in one study were optimistic about the benefits of service user involvement, a smaller group were "rationalist" (looking for specific, limited contributions), while the remainder were skeptical (Summers 2003). One study found that mental health nurses were feeling disempowered themselves, which made them more hostile to user involvement (Rutter et al. 2004).

Key to both Tojisha Kenkyu and Recovery Colleges is the notion of partnership, with the service user determining their course of action, in conjunction with professionals. Partnership is based around communication and cooperation. This has to start with a commitment to hearing the voice of the service user. Recovery means the professional letting go and allowing the service user to have more control. This brings with it the risk of tragic outcomes for the service user, such as self-harm or suicide, or becoming a victim or perpetrator of violence (Thornicroft and Tansella 2005;

Schwartz et al. 2013). However, the majority of people with mental health issues are not at such risk. The presumption should be that individuals are not at risk (see Grenier and Flood, Chapter 10, this volume). As with everyone, these individuals are innocent unless proven otherwise (Davidson et al. 2006:644).

If recovery is defined as learning to live with mental illness and working to achieve civil rights and community participation, rather than as a clinical recovery or cure (Pilgrim 2009), then this implies that persons affected by mental distress have experiences that parallel other persons with disabilities (Davidson et al. 2006), and that the role of the professional is to offer support and advice rather than to provide a heroic cure. This approach brings psychiatry into line with other specialties that support people with chronic health conditions (see Solvang, Chapter 7, this volume). The question becomes: how can people with mental distress live in the community, participate in society, earn a living, and be protected against discrimination? People with mental health conditions are among the final group of people with disabilities to experience this emancipation. Psychiatric expertise may be less relevant in this struggle than the skill sets of social workers and community activists. Mechanisms such as Recovery Colleges and Tojisha Kenkyu should be understood not primarily in terms of symptom control but as part of the process of transferring power from professionals to people who experience mental distress and disabling barriers. As Kiyoshi Hayasaki, one of the founding members of Bethel, has said:

> In the past, people with psychiatric disabilities would have been seen as out of the ordinary. But I think people with psychiatric disabilities are gold. (quoted in Nakamura 2007)

REFERENCES

Ando, S., and G. Thornicroft. 2012. "Attitudes to Mental Illness in Japan and Britain." In *Mental Health Care in Japan*, edited by R. Taplin and S. J. Lawman, 112–123. London: Routledge.

Beresford, P. 2000. "Service Users' Knowledges and Social Work Theory: Conflict or Collaboration?" *British Journal of Social Work* 30:489–503.

Crossley, M. L., and N. Crossley. 2001. "'Patient' Voices, Social Movements and the Habitus; How Psychiatric Survivors 'Speak Out.'" *Social Science and Medicine* 52:1477–1489.

Crowe, S., 2011. "The Case Study Approach." *BMC Medical Research Methodology* 11:100.

Davidson L. 2005. "Recovery, Self Management and the Expert Patient—Changing the Culture of Mental Health from a UK Perspective." *Journal of Mental Health* 14:25–35.

Davidson, L., M. O'Connell, J. Tondora, T. Styron, and K. Kangas. 2006. "The Top Ten Concerns About Recovery Encountered in Mental Health System Transformation." *Psychiatric Services* 57(5): 640–645.

Denzin, N. 2006. *Sociological Methods*. New Brunswick, NJ: Aldine Transaction.

Department of Health [UK]. 1991. "The Patient's Charter." London: Her Majesty's Stationery Office.

Department of Health [UK]. 2001. "The Expert Patient: A New Approach to Chronic Disease Management in the 21st Century." London: Her Majesty's Stationery Office.

Department of Health [UK]. 2010. "Equity and Excellence: Liberating the NHS." London: Her Majesty's Stationery Office.

Dooher J., and L. Rye. 2013. "The Impact of Cuts on Mental Health Services: Good Mental Health in Leicester?" *Mental Health Nursing* 33(6): 1–4.

El Enany, N., G. Currie, and A. Lockett. 2013. "A Paradox in Healthcare Service Development: Professionalization of Service Users." *Social Science and Medicine* 80:24–30.

Faulkner, A., and J. Kalathil. 2012. "The Freedom to Be, the Chance to Dream: Preserving User-Led Support in Mental Health." Together for Mental Wellbeing website. http://www.together-uk.org/wp-content/uploads/2012/09/The-Freedom-to-be-The-Chance-to-dream-Full-Report1.pdf. Accessed January 1, 2015.

Gillard, S. G., C. Edwards, S. L. Gibson, K. Owen, and C. Wright. 2013. "Introducing Peer Worker Roles into UK Mental Health Service Teams: A Qualitative Analysis of the Organisational Benefits and Challenges." *BMC Health Services Research* 13:188.

Imamura, I. 2012. "How Mental Hospitals Treat Their Patients." In *Mental Health Care in Japan*, edited by R. Taplin and S. J. Lawman, 73–82. London: Routledge.

Ishihara, K. 2015. "Learning from *Tojisha Kenkyu*: Mental Health 'Patients' Studying Their Difficulties with Their Peers." In *Disability Research Today: International Perspectives*, edited by T. Shakespeare, 27–42. London: Routledge.

Ito, H. 2012. "Mental Health Policy and Services: Where We Stand." In *Mental Health Care in Japan*, edited by R. Taplin R and S. J. Lawman, 36–56. London: Routledge.

Kemp, V., and A. R. Henderson. 2012. "Challenges Faced by Mental Health Peer Support Workers: Peer Support from the Peer Supporter's Point of View." *Psychiatric Rehabilitation Journal* 35(4): 337–340.

Kumagaya, S. 2013. "Itami kara Hajimeru Tojisha Kenkyu." In *Tojisha Kenkyu no Kenkyu*, edited by K. Ishihara, 217–280. Tokyo: Igakushoin.

Lammers, J., and B. Happell. 2003. "Consumer Participation in Mental Health Services: Looking from a Consumer Perspective." *Journal of Psychiatric and Mental Health Nursing* 10:385–392.

Lawman, S. J. 2012. "An Overview of the User Movement in Japan and Britain." In *Mental Health Care in Japan*, edited by R. Taplin and S. J. Lawman, 98–112. London: Routledge.

Lomas, J. 1997. "Reluctant Rationers: Public Input to Health Care Priorities." *Journal of Health Services Research & Policy* 2:103–111.

McCann, T. V., J. Baird, E. Clark, and S. Lu. 2008. "Mental Health Professionals Attitudes Towards Consumer Participation in Inpatient Units." *Journal of Psychiatric and Mental Health Nursing* 15:10–16.

Nakamura, K. 2007. *Bethel: Community and Schizophrenia in Northern Japan* (film). New Haven, CT: Department of Anthropology, Yale University.

Pilgrim, D. 2009. "Recovery from Mental Health Problems: Scratching the Surface Without Ethnography." *Journal of Social Work Practice: Psychotherapeutic Approaches in Health, Welfare and the Community* 23(4): 475–487.

Repper, J., and T. Carter. 2011. "A Review of the Literature on Peer Support in Mental Health Services." *Journal of Mental Health* 20(4): 392–411.

Repper, J., and R. Perkins. 2013. *Social Inclusion and Recovery: A Model for Mental Health Practice*. Edinburgh: Ballière Tindall.

Rush, B. 2004. "Mental Health Service User Involvement in England: Lessons from History." *Journal of Psychiatric Mental Health Nursing* 11:313–318.

Rutter, D., C. Manley, T. Weaver, M. J. Crawford, and N. Fulop. 2004. "Patients or Partners? Case Studies of User Involvement in the Planning and Delivery of Adult Mental Health Services in London." *Social Science and Medicine* 58:1973–1984.

Schwartz, R., O. Estein, J. Komaroff, J. Lamb, M. Myers, J. Stewart, L. Vacaflor, and M. Park. 2013. "Mental Health Consumers and Providers Dialogue in an Institutional Setting: A Participatory Approach to Promoting Recovery-Oriented Care." *Psychiatric Rehabilitation Journal* 36(2): 113–115.

Shepherd, A., O. Shorthouse, and L. Gask. 2014. "Consultant Psychiatrists' Experience of and Attitudes Towards Shared Decision Making in Antipsychotic Prescribing, a Qualitative Study. *BMC Psychiatry* 14:127–137.

Shepherd, G., J. Boardman, and M. Slade. 2008. *Making Recovery a Reality*. London: Sainsbury Centre for Mental Health.

Slade, M., M. Amering, M. Farkas, B. Hamilton, M. O'Hagan, G. Panther, R. Perkins, G. Shepherd, S. Tse, and R. Whitley. 2014. "Uses and Abuses of Recovery: Implementing Recovery-Oriented Practices in Mental Health Systems." *World Psychiatry* 13:12–20.

Smith-Merry, J., and S. Sturdy. 2013. "Recovery in Scotland: The Rise and Uncertain Future of a Mental Health Social Movement. *Society and Mental Health* 3(2): 114–132.

Soffe, J., J. Read, and N. Frude. 2004. "A Survey of Clinical Psychologists' Views Regarding Service User Involvement in Mental Health Services." *Journal of Mental Health* 13(6): 583–592.

Summers, A. 2003. "Involving Users in the Development of Mental Health Services: A Study of Psychiatrists' Views." *Journal of Mental Health* 12(2): 161–174.

Tait, L., and H. Lester. 2005. "Encouraging User Involvement in Mental Health Services." *Advances in Psychiatric Treatment* 11:168–175.

Taplin, R., and S. J. Lawman, eds. 2012. *Mental Health Care in Japan*. London: Routledge.

Tebeanu, A. V., and G. F. Macarie. 2013. "The Role of Education in Mental Health: Considerations of Professionals from a Psychiatric Clinic Regarding Its Implications in the Process of Community Integration for Former Patients." *Procedia—Social and Behavioural Sciences* 76:827–831.

Thornicroft G., and M. Tansella. 2005. "Growing Recognition of the Importance of Service User Involvement in Mental Health Service Planning and Evaluation." *Epidemiologia e Psichiatria Sociale* 14:1–3.

Tickle, A., D. Brown, and M. Hayward. 2014. "Can We Risk Recovery? A Grounded Theory of Clinical Psychologists' Perceptions of Risk and Recovery-Oriented Mental Health Services." *Psychology and Psychotherapy: Theory, Research and Practice* 87:96–110.

van der Meer, L., A. E. de Vos, A. P. M. Stiekema, G. H. M. Pijnenborg, M.-J. van Tol, W. A. Nolen, A. S. David, and A. Aleman. 2013. "Insight in Schizophrenia: Involvement of Self-Reflection Networks?" *Schizophrenia Bulletin* 39(6): 1288–1295.

Wallcraft, J., M. Amering, and J. Freidin et al. 2011. "Partnerships for Better Mental Health Worldwide: WPA Recommendations on Best Practices in Working with Service Users and Family Carers." *World Psychiatry* 10:229–36.

Wallcraft, J., and M. Bryant. 2003. "The Mental Health Service User Movement in England." The Sainsbury Centre for Mental Health Policy paper 2. London: Sainsbury Centre for Mental Health.

13

Tension and Balance in Teaching "The Patient Perspective" to Mental Health Professionals

▸ ERIK ERIKSSON AND KATARINA JACOBSSON

KNOWLEDGE TO GAIN! *Service User Involvement for Better Psychiatric Care* is the (translated) title of a Swedish book claiming that people with mental illness and their families have a unique, albeit overlooked, knowledge of care (Nordén 2008). From this perspective, patients are considered a resource for the renewal and development of welfare organizations, while professionals are encouraged to give up "old ways of working and thinking." The book describes a trend in which patients are regarded as "experts by experience" and professionals endeavor to learn from them.

In recent decades, the concept of "service user involvement" has grown increasingly popular in the political discourse and welfare practices of Western countries (Braye 2000; Branfield et al. 2006), including Sweden (Hultqvist 2008). Academic knowledge as the sole basis for practice is questioned, with some authors proposing that professional authority is outdated and must be adjusted to incorporate the service user's expertise (e.g., Glasby and Beresford 2006; Ferguson and Ager 2008; see also Alm Andreassen, Chapter 2, this volume). Patient organizations are now invited to participate in service planning within mental health care (e.g., Rutter et al. 2004; Tait and Lester 2005)—a great departure from the history of patient organizations advocating patients' rights from the outside, sometimes confrontationally (e.g., Forbes and Sashidharan 1997; Peck, Gulliver, and Towel 2002).

Influenced by the international psychiatric community and by demands from the service user movement, in 2006, the Swedish government published an official report emphasizing the importance of increasing patient influence within psychiatric care in Sweden (SOU 2006). This declaration was followed by a series of governmental requests for service user participation in policymaking at both the national and local levels (see Shakespeare and Collins, Chapter 12, this volume). In 2010, one of Sweden's largest regional psychiatric organizations—here called the Public Psychiatric Organization (PPO)—responded by announcing the need for service user involvement at all levels. To enact this new policy, a trained social worker was recruited from a nonprofit service user organization to act as an "involvement coordinator."

Over the following years, the involvement coordinator led the head office to initiate a variety of service user activities—some aimed at increasing patient involvement at the policymaking level (e.g., service user councils) and in other activities intended to influence staff members to work in a patient-centered manner. For the latter purpose, patients and former patients were invited to receive training for various assignments. For instance, a course was offered to train "attitude ambassadors" to combat negative attitudes toward people with psychiatric illnesses. One program specifically trained individuals to relate their personal experiences to staff during meetings and similar gatherings (Eriksson 2013), while another course trained patients and former patients as educators to teach "the patient perspective" in an in-house training program called the Increased Dialogue Initiative (IDI).

In this chapter,[1] we examine the IDI program to explore how the concept of service user involvement is realized in a local context within one of Sweden's public mental health care organizations (PPO). This organization has facilities throughout the area and provides care across the spectrum of mental health to both adults and minors. It employs approximately 3,000 people.

The material selected for the present analysis is part of a larger body of information compiled as part of independent doctoral research that is not tied to the PPO or IDI (Eriksson 2015). The total material includes observations of activities during fieldwork related to many user-involvement initiatives, including the IDI program. The data extracted for the present analysis mainly consist of interviews with project managers, field notes from the IDI training program, and field notes from an evaluation day during which all service user educators met with project managers after the first round of the program.[2] In addition to the two project managers, nine educators and 22 staff participants were present during the fieldwork. The analysis is most strongly focused on the project leaders, who played an important role in the evolution of the IDI program, and two educators who were part of the program that was most closely followed by the researcher.

In this particular setting, service user involvement was created through interplay between project managers, patients-as-educators, and staff-as-students. In analyzing the training sessions along with the recruitment process and subsequent efforts to revise the program, we hope to identify the discursive frames within which the IDI program takes place. Hence, the analysis is guided by the following questions: Who is recruited to become an educator? How are the traditional relationships between patients and professionals challenged or preserved? What future tendencies may be traced by examining the chosen direction for IDI program development?

IDI ORGANIZATION

The IDI is organized so that staff training is run solely by current or former psychiatric patients. All clinical staff are invited. Over the course of four two-hour sessions in the classroom, two patients act as educators and experts—teaching "the patient perspective" to a group of about ten mental health professionals, mainly mental health nurses, assistants, and social workers. Among the observed IDI sessions, only two participants were in management positions, and no psychiatrists or psychologists were in attendance.

Two project managers have been integral to the program design and coordination. Peter, the "involvement coordinator," is employed full-time at the head office and coordinates all user-involvement activities within PPO. He was recruited from a national organization of service users and has no personal experience with mental health issues. The second project manager, Anna, is a teacher by training and has a history as a psychiatric patient. She is employed part-time and works with the IDI program. Other patients and former patients were also involved in program development.

A core idea of the training is to reverse the relationship between staff and patients. In opposition to the traditional view of patients as passive recipients of care, here patients are viewed as knowledgeable subjects and equal partners, with as much expertise as the professionals. PPO highly values the notion that service users have much to offer mental health staff by sharing their experiences of psychiatric care (e.g., Balen, Rhodes, and Ward 2010; Hayward et al. 2005) and thus holds more or less explicit expectations of efforts to implement service user involvement. Staff members who complete the IDI program are expected to return to their daily work with a new—and better—attitude toward the patients. Ultimately, it is hoped that the IDI will alter the staff–patient relationship to align it with the service user's conceptualizations of good-quality care, with the overall intention that patients should become "involved partners" in their daily care. The project managers guide the development of content and teaching methods in accordance with these goals, and with the aim of conveying both the need for recovery-oriented work based on a "patient's perspective" and that psychiatric care may actually help. For this purpose, the patients' own stories are important, particularly when emphasizing the central theme of the patient's "turning point"—meaning when the patient started to feel better (Eriksson 2013). The educators are trained to draw on and convey their individual experiences, without speaking as representatives of their patient organizations (cf. Barnes 1999:79).

In addition to sharing their personal stories, the educators initiate and lead "valuation exercises." In these exercises, the educators ask the group questions such as "Do you think patients and staff are equal at your workplace?" and "If you were a patient [and not a staff member], would you like the idea of being treated at the ward where you work?" The participants are instructed to answer the questions by leaving their chairs and moving themselves to various areas of the room to visualize different responses. For example, the left corner of the room may symbolize "yes," the right corner "no," and so on. In other cases, the instructor may draw an imaginary line across the room and tell the participants that one end represents 100 percent and the other end zero, and that they should position themselves along the line to illustrate the extent to which they agree with a certain statement. The educators also lead seminar-like discussions and facilitate conversations regarding suggestions for improving patient care and increasing user involvement.

The IDI is coordinated and marketed from PPO's head office, and local care units are solicited to "purchase" the training program for their staff members. The purchaser (i.e., the local care unit) is expected to provide a venue at the local site and to arrange for coffee to be served at each IDI session. The head office pays the educators' wages. These wages are deemed important both because of the educator's investment of time in teaching the program and as a signifier of educator value, in accordance with research on service user involvement (e.g., Rutter et al. 2004; Beresford 2013).

Our observations indicated that local units do not always honor the manager's efforts to enhance the status of patient-led training. The venue provided for training can sometimes hamper a professional impression of the program. For instance, the allocated rooms were often different for all four training occasions, and were in many cases inappropriate—too small, partly used for storage, remotely located in the basement, and so on. One IDI educator testified that "on one occasion there was no room booked, so we had to run the session among the patients in the dayroom at the ward." Coffee was seldom provided. In one case, two participants (i.e., staff members) arranged coffee for the group at the final gathering.

We also noted that the educators did not seem entirely comfortable with their new position at the hospital. In many cases, the "patient" identity seemed to overshadow the "paid educator" identity. For example, in one instance when the classroom key was to be picked up at the hospital reception desk, one of the educators waited in the long patient line instead of immediately announcing her need as an educator.

The IDI program that we followed most closely—with Sara and John as educators—was later considered particularly successful. After the last session, the participants brought Sara and John bouquets of flowers to thank them. During the same period, five other IDI programs were administered in other parts of PPO. Some of these programs were harshly criticized by participants, who made comments such as "What's the point?" and "Lack of structure!" Moreover, some patients had such bad experiences in their first attempts as IDI educators that they declined further engagement. During the following semester, PPO initiated an additional 10 to 15 revised training programs. We will discuss the revisions that were made to the program following our analysis of the recruitment process, and how the educators managed to convey "the patient perspective."

SELECTING AND DIRECTING THE SERVICE USER EDUCATOR

Not every expert by experience was accepted as an IDI educator. All selected patients were trained, but to be considered at all, they had to apply and to be approved. The project managers already knew several of the candidates. One of the project managers, Peter, is engaged in PPO's overall administration of service user activities. His colleague Anna explained that "Peter already had a pool, so to speak, with attitude ambassadors[3] and informants. So, we had them to choose from." In addition to the already known service users, IDI educators were also recruited from patient organizations.

The candidates had to meet certain requirements. During an interview, the researcher asked project manager Anna what those requirements were. She answered:

> That they had personal experience [of mental illness]; that they had reflected on it all. That even if it had been like crap when they were in care, they're still able to reflect a little: What was the reason? Why was that? What was my part in it? How might I have interpreted it? That you have a healthy mindset around it; that you're not out on some kind of rampage for revenge.

To detect and dismiss applicants who were "out for revenge," all candidates had to complete a form that asked about their "strengths and weaknesses" and their motives for becoming IDI educators. During the recruitment process, suitable candidates are chosen and thereby become *selected* experts by experience. As odd as it may seem, the requirement to "think healthy" about one's experiences of mental illness and psychiatric care was deemed vital for legitimacy. In this case, "thinking healthy" means that the candidate educator must not be unreasonably upset about the care they received and should be able to acknowledge that part of the care experience can be attributed to the patient. Educators must not be too harsh in their critiques, as this would likely thwart the aim of generating dialogue—a view that is in line with some psychological literature (e.g., Hayward et al. 2005).

Once selected as suitable educators, the recruits are trained. This training is administered by the project manager, Anna, and consists of four sessions, in which the recruits learn the IDI concept and receive instruction in "telling your story." It is widely acknowledged that patients practicing service user involvement might require training to participate adequately (e.g., Branfield et al. 2006; Rea 2004). In some instances, this training may focus on helping representatives to advocate for patient organizations (e.g., Alm Andreassen, Breit, and Legard 2014). In the presently described case, the training was more focused on promoting the thinking of the Public

Psychiatric Organization (PPO) and on directing performance (Eriksson 2013). There was a perceived need to model the narrative of the patient's experience (cf. Marvasti 2002). Anna describes these efforts:

> And we've tried to, well, limit the story, to put it simply. Because there's so much to tell, but you have to choose a little to tell, plus you have to think about what tone you use. Because getting out there and having an accusatory style, you'll kind of lose the staff at once. Then they won't listen. At the same time, one must also be allowed to talk about what has actually been bad. But naturally to emphasize what has been good!

Furthermore, all the educators receive an identical manual (called "The Folder" or, in Swedish, "Pärmen") to follow when executing the IDI training program. The Folder constitutes a binder with an index containing the structure of the training, tips regarding how to be a leader, facts to be used as background information, and various exercises for the staff participants. The Folder guides the educators on how to act and what to say—with an orientation toward user involvement as stipulated by public policy and administration. Through this selection and training, "the patient perspective" is carved out with regard to content, form, and style. A more suitable description of the "experts by experience" concept would be "selected experts by guided experience." However, in practice, we find that the educators do not follow The Folder to the letter.

SWITCHING BETWEEN SCRIPTED AND NARRATIVE PERFORMANCES

The IDI program that we followed most closely was taught by Sara and John, two former patients. Sara has been in and out of psychiatric care over many years, and John has personal experiences with PPO as both a patient and as a patient's family member. Throughout the program, Sara and John taught the patient perspective by alternating between two different methods of teaching performance: narrative performance and scripted performance. Here we use the term "performance" to describe the teaching occasion, including the audience's responses and coconstruction of the event (Hall and Matarese 2014; Riessman 2013:176ff.). Narrative performance refers to when educators frame their experiences and opinions as a story. This style was balanced with scripted performance, which more closely resembles "formal" teaching. Scripted performance refers to when educators explicitly use material (exercises, wordings, idioms, etc.) from The Folder and do and say things specifically from their training. Another characteristic feature of the two performance styles lies in the staff participants' responses to these different teaching formats: they are students during formal teaching and attentive listeners when stories are told, thus coconstructing the occasion.

The labels "scripted" and "narrative" denote different styles of teaching the patient perspective, as more or less instructed by the project managers. However, we are not suggesting that the two styles are entirely different from each other. Scripted performance is not exclusively dictated, and storytelling includes some organizational constraints—in fact, the educators' stories are as organizationally embedded as the formal teaching. In the words of Jaber Gubrium and James Holstein (Gubrium and Holstein 2009:174), "the big story" of PPO—emphasizing recovery through psychiatric care—sets the narrative agenda for the educators' own (little) stories.

Handling "The Folder"

The educators performed various tasks that were similar to formal teaching, including sharing "facts," initiating discussions with the participants, and leading various exercises. In turn, the participants played the role of students by taking notes, raising their hands, and asking questions at appropriate times. However, despite the educators' training and access to The Folder, scripted performance was often rather difficult or awkward for all parties involved compared with the ease and authority with which educators told their stories.

Consider the following extract from the field notes regarding an instance during which Sara and John led the participants through a "valuation exercise" to facilitate reflections and discussions on psychiatric care. One corner of the room was marked as a space for the answer "yes" and another corner for "no," with the space between the corners representing an "either-or" answer. The participants were instructed to physically move to the space that symbolized their answers to a given question. As stated in The Folder, Sara emphasized that there were no right or wrong answers and that the participants could change positions during the discussion. However, at the same time, The Folder is quite clear about what the "right" message is—what

Sara as an educator is supposed to convey to the participants. This situation presents the challenging task of leading the discussion in a certain direction, making sure the group ends up with opinions that are less prejudiced. As the following reconstruction from field notes indicates, Sara seemed to be stressed by the task:

> Sara rapidly moves on to the next question, reading directly from The Folder: "Do you feel that there are structures at your workplaces that could be stigmatizing for the patients?" People start walking towards "no" but they have only just started to move before Sara poses the next question from The Folder. One of the participants (a social worker in a management position) interrupts, saying: "But wait! I barely had time to think!" Thoughtfully she moves towards the space for "yes," declaring that there might actually be such structures. Other participants get involved in the topic and a discussion evolves.

We observed that the educators struggled to lead the valuation exercise, often failing to establish themselves as leaders, experts, and educators. Instead, as in the preceding example, it was common for one of the participants to gain control and steer the situation away from complete failure. The desired reversal of relationship—where the patients are meant to be the experts—is contested when the staff participants resume the role as the "true experts." Still, it is noteworthy that the "takeovers" often happened in subtle and implicit ways, such that the intended purpose was still achieved. In the preceding example, the participants started to discuss the meaning of "structure" and, toward the end, several more people joined the social worker closer to "yes."

Storytelling

When the educators engage in telling their own personal stories, the situation shifts dramatically, with the educators speaking more freely as they depart from the exercises and statements stipulated in The Folder. The practice of inviting service users to tell their stories has become institutionalized within the psychiatric organization—now constituting a regular feature on a number of occasions. Consequently, there is no need for an elaborated story preface in order to "create an agreement to talk for an extended period without an interruption" (Hall and Matarese 2014:85). In this example, reconstructed from field notes, Sara gets away with providing a rather blunt story preface:

> After the valuation exercise, Sara says without further explanation: "Now it's time for me to tell my story." She starts off by saying that today she feels fine and that she is in love with life again. Sara reads from her personal notes. She sounds insecure with a forced tone to her voice. But quite soon she stops using her notes, and with self-confidence she describes her first contacts with PPO. She tells about her brother's sudden death, and when she cut herself for the first time using a kitchen knife. The participants are silent, attentively listening to Sara without interruptions.

In this instance, Sara's story continued for about 20 minutes. Some passages are quite terrifying. She describes abuse in her home when she was a child, severe self-harm, and her subsequent experience of downright malpractice from psychiatric staff. The participants shake their heads in dismay, they sigh or gasp to signal what they find horrifying, and they make other confirming sounds to show their regret and support for Sara. The researcher wrote the following field notes:

> The atmosphere changes during Sara's narrative. Now everybody is attentive, and the vague feeling of puzzlement, the nervousness and unease from the earlier valuation exercise, disappear and are replaced by what seems like genuine interest. . . . When Sara falls silent, I feel deeply affected by her intense and intimate account. The other participants seem to feel equally shaken. Nobody moves, or says anything. Some nod slowly and thoughtfully. "Do you have any questions?" Sara finally asks. "Or, is it time for a break?" John says that a break is scheduled, but if anyone has any questions or thoughts, perhaps it's best to raise them right away.

At this point, the participants immediately asked Sara for additional details, and about what kind of care she believed would have helped her to avoid such a prolonged recovery. Then they asked for her opinion on common (negative) ideas about inpatient mental health care, psychiatric diagnoses, and much more. The planned coffee break was apparently forgotten.

Our observations suggest that when the educators shift to personal stories, they gain the participants' full attention and stand out as experts, in contrast to during their less convincing scripted performance. It is reasonable to believe that experience will lead to improvements in the educators' skills and competencies in both telling their stories and handling The Folder. Still, it seems that the specific educational situation itself is crucial for evoking respect for the service user's story and ascribed expertise. During another IDI program, Mary and Eva (two participants) discussed why they appreciate the educators' stories so much when they have heard numerous stories over the years in their capacities as mental health professionals. "What is the difference?" they asked themselves. "The tables are kind of turned here," said Mary. Eva agreed and continued, "Perhaps it's because you don't keep thinking about what to ask and how to help. You have the opportunity to just listen and think about what is said."

The narrative frame is also used for purposes beyond the sharing of experiences of living with mental illness. Educators also switch to storytelling when they shift their focus to offering tips for how staff can be more humane, so to speak. Their suggestions for humane patient treatment are generally rather modest, along the lines of "seeing the person—not just a patient." Sara gave a number of examples, including being served a cup of one's favorite tea, even though the kitchen is closed for the night, and having the bedsheets folded in a particular way because the staff knows a patient's preferences. In this situation, each example is framed in a storytelling manner that begins with a "story preface" (Hall and Matarese 2014), such as "I remember once when . . ." or "Let me tell you about a friend of mine. . . ."

Educators may also tell a story of an unpleasant experience of care (e.g., being put in restraints by five rough men laughing scornfully) and contrast it with a good story (e.g., staff staying while a patient is restrained and holding the patient's hands). The stories can trigger discussions about the importance of "seeing the person behind the patient." The participants make a number of suggestions, including that it might be a good idea to put off reading a patient's records before meeting with the patient, in order to preclude preconceived ideas.

A lively discussion ensued after an educator's story on "the right to be different," with staff participants expressing rather radical views on psychiatric diagnoses—for instance, regarding the desire to avoid medicating a patient with harmless delusions. During such discussions, the participants also share stories, including sad stories about patients they have met who were mistreated "by the system." The most common stories shared by participants relate the difficulties in "doing a good job" (i.e., having a patient-centered approach) because of the rules and regulations. The audience generally expresses signs of sympathy while listening to these accounts.

Questioning "The Folder"

Our data showed that experiences, opinions, and principles presented in the form of a personal story seemed to generate engaging responses from the participants, whereas educators' formal teaching often led to abrupt and awkward situations (sometimes rescued by the participants). Educators were generally careful to follow the manual, but they sometimes seemed to disagree with or resist its doctrine. For instance, PPO emphasizes the necessity of involving a patient's family, but one educator strongly advised against this with reference to his own negative experiences. This case demonstrates how educators can question prescribed guidelines of the IDI program by using the equally legitimate narrative form. In another example, one educator ridiculed what he claimed was required reading in The Folder, reciting it loudly with a dramatic and ironic voice. On another occasion, as field notes convey, the very term "service user" was contested:

> John reads a question for the valuation exercise from The Folder: "How would you feel about having a former service user as a colleague?" In fact, he comments, he doesn't really like the term "service user." He uses it only because it is the word used in The Folder. He says: "It sounds like a bureaucratic invention." Sara says that she agrees, and some of the participants do as well. "Perhaps we should decide to use the term patients then," John says.

This skepticism, shared by the IDI participants, is not unique. The disability movement has stated that "service user" is a stigmatizing designation that re-creates subordination (see Gubrium, Chapter 1, this volume). In Sweden, the term "service-user" was adopted with the aim of avoiding stigmatization and suggesting extended agency (e.g., Möller 1996), but it has been criticized by researchers as implying unrealistic freedom of choice (Järvinen 2002; McLaughlin 2009; Jacobsson, Thelander, and Wästerfors 2010). Within Swedish psychiatric care, the term "patient" is still commonly used in everyday language, while "service-user" is a term stemming more from the policy vocabulary.

EVALUATION DAY

Following the completion of six IDI programs at different locations, the project managers Anna and Peter called for an evaluation day with the educators. Eight out of 11 educators attended. The aim of the meeting was to use the evaluation forms that had been completed by participants in order to improve the IDI program. These forms included some complaints about a "lack of structure" during the sessions and about ambiguity concerning the program goal. Some IDI educators had expressed similar concerns.

More Scripts and Shorter Stories

At the start of the evaluation day, the educators formed two smaller groups to discuss their suggestions for improvements to future IDI programs. After an hour-long discussion, the groups came together and reported two fairly long lists of suggestions. Upon completion of this reporting, Anna stated that none of the suggestions was new to her and, somewhat surprisingly, the project managers described their own proposal for a revised version of the program, with the aid of a PowerPoint presentation. This action made the educators' previous work to define weaknesses and propose improvements seem superfluous.

While the program's agenda had previously been partly determined by requests from the IDI participants, the managers now suggested a fixed theme for each of the four meeting occasions:

1 Establishing an alliance
2 Becoming partners
3 Working on recovery
4 This is what we want to change!

Another proposed change was that the educators would use a PowerPoint presentation to guide participants through each theme. In the new format, each theme would be introduced "theoretically" by referring to research in order to "construct a foundation that is not exclusively based on the educator's own story," as Peter put it. Furthermore, it was proposed that the life stories should not be shared at full length at the first meeting occasion but should rather be divided into four shorter stories with content fitting the current theme. This news caused some distress among the educators:

> Sara says: "But it's very different to tell your story in 15 minutes or in two hours!" Carl, another patient educator, asks with a tone of voice that seems annoyed or confused: "But are we supposed to include everything, or what?" The project manager Peter answers: "That's the thing! You don't have to [tell everything]!" Sara objects: "But the participants are too curious just to tell a part of it!" Peter concludes the exchange by stating: "Well, it's good if they continue to be curious until the next meeting as well!" (reconstructed from field notes)

IDI participants as well as educators had described the need for a more defined structure and a clearer purpose for the program. Paradoxically, in trying to meet this request, the revised program toned down the contribution of the educators' experiences of psychiatric illness and care—the main reason for engaging patients to run the program. The revised program resembles a more traditional lecture, with a presentation depicting various "models," highlighting previous research, and so on. This is often unfamiliar territory for the IDI educator, whereas "telling my story" is performed with a fair amount of confidence.

Evaluating for Evidence

Within contemporary public welfare administrations, solid knowledge ("evidence") is to a large degree equated with measurements, standards, and quantitative assessments (Timmermans and Berg 2003). In this spirit, Anna and Peter presented a new model for evaluating the IDI program. The initial evaluation form used had been constructed jointly by the educators and project managers but was now replaced by a "pre- and post-test" evaluation designed by researchers from a university-based "center for evidence-based psychosocial interventions." The new evaluation represents part of a government initiative to measure the effects of service user involvement—in other words, whether the IDI program really changes the staff members' attitudes as desired. Anna presented this news to the educators cheerfully and with pride: "Listen to this! We've got an evaluation linked to the IDI program!" However, the educators were not impressed, and rather insisted on keeping "the old" questionnaire that they helped to create:

> Sara asks: "What will happen to our own questionnaire now? Will it be distributed at the same time? This new one is all about change in the staffs'

> attitudes, while the old one can be used to improve our own performance." "I'm afraid the first questionnaire won't be distributed," says Anna regretfully. John says: "But it's the first one that is important for us!" A loud discussion follows, and the common opinion among the educators is that they must keep the first questionnaire. Anna and Peter continue to defend themselves. They acknowledge the importance of the first questionnaire, but finally conclude "you can't have it all." (reconstructed from field notes)

This was the only time during the entire evaluation day that the educators voiced an opinion that clearly contradicted the changes proposed by the project managers. Hence, the educators' only serious attempt to alter the proposed development of the program was unsuccessful.

TENSION AND BALANCE IN TEACHING PERFORMANCES

So far, we have discussed the management's efforts to support the educators yet control the content and form of the training sessions. We have also established that the educators seem to enjoy the sought-after expert role to a greater extent when they engage in storytelling rather than scripted performance. Paradoxically, efforts to develop the program include a shift toward reducing or fragmenting the narrative elements in favor of a more traditional lecturing style. In conclusion, we will consider this course of events with a discussion of why the service user story is particularly powerful in this context, why there seems to be little faith in educators' competence to handle their tasks, and the implications of the chosen direction of the revised program.

Toward the end of the IDI program, the educators are instructed to ask the participants what they have enjoyed the most. "Your stories!" is by far the most common answer. The participants state that these stories allow them to see "the person behind the diagnosis" as well as to learn more about the good and bad ways that staff can treat patients. The institutional framing of "service-user involvement" offered in the program, with the explicit narrative right given to the educator (Atkinson and Delamont 2007), lends the stories a different impact compared with stories told during the normal workday. For example, an intake interview is necessarily focused on the practical purposes at hand (cf. Holstein and Miller 1993), such that "seeing the person behind the diagnosis" is subordinate to a different set of problems:

what questions to ask, what to document in the medical file, and what decisions to make.

In this chapter, we have paid more attention to the act of storytelling than to the stories per se. We have highlighted how the educators alter and balance between scripted and narrative performances, and how these performances are received by the audience. The implementation of service user involvement within the presently examined setting is rhetorically colored by consensus, with few examples of the staff–patient relationship portrayed in terms of conflict. Within this context with a strong emphasis on mutual understanding, storytelling seems particularly well suited for encouraging "harmonious dialogue." When educators described maltreatment, the criticism of the psychiatric organization was softened, since it was embedded in the story (see also Eriksson 2013). Lessons learned from such service user experiences are easy to agree on (see Alm Andreassen, Chapter 2, this volume). Furthermore, in addition to passively listening to the service users' stories, the staff members also share stories—often describing cases where rules and regulations have prevented them from doing a good "patient-centered" job. Such accounts attract sympathy from the listeners (participants and educators) and support the joint blame of a diffuse agent, such as "the system" or "the law."

Despite the fact that the educators' stories were generally appreciated, the project managers expressed concern that educators would fail to "reach" the staff (both before and after the first run of the program). They are anxious regarding the educators' abilities to successfully convey their experiences to the staff. Such concerns were shared by the fieldworker, Erik, who made several notes about his own worries and nervousness that the educators would fail to present themselves or the program in a manner that captured the staff's interest and concern. This fragile confidence in the educators' skills and expertise could reflect a general assumption that the psychiatric patient is ignorant, incompetent, and incapable of the task—indeed, the very image that the program aims to refute. However, it seems more reasonable to link the lack of trust to the tensions inherent in the staff–patient relationship, and some misgivings regarding whether the IDI program can successfully recast the roles. Will the staff acknowledge the patient as an expert? Will they accept guidance from the patient? From this point of view, it can be said that there is also little confidence in the ability of staff to adopt the student role.

The eagerness to support a successful exchange between patients and staff is visible in the project managers' efforts to encourage and coach the educators toward finding a middle ground. It is specifically stated that the educators must not be too harsh in their critiques of psychiatric care, as an accusatory style will lead educators to "lose the staff at once." The names given to service users ("ambassadors") and involvement activities ("dialogue") are instructive, suggesting a diplomatic approach in the original sense of the word—reflecting the need for a messenger between people to transmit messages, make requests or demands, or encourage concessions on various issues. This approach implicitly acknowledges potential conflicts of interest between patients and staff. By engaging "selected experts-by-guided-experience," conflicts may be kept to a minimum, thereby paving the way for a dialogue to reach common understandings.

In developing the program, complaints about a lack of structure were immediately met with a stronger reliance on conventional forms of education and traditional sources of knowledge. However, increasing the formal dimension of the IDI program is likely to be counterproductive—presenting a risk of creating even more ambiguities as it further distracts the educators from their core expertise of telling their stories. Another consequence may be a more narrow selection process of articulate and educated patients, which will ultimately lead to a professionalization of the service user (cf. El Enany, Currie, and Lockett 2013). The program managers' suggestion to divide the educators' personal story into four "episodes" may further complicate the educators' task. More importantly, the fragmentized story may lose its impact as a particularly useful method for staff and patients to communicate in this form of service user involvement (in-house training).

Although our findings highlight the educators' narrative performance as successful (and their scripted performance as more troublesome), this does not imply that storytelling is the more "true" or "authentic" way to enact service user involvement (cf. Atkinson and Delamont 2007; see Carr, Chapter 4, this volume). As we pointed out earlier, the educators' stories are constrained by a given narrative agenda, no less organizationally embedded than the more formal teaching. However, our findings do suggest that for the specific purpose of recasting the roles—turning the experts into students and the patients into experts—storytelling appears to be a promising and powerful teaching method.

NOTES

1 Much appreciation is given to Anna Meeuwisse, Malin Åkerström, and the editors for their helpful comments on previous versions of this chapter, and to the Swedish Foundation for Humanities and Social Sciences for partial funding.

2 The interviews were transcribed verbatim. The quotations presented in this chapter have been translated into English in a manner that preserves the original meaning and style. Field notes were taken in Swedish. Speech quoted in the field notes is not exact utterance but is used to facilitate reading. Names of people and of the program, along with other revealing details, have been altered to preserve anonymity.

3 The Attitude Ambassadors are a nationwide educational effort similar to IDI, focusing on counteracting stereotypes and fighting general negative attitudes toward people suffering from mental illness.

REFERENCES

Alm Andreassen, T., E. Breit, and S. Legard. 2014. "The Making of 'Professional Amateurs': Professionalizing the Voluntary Work of Service User Representatives." *Acta Sociologica* 57(4): 325–340.

Atkinson, P., and S. Delamont. 2007. "Rescuing Narrative from Qualitative Research." In *Narrative—State of the Art*, edited by Michael Bamberg, 195–204. Amsterdam: Benjamins.

Balen, R., C. Rhodes, and L. Ward. 2010. *Social Work Education* 29(4): 416–426.

Barnes, M. 1999. "Users as Citizens: Collective Action and the Local Governance of Welfare." *Social Policy and Administration* 33(1): 73–90.

Beresford, P. 2013. *Beyond the Usual Suspects*. London: Shaping Our Lives.

Branfield, F., P. Beresford, Eamon J. Andrews, P. Chambers, P. Staddon, G. Wise, and B. Williams-Findlay. 2006. *Making User Involvement Work: Supporting Service User Networking and Knowledge*. York: Joseph Rowntree Foundation.

Braye, S. 2000. "Participation and Involvement in Social Care: An Overview." In *User Involvement and Participation in Social Care*, edited by Hazel Kemshall and Rosemary Littlechild, 9–28. London: Kingsley.

El Enany, N., G. Currie, and A. Lockett. 2013. "A Paradox in Healthcare Service Development: Professionalization of Service Users." *Social Science and Medicine* 80:24–30.

Eriksson, E. 2013. "To Tell the Right Story: Functions of the Personal User Narrative in Service User Involvement." *Journal of Comparative Social Work* 8(2): 1–32. http://jcsw.no/?page=issueContent&issue=issue12&section=articleContent&article=06.

Eriksson, E. 2015. *Sanktionerat motstånd. Brukarinflytande som fenomen och praktik.* Doctoral dissertation. Lund: Socialhögskolan, Lunds universitet.

Ferguson, I., and W. Ager. 2008. "Ways of Knowing." In *Service User and Carer Involvement: Beyond Good Intentions*, edited by Mo McPhail, 60–71. Edinburgh: Dunedin Academic.

Forbes, J., and S. P. Sashidharan. 1997. "User Involvement in Services—Incorporation or Challenge?" *British Journal of Social Work* 27:481–498.

Glasby, J., and P. Beresford. 2006. "Commentary and Issues: Who Knows Best? Evidence-Based Practice and the Service User Contribution." *Critical Social Policy* 26(1): 268–284.

Gubrium, J. F., and J. A. Holstein. 2009. *Analyzing Narrative Reality.* Thousand Oaks, CA: Sage.

Hall, C., and M. Matarese. 2014. "Narrative." In *Analysing Social Work Communication: Discourse in Practice*, edited by Christopher Hall, Kirsi Juhila, Maureen Matarese, and Carolus van Nijnatten, 79–97. New York: Routledge.

Hayward, M., S. West, M. Green, and M. Blank. 2005. "Service Innovations: Service User Involvement in Training: Case Study." *Psychiatric Bulletin* 29(11): 428–430.

Holstein, J. A., and G. Miller. 1993. "Social Constructionism and Social Problems Work." In *Reconsidering Social Constructionism—Debates in Social Problems Theory*, edited by J. A. Holstein and G. Miller, 151–172. New Brunswick, NJ: Transaction.

Hultqvist, S. 2008. *Om brukardelaktighet i välfärdssystemen—en kunskapsöversikt.* Växjö: Växjö University Press.

Jacobsson, K., J. Thelander, and D. Wästerfors. 2010. *Sociologi för socionomer: En stående inbjudan.* Malmö: Gleerups.

Järvinen, M. 2002. "Mötet mellan klient och system: Om forskning i socialt arbete." *FORSA Information* 7:8–14.

Marvasti, A. B. 2002. "Constructing the Service-Worthy Homeless Through Narrative Editing." *Journal of Contemporary Ethnography* 31(5): 615–651.

McLaughlin, H. 2009. "What's in a Name: 'Client,' 'Patient,' 'Customer,' 'Consumer,' 'Expert by Experience,' 'Service User'—What's Next?" *British Journal of Social Work* 39:1101–1117.

Möller, T. 1996. *Brukare och Klienter i välfärdsstaten: Om missnöje och påverkansmöjligheter inom barn- och äldreomsorg.* Stockholm: Publica.

Nordén, H. 2008. *Kunskap att hämta: Brukarmedverkan för en bättre psykiatri.* Stockholm: Gothia Förlag.

Peck, E., P. Gulliver, and D. Towel. 2002. "Information, Consultation or Control: User Involvement in Mental Health Services in England at the Turn of the Century." *Journal of Mental Health* 11(4): 441–451.

Rea, D. M. 2004. "Changing Practice: Involving Mental Health Service Users in Planning Service Provision." *Social Work in Health Care* 39(3–4): 325–342.

Riessman, C. K. 2013. "Analysis of Personal Narratives." In *Qualitative Research in Social Work*, second edition, edited by Anne E. Fortune, William J. Reid, and Robert L. Miller Jr., 168–191. New York: Columbia University Press.

Rutter, D., C. Manley, T. Weaver, M. J. Crawford, and N. Fulop. 2004. "Patients or Partners? Case Studies of User Involvement in the Planning and Delivery of Adult Mental Health Services in London." *Social Science and Medicine* 58:1973–1984.

SOU. 2006. *Ambition och ansvar. Nationell strategi för utveckling av samhällets insatser till personer med psykiska sjukdomar och funktionshinder* [Official reports of the Swedish government].

Tait, L., and H. Lester. 2005. "Encouraging User Involvement in Mental Health Service." *Advances in Psychiatric Treatment* 11:168–175.

Timmermans, S., and M. Berg. 2003. *The Gold Standard: The Challenge of Evidence-Based Medicine and Standardization in Health Care.* Philadelphia: Temple University Press.

14

Reimagining the Doctor-Patient Relationship

▸ *IAN GREENER*

DOCTORS, ALONG WITH PERHAPS LAWYERS AND CLERICS, are the archetypal professionals. As far as the values of service and care are concerned, their relationship with patients in many ways has flagged the human service relationship in general. Those of us born well before the twenty-first century are familiar with role models of friendly but authoritative men (and they were all men) saving lives through the application of their encyclopedic scientific knowledge, provided to the grateful, deferent patient before them (Dingwall and Lewis 1983). Doctors were at the pinnacle of the career ladder, the scaling of which required the highest academic performance, which was rewarded by both high social status and good pay. We looked to doctors to make us well or whole in our hours of need, and held them in the greatest respect (Porter 2002).

However, this does not really tell the whole story (see Alm Andreassen, Chapter 2, this volume). Since the 1960s, a range of countervoices has emerged to challenge the role and the behavior of doctors in our health care and society, suggesting that those they are treating should be more critical and even suspicious in their encounters with medics (Gabe, Kelleher, and Williams 1994). Women in the 1960s and 1970s began to take a critical look at the way they were treated when in the care of doctors, often male, and presented strong evidence that often they were not being well served. Criticisms of childbirth processes and their apparent medicalization extended to include medical behavior, which to many women appeared to be patronizing and arrogant, and led to new movements that sought alternative answers to understanding women's bodies and health needs (Ruzek 1978). Disability rights groups began to campaign against attempts to "normalize" bodies through the use of often-painful prosthetics, and demanded that the societal environment be modified to grant fair access to everyone (Clarke 2004; Welshman and Walmsley 2006; see Solvang, Chapter 7, this volume). The view that disability is an individual medical problem was challenged and undermined (Oliver 1990). The psychiatric survivor movement challenged the often-dominant view of mental health professionals, emphasizing the injustices and inequalities it led to (Morrison 2009; see in this volume Eriksson and Jacobsson, Chapter 13, and Shakespeare and Collins, Chapter 12). Social scientists began to explore empirically the provision of health care and found power relations that often appeared to be more about preserving professional or class status than helping others (Freidson 1988; Larsen and Rootman 1976). Patient groups, often taking inspiration from feminist and disability rights campaigners, began to campaign for more general consumer-type rights (Allsop, Baggott, and Jones 2002).

Doctors have also found themselves accused of negligence or even cruelty. Their regulatory systems have sometimes been found wanting when it comes to protecting patients (Smith 2002) or in ensuring doctors keep up-to-date with their knowledge and practices (Walshe 2003). We have become increasingly aware of entrenched inequalities in health and health care (Bambra 2011), and there are also important senses in which medicine has "e-scaped" (Nettleton and Burrows 2003). As medical knowledge has become more widely available through its publication and accessibility through the Internet, this has led patients to be much more prepared to self-diagnose and challenge the expertise of doctors. Although doctors remain among the most powerful and trusted of professionals (Salter 2004), the relationship of the profession both to the state and to its patients has changed considerably (Moran 1999), leading to the opening up of a range of newer possibilities. At the same time, however, the ability of different groups to take up these new possibilities is uneven in that it depends not only on the resources available to patients and doctors but also on their interpersonal rapport and the empathy and trust each is able to bring to the relationship—their "cultural health capital" (Shim 2010). This is a crucial consideration, to which we will return.

RESPONDING TO THE CRITIQUES OF DOCTORS

Doctors, in response to this sustained critique, have given some ground. The General Medical Council (GMC) in the United Kingdom has attempted to redefine what professionalism means to their members through a series of "Good Medical Practice" publications (the most recent being General Medical Council 2013). Good Medical Practice attempts to fight a rearguard action against the criticisms of the profession by relocating doctor-based professionalism in terms of doctors being recognized as holding expertise, based especially on evidence-based medicine, but with their duty to serve their patients. Their patients, in turn, have been recast away from the very passive role of the past to being instead clients with their own individual needs to be met.

Some doctors have tried to draw lines in the sand, suggesting that most of their peers are doing a good job and need our support but that the profession is now confronted by an increasingly hostile media and a public who consider themselves consumers of health care rather than patients (Tallis 2005). Even Eliot Freidson, whose work was at the vanguard of criticism of doctors in the 1960s, seemed to be suggesting toward the end of his career that we had to respect professionals such as doctors, as their roles occupied a "Third Logic" (in contrast to market or bureaucracy) that we could not do without (Freidson 2001). But it is very clear that there is little danger of doctor–patient relationships going back to how they were in the 1950s—we have come too far from there and have reached a point where patients, for the variety of reasons outlined, will not be as compliant or deferent again. Indeed, doctors may find themselves in situations where, should they need to challenge patients about their lifestyle choices in respect to, for example, diet, smoking, or drinking, may expect to find their patients noncompliant or even aggressive about being questioned.

In many respects, policymakers are to blame for patients behaving so differently, in that they have been actively redescribing patient roles in terms of consumer or shopper terms (see Jensen and Villadsen, Chapter 11, this volume). They have increasingly suggested that doctor–patient relationships should be based on a consumer-driven model in which health care is like any other good (Secretary of State for Health 2000). In this model, in the same way as consumers do not need to know how their smartphones were designed and made but must simply be able to choose the one that serves their needs best, patients do not need to understand that much about health care, just be able to buy the services of a doctor who is best able to meet their requirements. The consumer model casts care as a contract between patient and doctor, with that contract being freely movable to the professional judged to be providing the best service. This change to a contract-based model of care is meant to act as a driver for health services more generally to improve their responsiveness to patient need (Greener and Powell 2009) and therefore to a general improvement in standards for everyone through the workings of the invisible hand of the marketplace.

A key, but often overlooked, element in the consumerization of medicine is the growth in use and availability of complementary and alternative medicine (CAM). Many CAM practices have something in common with the feminist movement, especially its rejection of male-dominated, science-led treatments, but this is not the driver of their expansion. That expansion presents us with an initial paradox: how is it that when conventional, what we might term science-based, health care in developed countries has become more widely available than ever before, people are looking instead to homeopathy, Chinese medicine, or the hundreds of other treatments that together present themselves as alternatives? Two answers are that conventional medicine has limits, and as consumers we dislike having such limits imposed on us, and that CAM therapists are often able to devote significantly more time and individual attention to patients than conventional medicine practitioners are able to.

Conventional medicine has bumped up against two limits from which we can learn. First, after a period of optimism in which it appeared we might soon expect modern medicine to be able to cure any disease, we have discovered that the pace of dramatic innovation has slowed (Le Fanu 1999). Our expectations of medicine, driven by the extraordinary period of postwar innovation around antibiotic discovery and transplantation, are extremely high, and we continue to look to doctors to be able to find miraculous cures for whatever ails us. But we have seen a rise in long-term conditions that, by their nature, are likely to be incurable into the foreseeable future. We have not found a cure for all cancers, and are experiencing a rise in conditions such as type 2 diabetes and obesity, which are linked to lifestyle. Equally, there often appears to be conflicting or even contradictory advice from our authorities regarding how we can avoid such diseases (Taubes 2008). We often find ourselves disappointed when modern medicine cannot miraculously cure us, but we are also confused as to what it is asking us to do to avoid disease in the first place.

Second, modern medicine has often become standardized to a point where it can become transactional and lose the sense of being personal (McCartney 2012), as it becomes increasingly based around checklists and automated cues to check with patients rather than around listening to their stories (see Pösö, Chapter 9, this volume). As the practice of medicine has become increasingly standardized through the use of care protocols and frameworks, and increasingly scrutinized through the recording and comparison of clinical data, there are dangers that we will overlook the fact that doctor–patient relationships are, as the name suggests, relationships, and need to be thought about as such. In many respects, complementary medicine has been able to directly address this concern by offering longer appointments and a more personalized experience, even if there remains little evidence (in the sense of evidence-based medicine) in support of many of the practices that it offers.

The problem with the consumer-driven model of health care is that it is not at all obvious that patients have the ability to choose the best provider of care, even if they are not required to know about health care themselves to make the model work (Greener 2008a). Equally, when we consider the huge public health problems that industrial nations now face—not least with respect to conditions such as obesity and alcohol consumption, where the public has been bombarded with information about diet and drinking advice for decades—it would seem that many of us struggle to make choices that would improve our health, even if we know that what we are presently eating and drinking is not good for us. This seems to indicate that, as far as health care goes, we are flawed consumers—choosing the wrong things for ourselves and struggling to make the right choices in terms of which health professional we would like to see to discuss our health problems. Equally, in a less-than-rational marketplace, it is not clear how casting doctors as service providers like any other is meant to work—if patients do not make the right choices, then that would, without strong regulation, appear to create the space for charlatans and quacks with good sales skills and a sympathetic bedside manner to flourish.

Building on the insight that our rationality in decision making is often less rigorous than standard economic textbooks might suggest, "nudge" thinking (Thaler and Sunstein 2008) on health care accepts that at least our "default" choices can be changed through "decision engineering" to get us to look after ourselves better. If supermarkets put chocolate next to the tills, when our willpower is low and we are waiting to pay, we may find ourselves buying food that we had no intention of purchasing when we entered the store. Moving temptation away, or replacing chocolate with fruit in the payment waiting areas, might lead to a very different outcome. The "nudge" approach recasts patients as being more easily led than in the consumer model while at the same time still allowing choices, albeit ones that are heavily influenced by the "default" option engineered within them. Doctors within the nudge approach become expert advisers as to what the default engineered into our everyday life ought to be while at the same time being encouraged to act as decision engineers for their patients, configuring their choices in such a way that they are led toward a healthier diet or drinking less. Doctors might "nudge" patients who are overweight by getting them to use pedometers and sharing their data electronically so they become more aware of their own levels of activity, as well as seeing how they compare to an ideal or peer group. The current default, which might involve a lack of movement, moves from activity being largely invisible to being explicitly measured and compared. Patients can overrule the defaults or decide not to comply with them, but the healthy option is one that doctors might try and move into the foreground of decision making for their patients. In setting these defaults, doctors use evidence-based medicine to find both treatments and areas of health care where nudging their patients will generate the biggest benefits. By so doing, doctors emphasize their roles as experts and interpreters of evidence as well as engineers of decision-making processes on behalf of their patients.

The nudge approach, then, accepts the limitations of health care (or other areas where the state wishes to intervene, such as pensions) as a consumer good and of patients as choosers, even if it preserves their right to opt out of the state-sanctioned default. Patients are flawed consumers, but we work with those flaws to try and come to the societally best outcomes. Doctors are regarded as experts capable of working out what that best outcome is from evidence-based medicine, as well as then looking to further scientific studies to find the means for engineering decisions for their patients so that their defaults are set in a way that leads patients to choose them. There are two obvious flaws here—one on the consumer side and one on the producer side.

The flaw in nudge thinking on the consumer side comes in its critique of the rational consumer model, in that it accepts that people make what look like suboptimal decisions and need to have their decisions engineered to change the defaults to allow them to make better choices but at the same time allows the same flawed consumers to opt out of those "right," default choices if they wish to. It is as if we still want people to have choices in a consumer form but recognize that they are not very good at making them. This seems like a rather unsatisfactory, muddled middle ground. In defense of this view, writers such as Ariely (2008) suggest that we are "predictably irrational," so, even though we seem to make poor decisions if left to our own devices, those decisions are at least predictably flawed. But this is still a considerable distance from justifying increased consumerism on the grounds that we might be able to correct for it by engineering default choices so that they are healthier.

On the producer side, the nudge approach seems to assume that health professionals are unproblematically able to come up with the evidence to show what people ought to be doing by default to improve their health care by carefully assessing evidence, and this may not be the case either. Advice on diet has changed a great deal over the last 20 years (Taubes 2008), and today we seem confused as to whether our biggest dietary concern ought to be fat or sugar intake. Whereas there is a durable antismoking consensus in place, it is less than clear what alcohol intake level we ought to be steering people toward. Whereas we can come up with some broad principles on which there is consensus (maintain a healthy diet and weight, do not smoke, drink only in moderation), anything beyond this seems open to remarkable amounts of contestation. If we are to change defaults by nudging patients to improve their health, there are not many nudge situations we can actively engineer that are supported by a strong scientific consensus.

A third model of doctor–patient relationships we have seen emerge recasts them in another way. The "expert patient" (Department of Health 2001; Wilson 2001; Greener 2008b; see also Solvang, Chapter 7, this volume) approach was originally rooted in the care of long-term conditions (Lorig et al. 2001), and it suggests that patients, through their individual engagement with doctors and treatments, can develop their own form of expertise from their personal experiences of looking after themselves and from the care they have received. As it is based on the individual experience a person has of his or her own body, albeit one that is increasingly shared via support groups in both the real and virtual worlds, this model of what it is to be a patient may or may not correspond to the way that patient is categorized in evidence-based medicine. This is because our own narratives, explanations, and experiences may not conform to the trials-based approach of modern medicine, with its emphasis on average results and significant effects. Doctors, in consultation with expert patients, may suggest new treatments through a process of negotiation and discussion, but recognizing the experiential knowledge of the patient, who becomes an active partner in the care process. Doctors' expertise is recognized and acknowledged, but it is not the final arbiter of the direction in which care should go, as that comes through a partnership with patients.

The expert patient model shows that engaging patients in their own care can offer a means by which they can acquire expertise and knowledge, but it often appears to be supported by policymakers in a context where it is being used as a means of trying to save money. This ignores the huge initial investment that making patients "experts" requires, whether such a model can be extended out of the context of long-term conditions, and the need to make it clear that doctors have to change their practices in line with this radical new model of doctor–patient relations. Although the expert patient model goes beyond consumerism in terms of empowering patients and asking them to lead their own care, it falls down if it is not adequately supported by health professionals or if policymakers do not appear to understand the considerable initial investment in changing practices that it requires from both doctors and patients.

We therefore find ourselves in a position where old relationships between doctors and patients have broken down but without a clear idea of what we need to replace them. Although these relationships may still exert a hold over us in situations where we are extremely ill or badly injured and are therefore prepared to forego our claims of agency, in most dealings with doctors, patients have come to demand a stronger voice. However, we have yet to work through the implications of the gains in agency that feminism, disability rights campaigners, consumer rights organizations, and expert patient advocates have given us, while acknowledging that we may actually be pretty poor at making decisions about our own daily health care. How can we reimagine doctor–patient relationships to take account of the destabilization of health professionalism while accepting the limits to patient rationality and acknowledging the real public health challenges we face?

ROLES IN THE LOGIC OF CARE

To reimagine doctor–patient relationships and extend the expert patient model to other care settings, we need to start with why they exist—what Annemarie Mol has called "the logic of care" (Mol 2008). In Mol's view, but in common with other work (Lewis and West 2014), care is a relationship—a value and open-ended commitment by both doctor and patient to try and make things better (see Gubrium, Chapter 1, this volume). In this view, care cannot be broken down into units or made subject to a contract, as it is unpredictable and not easily made subject to any kind of standardization. Doctors (and other health professionals) are there as experts, but not in a prescriptive sense. Instead, doctors are positioned in roles where they work in long-term partnership with patients (as in the expert patient model), with both sides making a commitment to try to make things better for the patient. This is not the consumer model, which is based on care being standardized, exchanged, and paid for, and Mol explicitly rejects the idea of care being provided in that narrow way, as it directly contradicts the logic she presents. In the context of health services, care functions not because of staff doing what it says in their job descriptions, or because they treat care as a contract, but because they are prepared to go much further, forming relationships with patients and finding out their specific needs so both doctor and patient can work together to try and improve the situation.

Expecting care to happen in the manner suggested by Mol sets the bar extremely high, and perhaps it can be achieved only as an ideal. It demands a huge amount of the doctor in terms of knowledge and patience, challenging the view of professionalism in which they may have been trained and where they expected patients to simply do as they are told. Instead, doctors need to think about their roles so they are working through the options for individual patients with them and are committed to helping their patients achieve their goals, which has already been advocated by some doctors (Tudor-Hart 1988). Here, care is regarded not as an individual transaction but as an ongoing commitment.

Asking doctors to rethink their roles in care is also hugely demanding on patients, moving them away from a view of their interactions with doctors as being only necessary when they are ill and where they might expect a miracle cure through a drug or operation that allows them to continue to live their lives without any changes. It requires patients to take seriously their own health and well-being, both physical and mental, and to be prepared to work toward their improvement in partnership with doctors and other health experts. It requires them to invest in their cultural health capital, not only by acquiring better knowledge of the way their bodies work but also by being prepared to engage with health professionals in ways they may not be used to. There is evidence that doctors tend to treat better those patients they regard as being more attractive (often based on socioeconomic status) (O'Reilly et al. 2006), and this is necessarily tied to the cultural health capital attached to the relationship between particular doctors and patients. This will be hard to challenge and to move toward a situation where the same high level of treatment might occur in every doctor–patient exchange.

STEWARDS AND GUARDIANS

Mol's view of care, then, asks both doctors and their patients to commit themselves to a longer-term relationship and a long-term goal: the patient's well-being. This means considering patients not as passive receivers of medical advice or as consumers, or even flawed consumers or "expert" patients, but instead as what we might think of as stewards. Patients are stewards in the sense of holding stewardship of their body and mind, both of which will be needed by their future selves. Some views of postmodernism might reject this view out of hand, suggesting that we have no commitments to our future selves, who may be very different—that we are (following Deleuze) "rhizomic" and thus should celebrate change in ourselves rather than continuity (Linstead and Pulleyn 2006). But accepting that we change over our lives does not mean that we do not have commitments to our future selves: if we drink to excess and abuse our bodies today, it is likely to have consequences we will have to deal with at some point. If we pay no attention to our mental health, that also is likely to bring us to account eventually. To view ourselves as stewards is not to reject the notion of the decentered self, which has been the direction of social theory since at least the 1970s, but it is, following Ricoeur, to accept that the commitments and promises that we make, and our ability to honor them despite the changes we go through in our lives, are what make us who we are (Ricoeur 1995).

The importance of our commitments expands the notion of stewardship beyond our own bodies and minds to others as well. None of us exists alone—we can meaningfully make promises to ourselves and honor them (Searle 1983), but we routinely have to make commitments to others, and through friendship and a variety of other relationships, we seek to honor those commitments despite the best efforts of time to interfere with them. In this sense, we are also stewards of our relations to others—we seek to maintain some relationships throughout our lives and to begin new relationships with others. Those relationships often depend on our maintaining material networks and resources (such as homes or families), and these also make commitments of which we are stewards. Some of us wish to go further still and wish to be stewards of institutions such as universities or the environments in which we live, making a commitment to preserve those as well.

Considering our relationship to ourselves and to others through stewardship of our bodies and minds goes directly against the consumerist ethos that pervades many of our relationships at present. Consumerism is a focus on the satisfaction of needs in the present only—there is considerable evidence that our decisions heavily discount the future, even if such a view ignores the problems this is likely to lead to in terms of our own future physical and mental health (Barber 2007). Following Ricoeur, we do not have to claim that our selves never change in order to make a commitment. All we have to do is acknowledge that we have a commitment both to ourselves and to others in the future, and as such we must act against the change that surrounds us in order to honor those commitments. Perhaps, in a postmodern world, we do not have to honor commitments either to ourselves or to anyone else. But, in such a world, it is hard to see how any kind of society or social fabric holds up at all—if we acknowledge the ontology of commitment or promise, then we accept, along with Searle (2010), that it is possible to derive an "ought" from an "is" because it is intrinsic to the function of a promise that it be honored, for without its honoring, a promise makes no sense conceptually. If we believe promises are necessary in order to form relationships with others, then we have to accept that such relationships come with deontic powers, with commitments being made on both sides, and that those commitments require our stewardship through honoring them.

Equally, we have to accept that we only get one body. Even if we are increasingly able to replace parts of our bodies with artificial or alternative replacements, we are still some distance from those parts being as viable as our original limbs, so we have a duty to maintain what we have (or even try and improve their condition) as a commitment to our future selves. It makes no sense to form commitments to others that are based on an expectation that we will be available to them in the future if we do not believe that we will be able to honor those commitments. We have a commitment both to our bodies and to our minds to maintain them as well as we are reasonably able—we are stewards of both.

The expert patient model begins to embrace the idea of the patient as steward, but at its core, it is framed through the notion of self-management rather than the idea of commitment to ourselves and to others. By placing such an emphasis on management, expert patients are encouraged to be "self-managing," lessening their dependence on clinicians while increasing their self-monitoring to understand how they may better manage their conditions (Wilson 2001). This approach implies a commitment to the future self but does not carry it through as a relationship, instead reducing it to a self-management issue only. At the same time, the expert patient risks reducing relations with doctors to a fallback—something the patient only considers if their self-management fails. Instead, we need to think differently not only about patients as stewards but also about the role of doctors.

In the logic of care, doctors are not solely experts, although their roles do demand expertise. Instead, they are guardians, acknowledging that patients as stewards cannot know everything they need to know to look after their bodies and minds. Thinking of doctors as guardians locates them in a role of having responsibilities to patients that go beyond single interactions to a longer-term commitment to working with the patient as steward to try to improve their physical and mental health. Reimagining the doctor as guardian does not mean that doctors should prevent patients from being allowed to fail or fall short of the expectation that they try to improve their health if they wish to pursue paths that do not recognize medicine as having a positive contribution to care. Neither does it mean that patients cannot be allowed to make mistakes, as it may take several attempts to find the right balance between self-care and medical consultation, or several attempts to find the right balance of medications and exercise (for example). Instead, the reimagined relationship asks that failures and mistakes such as these occur in a context of positive experimentation, a long-term relationship where both parties are accountable to one another in terms of the longer-term goal of improving the health of the patient. In a long-term relationship of experimentation, both parties can try and improve health, with care the medium through which this goal is pursued. This requires an acceptance on both sides that there are no magic answers, no shortcuts, and that improving care and health alongside it is something that has to take place across a lifetime.

Reimagining the doctor as guardian, as well as thinking of the role as forming a long-term partnership with patients, also asks doctors to think of themselves as being part of a wider care team. Patients, over their lifetimes as stewards of their bodies and minds, will require a far broader range of support than any individual alone is able to provide. Doctors must take responsibility for linking with networks of other clinicians or carers in order to act as a gateway to other kinds of services when their patients require them. This does not mean allowing the guardianship responsibility to be passed on—doctors will still need to provide oversight and to work with their patients because of the long-term commitment doctors and patients need to make to one another—but it does acknowledge the complexity of care, and the fact that providing good care often occurs as part of a team rather than being the responsibility of an individual clinician, no matter how knowledgeable or competent he or she might be.

This analysis also requires that patient appointments with doctors be reorganized and rethought. At present, at least in the United Kingdom, the most likely way patients will contact a doctor is through their local general practitioner, and that appointment is likely to last less than ten minutes. Their local general practitioner, in turn, is likely to be located in a team of other general practitioners, with no particular guarantee that individual patients will get to see the same doctor twice. This model of care depends on information systems to provide the continuity of care between doctors and patients, and for patients to go to their general practitioners with only one problem at any one appointment—otherwise they are likely to run out of time. Any doctor will need a good information system, but instituting continuity of care requires more than such a system—it requires continuity in the relationship between doctor and patient. Equally, it requires that patients be able to access their medical records and be able to add to them and review them in order to keep them current so their doctors have access to the best possible information about their present health.

There have been a range of pilot projects (e.g., Palen et al. 2012) that attempt to deal with this, and the confidential nature of health records creates significant issues about security and confidentiality, but these barriers must be overcome if patients are to be able to record, as stewards, their health status beyond their occasional contacts with health professionals. The potential for linking health records to new "wearable" technologies is clearly huge but also requires careful thought lest such information in health records be used against patients in decisions about the provision of care or insurance. It also requires that doctors take their share of responsibility for ensuring that the same opportunities to receive care occur for all their patients.

• • •

In practice, we will all fall short of our idea of being a steward for our body and mind, but we need a narrative within which we should organize our lives and health care, and we need to make a long-term commitment to our future selves, as well as to those we love and to those whose communities we share, to try to improve things. The challenge is equally difficult for clinicians, who will have to accept that we no longer owe them obedience and deference and accept that the structure of our meetings with them will have to become more discursive and negotiated than it has often been in the past (a change that also puts demands on patients to be prepared for such meetings as well). Patients need the support not of remote professionals who are there to censor, castigate, or patronize them but who work with them toward the goal of good health, providing help, support, and expertise along the way.

This reimagining is a deeply challenging one. By positioning us as stewards of our physical and mental health, it rejects the idea that health care is there to "fix" us and that we should have little regard for how we eat or how little we exercise. In direct contrast to the consumer-driven model that confronts us at present, it suggests that we have responsibilities to ourselves and to others that we should try to live up to. At the same time, it positions doctors as guardians—our partners, with whom we should work toward longer-term goals. The emphasis on the guardianship role suggests that patients as guardians should not automatically defer to doctors but should instead enter into a longer-term relationship requiring negotiation and justification on both sides.

If we can think of care in this way, then we really will have reimagined relationships between doctors and patients, and the human service relationship in general, remembering the contribution professionals can make to our lives but also accepting that we have responsibilities to ourselves (our selves) as well.

REFERENCES

Allsop, J., R. Baggott, and K. Jones. 2002. "Health Consumer Groups and the National Policy Process." In *Consuming Health*, edited by S. Henderson and A. Peterson, 48–65. London: Routledge.

Ariely, D. 2008. *Predictably Irrational: The Hidden Forces That Shape Our Decisions*. London: HarperCollins.

Bambra, Clare. 2011. *Work, Worklessness, and the Political Economy of Health*. Oxford: Oxford University Press.

Barber, B. 2007. *Consumed: How Markets Corrupt Children, Infantilize Adults and Swallow Citizens Whole*. London: Norton.

Clarke, J. 2004. *Changing Welfare, Changing Welfare States*. London: Sage.

Department of Health [UK]. 2001. *The Expert Patient: A New Approach to Chronic Disease Management for the 21st Century*. London: Department of Health.

Dingwall, R., and P. Lewis. 1983. *The Sociology of the Professions: Doctors, Lawyers and Others*. London: Macmillan.

Freidson, E. 1988. *Profession of Medicine: A Study of the Sociology of Applied Knowledge*. Chicago: University of Chicago Press.

Freidson, E. 2001. *Professionalism: The Third Logic*. Oxford: Polity.

Gabe, J., D. Kelleher, and G. Williams. 1994. *Challenging Medicine*. London: Routledge.

General Medical Council [UK]. 2013. *Good Medical Practice*. London: General Medical Council.

Greener, I. 2008a. "Choice and Voice: A Review." *Social Policy and Society* 7(2): 255–265.

Greener, I. 2008b. "Expert Patients and Human Agency: Long-Term Conditions and Giddens' Structuration Theory." *Social Theory and Health* 6(4): 273–290.

Greener, I., and M. Powell. 2009. "The Evolution of Choice Policies in UK Housing, Education and Health Policy." *Journal of Social Policy* 38(1): 63–81.

Larsen, D. E., and I. Rootman. 1976. "Physician Role Performance and Patient Satisfaction." *Social Science and Medicine* 10(1): 29–32.

Le Fanu, J. 1999. *The Rise and Fall of Modern Medicine*. London: Abacus.

Lewis, J., and A. West. 2014. "Re-shaping Social Care Services for Older People in England: Policy Development and the Problem of Achieving 'Good Care.'" *Journal of Social Policy* 43(1): 1–18.

Linstead, S., and A. Pulleyn. 2006. "Gender as Multiplicity: Desire, Displacement, Difference and Dispersion." *Human Relations* 59(3Q): 1287–1310.

Lorig, K., P. Ritter, A. Stewart, D. Sobel, B. Brown, A. Bandura, V. Gonzalez, D. Laurent, and H. Holman. 2001. "Chronic Disease Self-Management Program: 2-year Health Status and Health Care Utilization Outcomes." *Med Care* 11:1217–1223.

McCartney, M. 2012. *The Patient Paradox: Why Sexed Up Medicine Is Bad for Your Health*. London: Pinter and Martin.

Mol, A. 2008. *The Logic of Care: Health and the Problem of Patient Choice*. Oxford: Routledge.

Moran, M. 1999. *Governing the Healthcare State: A Comparative Study of the United Kingdom, the United States and Germany*. Manchester: Manchester University Press.

Morrison, L. J. 2009. *Talking Back to Psychiatry: The Psychiatric Consumer/Survivor/Ex-Patient Movement*. Palgrave: London.

Nettleton, S., and R. Burrows. 2003. "E-scaped Medicine? Information, Reflexivity and Health." *Critical Social Policy* 23(2): 173–193.

Oliver, M. 1990. *The Politics of Disablement*. Basingstoke: Palgrave Macmillan.

O'Reilly, D., K. Steele, C. Patterson, P. Milsom, and P. Harte. 2006. "Might How You Look Influence How Well You Are Looked After? A Study Which Demonstrates That GPs Perceive Socio-economic Gradients in Attractiveness." *Journal of Health Services Research and Policy* 11(4): 231–234.

Palen, T., C. Ross, D. Powers, and S. Xu. 2012. "Association of Online Patient Access to Clinicians and Medical Records with Use of Clinical Services." *Journal of the American Medical Association* 308(19): 2012–2019.

Porter, R. 2002. *Blood and Guts: A Short History of Medicine*. London: Penguin.

Ricoeur, P. 1995. *Oneself as Another*. Chicago: University of Chicago Press.

Ruzek, S. 1978. *Women's Health Movement: Feminist Alternatives to Medical Control*. New York: Praeger.

Salter, B. 2004. *The New Politics of Medicine*. London: Palgrave.

Searle, J. 1983. *Intentionality: An Essay in the Philosophy of Mind*. Cambridge: Cambridge University Press.

Searle, J. 2010. *Making the Social World: The Structure of Human Civilization*. Oxford: Oxford University Press.

Secretary of State for Health [UK]. 2000. *The NHS Plan: A Plan for Investment, a Plan for Reform*. Vol. Cmnd 4818-I. London: HMSO.

Shim, J. 2010. "Cultural Health Capital: A Theoretical Approach to Understanding Health Care Interventions." *Journal of Health and Social Behaviour* 51(1): 1–15.

Smith, J. 2002. *The Shipman Inquiry: First Report, Volume One: Death Disguised*. London: HMSO.

Tallis, R. 2005. *Hippocratic Oaths: Medicine and Its Discontents*. London: Atlantic.

Taubes, G. 2008. *The Diet Delusion*. London: Vermillion.

Thaler, R., and C. Sunstein. 2008. *Nudge: Improving Decisions About Health, Wealth and Happiness*. London: Yale University Press.

Tudor-Hart, J. 1988. *A New Kind of Doctor*. London: Merlin.

Walshe, K. 2003. *Regulating Health Care: A Prescription for Improvement?* Maidenhead: Open University Press.

Welshman, J., and J. Walmsley. 2006. *Community Care in Perspective: Care, Control and Citizenship*. London: Palgrave.

Wilson, P. 2001. "A Policy Analysis of the Expert Patient in the United Kingdom: Self-Care as an Expression of Pastoral Power?" *Health and Social Care in the Community* 9(3): 134–142.

15

Who's Who and Who Cares?

PERSONAL AND PROFESSIONAL IDENTITIES IN WELFARE SERVICES

▸ MARIAN BARNES

AN EARLY EXAMPLE OF A STRATEGIC INITIATIVE designed to strengthen the voices of those who use social care services was a project called the Birmingham Community Care Special Action Project (CCSAP). I evaluated this project, and I have written about aspects of it in different places (e.g., Barnes 1997). It was my first significant exposure to issues and initiatives that would form a major focus of my research for the next 25 years.

As I was thinking about this chapter, I remembered an exchange between members of what was called the Search Team—a group of service users (disabled people, people with mental health problems, older people) and carers who were constituted to ensure a continued impetus for work that had been started by CCSAP. The Search Team was unusual in having terms of reference that included different user groups and also carers. It allowed for some representation from voluntary organizations that campaigned on behalf of those groups, but it excluded anyone who worked for the city council, at that time the major provider of social care services. However, during one discussion, it occurred to group members that some carers (e.g., parents of disabled children, adult children of aging parents) could and did work for the city council. This resulted in a lively discussion about whether such people could become members of the Search Team. It was concluded that "frontline staff," including home helpers, refuse collectors, and housing officers who were also carers, would be allowed to join but that senior managers would not. The group, established to contribute to the "empowerment" of service users and carers, drew a distinction based on assumptions of power within professional or bureaucratic roles to define the limits beyond which they were not prepared to extend membership.

This incident provides a jumping-off point for the issues I want to explore in this chapter. Firstly, there is no essential dichotomy between those who provide health and social care services and those who use them. People can and do occupy both positions at the same or different times. Secondly, from a theoretical perspective, we need to understand how different identities interact to result in people being positioned differently at different points in their lives or in different social contexts (see Newman, Chapter 16, this volume). And thirdly, we need to recognize the significance of power as a key dimension of these processes. Running through all these questions is the significance of epistemology: whose knowledge is recognized as legitimate and valuable in shaping encounters between services and those who use them? This is an issue also addressed by others in this book (e.g., Alm Andreassen, Chapter 2).

I will explore these issues through consideration of different contexts within which similar issues have emerged as a point of personal or political tension for individuals seeking to shift or transform relationships between "officials" (a term I use to encompass professionals and other frontline workers, managers, providers, and commissioners of services) and those who use public services. I will also suggest how different bodies of theoretical work, in particular feminist care ethics, might offer ways of understanding how such relationships are worked out between people occupying different positions within welfare services. I will suggest the potential of care ethics in terms of creative responses to the conflicts and tensions that can arise and what this suggests about broader political and ethical questions about "who cares" and how responsibilities for care are allocated and resisted.

The concept and practice of "care" has been a site of dispute in the emergence of disability movements protesting poor treatment within welfare systems as well as exclusion from mainstream social and economic life (e.g., Beresford 2008). The language of rights and citizenship rather than that of care and welfare has been important in framing the claims of disabled people, those living with mental health problems, and others seeking recognition and representation within policy and service decision making, as well as control over personal support services (see in this volume Gubrium, Chapter 1; Solvang, Chapter 7; Shakespeare and Collins, Chapter 12;

Miller and Kontos, Chapter 8). Collective action generating an "oppositional consciousness" (Mansbridge and Morris 2001) has contributed to important successes in the transformation of relationships between providers and users of services, but I want to argue that we should think in terms of "rights *and* care" rather than "rights *not* care," and that we need to complicate assumptions underpinning binary oppositions between users and officials.

My starting point is empirical research that has explored, in rather different ways, how relationships between users and professionals are being renegotiated. The sites of such negotiations include frontline interactions at the point of service use, spaces in which users, providers, and policymakers come together to deliberate, and research designed to generate new knowledge that can inform policy, service design, and delivery. I use theoretical work to reflect on what we can learn from lived experience and what this suggests not only about how we can conceptualize such relationships but how they might be transformed. Most (but not all) of the research I draw on is from the United Kingdom and is located in different service and policy contexts over a number of years. My argument here is not primarily focused on any particular policy or service context but on how we might think about such relationships and how they might be improved.

WHO AM I TODAY?

As we have seen from the preceding discussion, public officials can also be carers. They can also be disabled, users of mental health services, or share other aspects of identity with people who use the services they provide and/or are engaged in collective action to challenge, oppose, or influence policies and practices in which they are engaged.

For research on public participation, my colleagues and I interviewed a woman who worked for the city council and had a formal responsibility for facilitating relationships between the council and an organized campaigning group on environmental issues. Speaking of the dilemma she faced as an environmental activist who worked as a public official but was also being encouraged by activist colleagues to take part in neighborhood forum campaigning on similar issues, she said:

"Who am I? What's my role here?" They say just come as a resident. Well I am, but they won't know where my views are coming from, one moment I'll be Ms Council and the next Ms Resident. (Barnes 2009:45)

Another woman, in this case a Hindu working for an NHS (National Health Service) trust, whose role included facilitation of a minority ethnic group council designed to improve accessibility of health services for people from diverse ethnic groups in the area, was clear about how she should separate different aspects of her identity:

I'm biased. I'm the XXX Trust, I'm not a community member and that has to be very clear in my head. And that's the only way I can do this kind of work or the boundaries will get fudged, and I can't let that fudge my thinking process because then I'd become judgemental as well in how I work with the communities and so a line has got to go up. (Barnes 2009:43)

Exploring identities per se was not the purpose of the research that generated these reflections, but as we interviewed both "community members" and "officials" engaged in participatory initiatives in two English cities, it became clear that working out how to do participation also involved working out identities with respect to others engaged in these processes. Our research included examples of public service professionals occupying roles as community members in participation initiatives who adopted fundamentally different strategies in relation to this (Barnes 2009).

Shona Hunter offers a specific focus on professional identity in relation to other dimensions of personal and cultural identities (Hunter 2009). She presents a detailed analysis of how another Indian health professional, in this case a male Sikh GP (general practitioner) named Navneen, grappled with his identity and positioning within the changing architecture and culture of the NHS. Navneen explores his own cultural and personal subjectivity in relation to stereotypical views of "older Asian GPs." Hunter argues the importance of paying attention to the multilayered and often amorphous elements of feeling and experience, as well as gendered and raced biographies, which shape the way in which professional relations are lived. In her more recent work, she develops this further to argue that the everyday "relational politics" of actions and practices bring into being not only individual identities but also the state itself (Hunter 2015).

There is an increasing number of personal reflective accounts from people occupying professional roles who also have personal identities that can and do position them as "service users" in other contexts. Claire Tregaskis constructs her account of researching "constructions of disability" via a study of interactions within a leisure center by approaching the issues from ten different perspectives that encompass who she is in this context (Tregaskis 2004). Book chapters are headed "Being a . . .": researcher; consultant; member of staff; friend; woman; white; body; disabled person; oppressor; and activist. Thus, Tregaskis is not only "reporting research findings" but also including herself in the research process by reflecting on how she was seen by those she was researching and on the dilemmas associated with this. One conclusion she draws is the need to take a critical perspective on the social model of disability and the tendency of disabled activists to focus binary oppositions around the able-bodied/disabled axis, to the exclusion of other differences.

Rachel Perkins is rather more selective in her analysis of the different positions she occupies in relation to mental health services. As a consultant clinical psychologist and a campaigner in relation to mental health services, in particular for heterosexual women and lesbians, embarking on a third "psychiatric career" as a recipient of mental health services was both different and challenging:

> It involved no positive choice on my part. . . . There are no guidelines about how to be a recipient of mental health services. No one tells you the rules as in a job description. Despite my long association with mental health services I found myself completely at sea, not really knowing what to do and feeling very alone. There were people around, but somehow I could not make contact with them as I usually did. An intangible barrier seemed to divide us. (Perkins 1999:135)

Perkins reflects that both her professional position (as a "radical" professional) and her user identity result in invitations to write and speak about mental health services. However, neither she nor her audiences can divorce the different aspects of her relationships with services. For her, as a professional, it was not an option to keep quiet about her need to use as well as provide services: "What would this say about the way I viewed those with whom I worked? What would it say about the 'them and us' divide, which blights mental health services?" (Perkins 1999:145).

How people work out who they are in the context of roles and identities that cross the user and provider divide is both complex and diverse. Tregaskis's delineation of these identities as distinct and capable of separate analysis may be hard to sustain. Nicki Ward cites a woman in her study of lesbians and social exclusion. Amy did not identify herself as a professional but was very clear that it was not possible to separate out other aspects of her identity:

> It's like other people are always trying to make you separate stuff out, not for you but for them. . . . You know are you doing this as a woman or as a lesbian or as somebody with a mental health problem or what and it's like but they are all me, they are all part of me. You know that's bloody where lies madness if you ask me. . . . People will try and go oh that's not relevant and that's not relevant but you can't sort people out into bits. (Amy, cited in Ward 2005)

Perhaps the only general conclusion we can draw is the need *not* to assume that identities relating to relationships with services are either dichotomous or fixed. While negotiating this fluidity may be uncomfortable, it can also open up spaces for change. As Hunter argues, individual subjects are never purely "inside" or "outside" the state (in this instance as policy maker and/or service provider), and it can be precisely this that may unsettle the status quo (Hunter 2015).

WORKING THE DIVIDE

Rejection of "disempowering" treatment by welfare professionals has resulted in successful campaigning on the part of many disabled people to achieve transformation through the "personalization" of services. Much has been written in support of and critiquing both the concept and practice of personalization (e.g., Barnes 2011; Leadbetter, Bartlett, and Gallagher 2008). Claims that personalization could, at the same time, succeed in reducing the costs of services and empower service users where other attempts to do so had failed have, unsurprisingly, been shown to be suspect. It is not my purpose here to review evidence about personalization in practice, but it is important to recognize the centrality of the concepts of "choice and control" to such service provision models and what this implies for the nature of the face-to-face interactions through which those who use services encounter those who provide them. It is also important to distinguish the rather crude assumptions that inform official policy discourse and both the analysis and practice of personalization in different contexts.

Early research into the implementation of personalization via individual budgets in the United Kingdom indicated that this was experienced less positively by older people than by younger disabled people (Glendinning et al. 2008). This is perhaps not surprising. One of the ironies of the drive toward this way of enabling people to access services was that it was intended to be user centered and responsive to the individual. But the model was based substantially on critiques from adult disabled people, and the same model was to be applied in very diverse contexts. While the services individuals might be encouraged to choose were up to them (as long as the budget could stand it), what could not be chosen was the model within which relationships between service users and the welfare system were to be constructed. Personalization embodies the dominance of the values of individualism. But, perhaps perversely, it is not able to respond to the diversity of older people's needs, particularly those seeking help when they face multiple health problems as they are nearing death (Lloyd 2010).

This reminds us of the importance of how people in different circumstances experience face-to-face encounters with those from whom they seek help. But what social care reforms have prioritized has been the systems and criteria that govern who is able to access services, and how decisions about help received are made. I am not arguing that such systems are not important; far from it. But what they neglect is that service use is experienced through the interactions between individuals and that those interactions are shaped both by the policy and institutional context in which they are embedded and by the relational dynamics of the encounter itself (see also Solvang, Chapter 7, this volume).

Thus, for example, a key role in the context of personalization is that of the personal assistant (PA), who works with individual disabled people and may be employed by them directly. This relationship is seen to enable service users to control the support they receive through a "purchaser–provider" or employer–employee relationship. In a nuanced study of interactions between people with learning disabilities and their PAs, Williams and her colleagues (Williams et al. 2009) highlight the "uses of shared references [that] appeared to foreground the 'friendly' nature of the relationship between the person with learning disabilities and their PA, rather than an institutional relationship, in which one person had greater rights than the other" (p. 620). During the encounters that formed the subject of this research, PAs moved between what might be considered "professional" identities and identities that were more "informal," and people with learning disabilities shifted between identities as "employer" and "friend."

Is the fluidity and potential that this offers in terms of enabling more empowering relationships between user and worker a result of the specific role and institutional context? Williams et al. (2009) suggest that such outcomes are not inevitable, and I suggest that they are neither determined by nor restricted to this context. Jenny Morris, a disabled feminist, challenges the way in which "care" and "dependency" have been excised from service discourse, illustrating her case with an insight from research on young disabled people in which she observed a young man in a day center (Morris 2001). Day centers have been the focus for much of the critique of services that separate disabled and older people from "mainstream" services, such as leisure centers. But here Morris notes a transformation in the way in which this young man participated in relationships within the center in comparison with his behavior in a residential school he had previously attended. In comparison with an absence of interaction with others in the residential school, in the day center he actively participated with staff and other service users and communicated his agreement and disagreement using nonverbal methods. This transformation, Morris argues, "had been brought about by a 'care' relationship which started with his human right to communicate and sought ways to make this possible" (p. 14). Thus, it is the nature of the relationship, a relationship that recognizes that care and human rights are linked, that makes the difference. It is not the role—day center workers as well as PAs are capable of working in a way that recognizes human rights, and it is not dependent on structuring relationships through the control exercised by an employer or purchaser.

Once we recognize the significance of the relationship between workers and service users, the priority accorded to choice and control as the basis on which to construct interactions must be questioned. Both offer little insight into the quality of interaction necessary to enable the achievement of rights. Neither recognizes the significance of care and the different logic that underpins care rather than choice (Mol 2008). But a relational perspective also reminds us that we need to attend to the position of workers as well as service users.

Care workers are usually poorly paid and have limited employee power. They are predominantly women, and they are often from minority ethnic groups and from the lower social classes. As the flexibility encouraged by personal support services has developed, alongside a retreat of direct provision by public authorities, there has been an increase in the number of care workers whose work is done almost exclusively in private homes. These workers are paid only for the direct contact time and may be on zero hour contracts if they do not know when or for how long they will work and thus how much they will earn each week. Many of these workers are migrants, and some of them live with an uncertain immigration status (Cangiano et al. 2009). As well as examples of positive relationships between care workers and those they cared for, the Cangiano et al. study revealed cases of exploitation of care workers by families who employed them directly. Similarly, in a study conducted in Naples, Lene Nare identified vulnerabilities experienced by care workers and care receivers in such contexts (Nare 2013).

Achieving justice for service users through transforming the nature of relationships between users and providers cannot be achieved at the expense of justice for those who work at care. We need other ways of theorizing such relationships besides those offered by neoliberal ideologies that see market exchanges as the route to shift the balance of power or by approaches based on competitive rights that advocate user rights while ignoring rights of workers.

CHANGING IDENTITIES

The development of diverse policies and practices intended to shift relationships between those who decide about, those who provide, and those who receive services has resulted in the emergence of different identities that are both ascribed to and claimed by service users. I have explored the dilemmas and opportunities associated with the opening up of identities such as "expert by experience," peer supporter, user governor, user researcher, and others in the context of mental health services (Barnes 2015). These are often in tension with more "activist" identities associated with collective action within the mental health user movement. I suggest that negotiations among service users and between users and professionals regarding identities "have been constructed around shifting discourses within statutory services concerning relationships between state, citizens and service users"

(p. 146). Their emergence means we need to understand how relationships are being transformed in contexts other than face-to-face service use. I will illustrate this point using recent work with older people.

Following participative research on older people and well-being, my colleagues and I worked on a "translational" project to apply findings from the research to develop learning materials for social care practitioners. This brought together a team comprising older people who had worked as co-researchers on the well-being project, older people who had not been part of that project but who were involved in older people's forums, social care practitioners from the voluntary and statutory sectors, and university researchers. In line with the expectations of funders of this project (the Economic and Social Research Council Follow On scheme), we described it in the grant proposal as a "knowledge exchange" project. In this proposal, we linked the different participants with different types of knowledge: experiential, practitioner, and research/theoretical knowledge. We argued that creating a space in which these different types of knowledge could come into dialogue with each other would enable us to produce output that was both relevant to practitioners and grounded in what we had learned was important to older people in order to sustain their well-being.

Like all such projects, it generated substantial learning through the process of doing. This prompted both structured reflection among the three of us who initiated the work (my colleague Lizzie Ward at Brighton University and Bea Gahagan at AgeUK Brighton and Hove) and a decision to analyze transcripts of selected team meetings of this project and from the previous research team meetings, involving older people but not practitioners. We wanted to compare the way in which issues regarding well-being, and in particular issues related to the significance of care, were talked about in these two rather different groups.

This analysis demonstrated that the ascription of different knowledge and identities on the basis of the roles allocated to different participants could not be sustained. Some of the older people had previously worked in jobs related to care services: one had been a nurse, another a social care manager, and another a magistrate, for example. For some, this meant that these forums held significance as spaces in which they could continue to apply knowledge or understanding gained from their working lives rather than spaces where they could emphasize their experience of being an "older person."

For one woman in particular, her involvement in the research project as a peer researcher was what provided her with the authority to contribute to the translation project. Thus, the knowledge she contributed to this work derived not only from her experiential knowledge of growing older but also from that gained as a researcher. As facilitators of these processes, Lizzie, Bea, and I sought to draw out general issues and make connections between different narratives within the groups. But, as discussions developed, this role was also played by others in the group, and we, too, told our stories based on knowledge of older relatives and, to some extent, our own reflections on what it means to grow older. And we thought we had been successful when practitioners started to reflect on their own personal experiences as well as to talk about the practice dilemmas they faced in their work.

It was not the case that differences based in the different positioning of participants became unimportant. Nor was the blurring of identities that I have suggested here unproblematic. Resistance to aging is well established in contemporary cultures, and at least one of the older women who took part used this deliberative space as an opportunity to draw on her previous professional work as a social care manager, resisting talking about her experiences of growing older. But this experience does offer a rather different perspective from some other accounts of sites that have been designed to enable deliberation between service users and officials (Ward and Barnes 2015).

Elsewhere I have discussed contexts in which mental health service users have been regarded as "rude" for expressing the pain associated with their experiences (Barnes 2008; Church 1996) or have had their words revised to avoid "frightening" doctors with their anger (Barnes and Wistow 1994). While these examples are now quite old, more recent research into mental health user involvement suggests that, while the discourse might have changed, it is still the case that *how* service users talk about things they are unhappy with affects the seriousness with which their experiences are acknowledged (MacDonald et al. 2014). While it is increasingly acknowledged that it is possible to be both a mental health service user and a professional, the fear and stigma associated with mental illness may make it harder to bridge the "them and us" divide that Rachel Perkins identified than it is to acknowledge that growing older is something that we will all experience if we survive.

The way in which deliberation between service users and officials takes place within the different contexts that have been developed to enable influence over policy and service design affects the extent to which different identities generate oppositional relationships or hold the potential for the formation of alliances and the transformation of both users and officials. I have argued elsewhere that this requires "deliberating with care" (Barnes 2008; Barnes 2012, chapter 8). In order to suggest what this involves, I will introduce the theoretical perspective that I find helpful in understanding this.

REIMAGINING SERVICE RELATIONSHIPS THROUGH AN ETHIC OF CARE

The assertion of distinct identities as disabled person, carer, and survivor was important in achieving recognition of the powerlessness of users in relation to services. But I am now suggesting that basing future practices on conflictual identities in this way is not a helpful strategy. I also suggest that theoretical developments enable us to offer a more creative reimagining than has been evident as a result of the unholy alliances between rights claims from user movements and neoliberalism.

One body of work relevant to this is that on intersectionality (Crenshaw 1991). Originally advanced as a way of understanding how both race and gender need to be thought of together in addressing how subordination works in practice, intersectionality has been applied to various contexts relevant to a consideration of transforming relationships between users and providers of welfare services (e.g., Krumer-Nevo and Komem 2013). It is also being linked to the main theoretical perspective I want to advance here: feminist ethics of care (Hankivsky 2014; Ward 2015). The critical perspective of intersectionality links to the transformative aims of feminist care ethics, and both require a conception of social justice that reflects the multidimensionality of identity.

Service user movement claims for transformation derived from experienced marginalization, injustice, and sometimes oppression. Too often, services nominally intended to help the situation exacerbated such experiences. But assuming that such injustices can be rectified through reconstructing user–provider relationships as either consumer or employee relationships implies a skewed concept of justice. It is more helpful to think of justice as necessitating transformative recognition and redistribution, as Nancy Fraser argues (Fraser 1997). This not only holds the possibility of unsettling the group differentiations that structure unequal social relations but also holds out the possibility of coalitions between social movements originally based in what were assumed to be distinct identities. I have previously argued the potential of this in relation to coalitions between mental health service user and carer movements (Barnes with Gell and Thomas 2010). But we can also suggest that alliances between care workers and service users hold a greater potential for achieving justice for both than do conflictual approaches that privilege one dimension of identity over others and thus do not recognize, as the example I started with suggests, that we can occupy both positions.

While early work on the ethics of care (Gilligan 1982) distinguished this from justice ethics, more recent work has instead sought to explore the necessary relationship between care and justice in conditions of vulnerability (e.g., Kittay 1999; Engster 2007). I have drawn on this work to argue the significance of an ethic of care to social policies and practices capable of enabling justice (Barnes 2012). So how can care ethics help here?

Among the important insights of the feminist ethic of care is that the need for care is universal (Tronto 1993). If we all need care, not only when we are infants, old, or ill but throughout our lives, then distinguishing people on the basis of identities as care givers or care receivers becomes problematic. The implications of this have been addressed in relation to lay care giver/care receiver identities (e.g., Ward 2011). Although less attention has been given to the implications regarding paid care workers, Bowden (1997) has acknowledged this in relation to the position of nurses, Manea (2015) has suggested that we need to recognize the needs of migrant doctors as care receivers, and Tronto (2010) has called for "caring institutions" that we might understand as recognizing the need of workers to experience being cared for in their work. It is certainly the case that current employment practices within welfare services (and other contexts) demonstrate little care for employees. Promoting the rights or interests of service users while not also protecting those of both paid and unpaid care givers should not be the way forward.

Accepting responsibility to act in response to attending to need is central to the ethics of care (Tronto 1993). But such responsibility cannot be limited to those at the front line who are engaged in face-to-face caregiving (Tronto 2013). Collective responsibility affects the preparedness to fund care services at a level that permits the possibility of good caring relationships rather than disaggregating the tasks of care (helping someone dress, eat, use the toilet, etc.) and allowing no "time to care" during domiciliary visits. Recognizing care as a moral and political issue as well as a relational practice means that the question "who cares?" is one in which we are all implicated. Caring about others is a necessary precursor to action to enable social justice (Sayer 2011). It is not enough to think about how we can transform frontline relationships. We must also consider how we can create a "caring democracy" in which solidarities are expressed through "caring with" others (Tronto 2013). In thinking about transformations, how policies get made is as important as how services are delivered.

The starting point for care is attentiveness that enables recognition of the needs of others (Tronto 1993). In the context of deliberative policymaking, I have argued that:

> Deliberative practices which enable dialogue about experiences deriving from the disadvantage and marginalisation resulting from disability, old age or mental distress, from experiences of giving and receiving care, of abuse, discrimination and marginalisation can encourage attentiveness to such experiences and give recognition to them. This implies a preparedness to listen and to hear what is being said, even if it is expressed in ways that fall outside communicative norms familiar to public officials. (Barnes 2012:161)

Such deliberation opens up possibilities for expansion of insight, understanding, and moral sensibility through dialogic processes.

Attentiveness is necessary in all contexts in which interactions between those who use services and those occupying other roles in relation to services take place. But the ethics of care recognizes that attention to care receiving is also necessary to enable the integrity of care. Recipients are not passive but contribute experiential knowledge and, through their responses, enable learning about what constitutes good care (Barnes 2012). This focus on the agency of the care receiver emphasizes the contextual nature of caregiving and care receiving and the necessity of understanding the sociocultural as well as personal dimensions of this context. This includes understanding the significance of unequal power and vulnerability that characterize many contexts in which care is given and received.

This is very different from a practice perspective that prioritizes empowerment through information giving and choice. Viewing information giving as a rational process that has a linear relationship with enabling "good care" fails to recognize the emotion-laden impact of much information, as well as the diverse contexts in which care happens (see Grenier and Flood, Chapter 10, this volume). This was very evident in a study of an information and support program for carers of people with dementia, where responses to information about the trajectory of dementia led to despair as well as better understanding (Barnes and Henwood 2015).

Transformative caring practice does not happen when practitioners "pass over" responsibility for decision making with the information they proffer but instead when they engage in dialogue about how good care can be achieved. The ethics of care offers a language within which such conversations can take place.

• • •

Personal accounts of those involved in caring relationships, and from those who have experienced an absence of care, give testimony to the way in which identity is forged through such interactions. Who we are is, in part, a consequence of how we are situated in relationships of care. While those occupying positions of power may claim "privileged irresponsibility" (Tronto 1993) and deny that they are implicated in care in any way, this does not exclude them from the reality that they were all "some mother's child" (Kittay 1999) and that their survival is dependent on the care of others. Those who provide services as well as those who currently use them cannot assume that these positions are fixed, and it is in the interests of all of us to ensure the availability of good care.

Evidence of the absence of such care has prompted oppositional action on the part of some service user movements. For some, this has involved arguing for "rights not care" and for solutions based on individualized models that rely on market mechanisms to transform relationships. One danger of this approach is that of disregarding the position of care workers, whose own rights are being undermined as austerity is used as an excuse to further worsen conditions of employment. The challenge now is to recognize who is "the opposition" and how we might achieve change that reflects broader acceptance of care as a value informing political decision making as well as frontline service delivery. Work on the ethics of care offers a framework within which we can understand what is necessary personally, politically, and in practice contexts to achieve transformative change.

REFERENCES

Barnes, M. 1997. *Care, Communities and Citizens*. Harlow: Addison Wesley Longman.

Barnes, M. 2008. "Passionate Participation: Emotional Experiences and Expressions in Deliberative Forums." *Critical Social Policy* 28(4): 461–481.

Barnes, M. 2009. "Alliances, Contention and Oppositional Consciousness: Can Participation Generate Subversion?" In *Subversive Citizens: Power, Agency and Resistance in Public Services*, edited by M. Barnes and D. Prior, 33–48. Bristol: Policy.

Barnes, M. 2011. "Abandoning Care? A Critical Perspective on Personalisation from an Ethic of Care." *Ethics and Social Welfare* 5(2): 153–167.

Barnes, M. 2012. *Care in Everyday Life, an Ethic of Care in Practice*. Bristol: Policy.

Barnes, M. 2015. "Survivors, Consumers or Experts by Experience? Assigned, Chosen and Contested Identities in the Mental Health Service User Movement." In *The Identity Dilemma, Social Movements and Collective Identity*, edited by J. Jasper and A. McGarry, 131–149. Philadelphia: Temple University Press.

Barnes, M., and F. Henwood. 2015. "Inform with Care: Ethics and Information in Care for People with Dementia." *Ethics and Social Welfare* 9:3.

Barnes, M., and G. Wistow. 1994. "Learning to Hear Voices: Listening to Users of Mental Health Services." *Journal of Mental Health* 3:525–540.

Barnes, M., with C. Gell and P. Thomas. 2010. "Participation and Social Justice." *Social Policy Review* 22:253–274.

Beresford, P. 2008. *What Future for Care?* York: Joseph Rowntree Foundation.

Bowden, P. 1997. *Caring: Gender Sensitive Ethics*. London: Routledge.

Cangiano, A., I. Shutes, S. Spencer, and George Leeson. 2009. *Migrant Care Workers in Ageing Societies: Research Findings in the United Kingdom*. Oxford: COMPAS.

Church, K. 1996. "Beyond 'Bad Manners': The Power Relations of 'Consumer Participation' in Ontario's Community Mental Health System." *Canadian Journal of Community Mental Health* 15(2): 27–44.

Crenshaw, K. 1991. "Mapping the Margins: Intersectionality, Identity Politics and Violence Against Women of Color." *Stanford Law Review* 43:1241–1299.

Engster, D. 2007. *The Heart of Justice: Care Ethics and Political Theory*. Oxford: Oxford University Press.

Fraser, N. 1997. *Justice Interruptus: Critical Reflections on the "Postsocialist" Condition*. London: Routledge.

Gilligan, C. 1982. *In a Different Voice: Psychological Theory and Women's Development*. Cambridge, MA: Harvard University Press.

Glendinning, C., D. Challis, J. Fernandez, S. Jacobs, K. Jones, M. Knapp, J. Manthorpe, N. Moran, A. Netten, M. Stevens, and M. Wilberforce. 2008. *Evaluation of the Individual Budgets Pilot Programme: Final Report*. York: SPRU, University of York, PSSRU, Social Care Workforce Research Unit.

Hankivsky, O. 2014. "Rethinking Care Ethics: On the Promise and Potential of an Intersectional Analysis." *American Political Science Review* 108(2): 252–264.

Hunter, S. 2009. "Subversive Attachments: Gendered, Raced and Professional Realignments in the 'New' NHS." In *Subversive Citizens: Power, Agency and Resistance in Public Services*, edited by M. Barnes and D. Prior, 137–153. Bristol: Policy.

Hunter, S. 2015. *Power, Politics and the Emotions: Impossible Governance?* London: Routledge.

Kittay, E. F. 1999. *Love's Labor: Essays on Women, Equality and Dependency*. London: Routledge.

Krumer-Nevo, M., and M. Komem. 2013. "Intersectionality and Critical Social Work with Girls: Theory and Practice." *British Journal of Social Work* 25(4):1190–1206. doi: 10.1093/bjsw/bct189.

Leadbetter, C., J. Bartlett, and N. Gallagher. 2008. *Making It Personal*. London: Demos.

Lloyd, L. 2010. "The Individual in Social Care: The Ethics of Care and the 'Personalisation' Agenda in Services for Older People in England." *Ethics and Social Welfare* 4(2): 188–200.

MacDonald, D., M. Barnes, M. Crawford, E. Omeni, A. Wilson, and D. Rose. 2014. "Service User Governors in Mental Health Foundation Trusts: Accountability or Business as Usual?" *Health Expectations*.

Manea, T. 2015. "Care for Carers: Care Issues in the Context of Medical Migration." In *Ethics of Care: Critical Advances in International Perspective*, edited by M. Barnes, T. Brannelly, L. Ward, and N. Ward, 207–218. Bristol: Policy.

Mansbridge, J., and A. Morris, eds. 2001. *Oppositional Consciousness: The Subjective Roots of Social Protest*. Chicago: University of Chicago Press.

Mol, A. 2008. *The Logic of Care: Health and the Problem of Patient Choice*. Abingdon: Routledge.

Morris, J. 2001. "Impairment and Disability: Constructing an Ethics of Care That Promotes Human Rights." *Hypatia* 16(4): 1–16.

Nare, L. 2013. "The Ethics of Transnational Market Familism: Inequalities and Hierarchies in the Italian Elderly Care." *Ethics and Social Welfare* 7(2): 184–197.

Perkins, R. E. 1999. "My Three Psychiatric Careers." In *From the Ashes of Experience: Reflections on Madness, Survival and Growth*, edited by P. Barker, P. Campbell, and B. Davidson, 134–146. London: Whurr.

Sayer, A. 2011. *Why Things Matter to People: Social Science, Values and Ethical Life*. Cambridge: Cambridge University Press.

Tregaskis, C. 2004. *Constructions of Disability: Researching the Interface Between Disabled and Non-disabled People*. London: Routledge.

Tronto, J. 1993. *Moral Boundaries: A Political Argument for an Ethic of Care*. London: Routledge.

Tronto, J. 2010. "Creating Caring Institutions: Politics, Plurality and Purpose." *Ethics and Social Welfare* 4(2): 158–171.

Tronto, J. 2013. *Caring Democracy: Markets, Equality and Justice*. New York: New York University Press.

Ward, L., and M. Barnes. 2015. "Transforming Practice with Older People Through an Ethic of Care." *British Journal of Social Work*, 1–17. doi: 10.1093/bjsw/bcv029.

Ward, N. 2011. "Care Ethics and Carers with Learning Disabilities: A Challenge to Dependence and Paternalism." *Ethics and Social Welfare* 5(2): 168–180.

Ward, N. 2015. "Care Ethics, Intersectionality and Post Structuralism." In *Ethics of Care: Critical Advances in International Perspective*, edited by M. Barnes, T. Brannelly, L. Ward, and N. Ward, 57–68. Bristol: Policy.

Ward, N. J. 2005. *Social Exclusion and Mental Wellbeing: Lesbian Experiences*. PhD thesis, University of Birmingham.

Williams, V., L. Ponting, K. Ford, and P. Rudge. 2009. "'A Bit of Common Ground': Personalisation and the Use of Shared Knowledge in Interactions Between People with Learning Disabilities and Their Personal Assistants." *Discourse Studies* 11(5): 607–624.

16

Border Work

NEGOTIATING SHIFTING REGIMES OF POWER

▸ JANET NEWMAN

"TRANSFORMATIVE CHANGE" HAS LONG BEEN the rallying cry of those with a stake in human service provision. It has been the call of social movement activists seeking enhanced rights and voice. But it has also been the demand of policymakers seeking to redraw the relationship between state and citizen (shifting responsibility, promoting resilience, and changing citizen behavior). My focus in this chapter is on how these different demands intersect and on the labor at stake in managing the contradictions that arise, especially in conditions of retrenchment and austerity. I address such questions by drawing on the idea of "border work." The focus on actors working the borders of contemporary policy and politics challenges the concept of "transformation" as a kind of epochal change. It draws attention to the transformative processes of reimagination and reflexive practice on the part of those working for change (see Gubrium, Chapter 1, this volume).

The idea of border work can be traced through a range of different literatures that variously conceptualize such workers as "boundary spanners" and "boundary crossers" (Lewis 2008; Milligan and Conradson 2006), "civic entrepreneurs" (Durose 2011), "exemplary practitioners" (van Hulst, de Graaf, and van den Brink 2012), "everyday makers" (Bang and Sørensen 1999), or "community organizers" (Wills 2012), all of which refer back to, and rework, the older conception of "street-level bureaucrat" (Lipsky 1980). Border workers face in multiple directions as both "state agents" and "citizen agents" (Maynard-Moody and Musheno 2000) or as "subversive citizens" within state bureaucracies (Barnes and Prior 2009) (see in this volume

Barnes, Chapter 15; Jensen and Villadsen, Chapter 11). But in contrast to much of the literature cited here, I do not view border workers as a special category of worker. Rather, I am concerned with those working the borders between different regimes of organizational, political, and social power: public and private, bureaucratic and civic, statutory and voluntary, state and market, governmental and social, activist and neoliberal.

The border work at stake in this chapter, then, is concerned not solely with individual professional–client relationships but with the wider articulation of different—and often contradictory—rationalities and practices. These might include:

- social movements, civil society activists, or user groups trying to influence policymakers;
- state and not-for-profit practitioners mobilizing the discourses of choice or personalization to challenge dominant organizational rationalities;
- community-based and volunteer agencies seeking both to survive and to find new spaces of influence following cuts and changes in the commissioning process;
- radical professionals and policy actors in state bureaucracies attempting to find spaces from which to pursue transformative agendas, such as "personalization" and "coproduction";
- organizations and managers, frontline staff, or social entrepreneurs seeking to align old and new rationalities to make emergent practices a new norm;
- policymakers and politicians trying to translate user movements and activist struggles in ways that resonate with political projects of state retrenchment.

It is evident from these examples that border work arises across political as well as organizational borders and is the work of social movements and activists as well as practitioners and policymakers. Many contemporary shifts draw on and appropriate social movement and activist commitments in order to legitimate new forms of rule (see Gubrium, Chapter 1, this volume). Border workers may struggle to reconcile the tensions that arise while struggling for what they and others view as progressive transformations and seeing those very transformations transmuted, hollowed out, and incorporated into dominant regimes. But they also use those same tensions to create new possibilities and opportunities. Border work, as such, has a generative potential.

This chapter begins by situating my arguments in an analysis of welfare reform, specifically the introduction of notions of choice, personalization, and coproduction. The second section considers the work of translation—working the borders between different meanings and discursive repertoires—while the third section explores the forms of embodied and affective labor at stake in negotiating multiple regimes of power. The final section explores the place of border work in the context, in many European states, of the rise of anti-welfare ideology and a politics increasingly dominated by austerity governance.

REFRAMING WELFARE REFORM

Coming out of feminism, my working life has witnessed a series of successful transformations of organizational life that seemed to respond to some of our demands (greater flexibility, more attention to human relationships in the workplace, equal opportunity policies, some acknowledgment of care responsibilities, and so on). Each of these was based on collective processes of reimagination (how might the world be different?) and action (making things visible, bringing issues to wider public debate, enacting new worlds within the confines of an often hostile present). But I have also witnessed the ways in which the political challenges of feminism have been deflected through a series of organizational technologies (the toothless action plan, the routinized "equal opportunity" training day, the bureaucratic architecture of human resources management). These processes of deflection can be linked to a broader analysis of how feminist demands have been incorporated into neoliberal transformations of the state and citizenship. For example, women's claims for independence (from patriarchal norms within the family and in employment, social security, and pension systems) were transmuted into the twin rationales of the gender-free "worker citizen" and marketized relations of care (Jensen 1999; Lister 2003). Both were highly compatible with the growth of neoliberal ideology and its transformations of both welfare and work. It is no surprise, then, that scholars now talk of the complicity of feminism and neoliberalism (Fraser 2009; McRobbie 2009).

Women were of course not the only group to demand both inclusion in and transformation of the welfare state. Disability activists challenged the oppressive nature of services based on a medical model of disability and promoted alternative models and forms of service innovation (Beresford 2012; see also Shakespeare and Collins, Chapter 12, this volume; Solvang, Chapter 7, this volume). Patient movements campaigned for access to new treatments and for more involvement in decisions made about individual care (Newman and Tonkens 2011). Mental health service users claimed rights to full citizenship rather than stigmatizing forms of treatment and incarceration (Barnes and Bowl 2011). Norms of care in old age were challenged by new forms of activism among the growing elderly population (Vabo 2011).

Three themes are evident in such claims. First, there is a demand for participation in decisions about one's own care or treatment, as well as in politics and policymaking. Second, there is a demand for recognition—as citizens, as members of the polity, and as people with authentic forms of expertise and experience. This is often coupled with a demand that so-called private issues—such as domestic violence, parenting, and caring—be recognized as public matters and thus legitimate objects of collective concern and public/state support. Third, there is a demand for more autonomy and choice: for the ability to shape one's own life and to be recognized as an independent person rather than a dependent subject (see Shakespeare and Collins, Chapter 12, this volume).

Each of these themes has prefigured new professional and organizational norms. But each has also been reworked in welfare reform discourses of active citizenship, choice, and responsibility that have tended to appropriate—and depoliticize—social movement claims. For example, studies of new welfare regimes in seven Western European nations (Newman and Tonkens 2011) trace how demands for choice were deflected and remade in the opening up of welfare markets but also how they helped transform stigmatizing and paternalistic welfare provision. The researchers traced how claims for recognition and voice were translated in the transformation of (some) services around norms of personalization, and how this offered expanded notions of the welfare subject while also detaching them from wider collective claims.

The researchers show how demands for inclusion were remodeled as duties and responsibilities: responsibilities for self-care and self-development, for the care of family and neighbors, and for community participation.

These were strongly supported by progressive professionals and policymakers but were also highly compatible with cuts to state-provided welfare and with the remaking of the meaning of welfare as policymakers turned to behavior change strategies and, in the United Kingdom, albeit briefly, norms of a "big society" (rather than a "big state").

As I write, a further set of transformations is taking place in human services around notions of "coproduction." This is an idea that seeks to transform borders—not only between practitioners and clients but also between the state and society. Coproduction is presented as an alternative to bureaucratic and market-based systems of delivery, neither of which takes adequate account of the importance of relationships to the effectiveness of service outcomes (Ostrom 1996; Cahn 2000; New Economics Foundation 2008). Such advocates argue that the contributions of patients, communities, and clients are at least as significant as the role of service deliverers to the achievement of positive outcomes. Coproduction seeks to tap into the "hidden resources" of communities, families, and networks in delivering services, rather than treating individuals as isolated clients or consumers.

Coproduction therefore is linked not only to transformations in human services but also to more fundamental shifts in the nature of the state itself. Like the shifts toward participation and choice, coproduction has its origins on the political left and among radical practitioners, social movements, and those searching for political alternatives to a discredited model of state provision. It is linked to critiques of traditional bureaucratic state forms and marketized state services, and its proponents offer a transformational image of a more relational, equal, and participatory social settlement. However, coproduction is also potentially aligned with a politics of state retrenchment in which communities and users are "responsibilized" to find personal and community resources beyond the state.

Such forms of analysis underscore the contested politics of welfare reform. They challenge singular, epochal narratives, whether of progress (personalization rather than bureaucracy, coproduction rather than dependence) or loss (the incorporation or co-optation of social movement demands into new regimes of rule). Narratives of progress point to the successful challenge to bureaucratic forms of welfare provision, the greater emphasis on the participation and involvement of service users, and enhanced autonomy and independence. Narratives of loss point to how struggles on the part of service users for greater independence and autonomy prefigured neoliberal attacks on the paternalistic "nanny state" and the expansion of marketization and consumer choice. This, many have argued, is associated with new forms of rule based on governmentalities of the self (Rose 1999; Cruikshank 1990): governmentalities that can be viewed as means of governing potentially unruly populations, rendering them compliant through the production of new forms of self-governing subjects.

However, narratives of co-optation and responsibilization have a rather conspiratorial tone and offer too generalized a picture of the workings of both governmental and corporate power. They tend to present welfare reform and organizational or professional change as unambiguous, flattening out complexity and rendering invisible the work of those managing the contradictions at stake. In contrast, ethnographic studies tend to highlight the ambiguity of new discourses and emphasize the role of social actors in mediating and translating new governmentalities. For example, the shift toward an emphasis on coproduction takes us back to the ambivalences around notions of choice, personalization, and responsibility. It is certainly the case that coproduction is all too readily aligned with the wider retreat of the state in favor of individual and community responsibility. But this does not detract from arguments about the benefits of coproduction (improved outcomes) and its capacity to reflect wider processes of social and political change.

A second qualification to grand narratives of progress or loss is the depiction of change they offer. Human service reform is not, I want to argue, a linear process in which new—or not so new—ideas and policies gradually come to displace more traditional organizational and institutional forms. Rather, a series of new or emergent policy discourses or reform narratives are actively translated as actors negotiate political, policy, and service relationships (see Gubrium, Chapter 1, this volume).

MAKING MEANING: THE WORK OF TRANSLATION

The analysis of new governmentalities of responsibility, choice, participation, or coproduction tends to focus on strategies, with little acknowledgment of how such strategies may be interpreted, refused, adapted, or perhaps remain unheard. Notions of *translation* offer a more extensive engagement with such processes than the grand narratives referred to earlier, and suggest something of the constitutive power of meanings in action (Clarke et al. 2015). Here, policy is not something that is handed down from a strategic center for execution by frontline practitioners but is something that is "drawn down" and imbued with meaning in specific contexts:

> The trope of translation is to emphasise the alternatives, and processes of re-transcription, which produces very diverse stories and voices in policy processes. Translation is also a dynamic framework to capture the fluidity of policy processes, with an emphasis on the constant (re)construction of issues, discourses, and actor networks, as part of real human agency. (Lendvai and Stubbs 2007:21)

My use of the term "translation" here is intended to suggest how border work is not concerned with the transgression of hard barriers or the breaching of impossible divides but rather is concerned with the negotiation of contested meanings of policy as it is enacted. The meanings that welfare workers, citizens, and service users bestow on the policies that shape their relationship with each other, with service organizations, and with the state have a constitutive force. It is through acts of translation that tensions between progressive and retrogressive forms of change are negotiated. Therefore, translation is a key element of border work.

I want to offer two examples that extend the focus of translation to encompass not only the making of meaning but also the articulation of meanings, politics, and power. The first is the study by Clarke et al. (2007) of the emergence of the citizen consumer as a policy subject in reforms to health, policing, and social care in the United Kingdom. Situated in the British tradition of cultural studies, this research drew on multiple methods: an analysis of policy texts and political pronouncements to identify the construction and legitimation of consumerism and choice in social welfare; interviews and textual analysis in three sectors undergoing change (health, policing, and social care); and survey data, focus groups, and interviews with citizens using those same services. Two sets of findings are of significance in terms of the arguments of this chapter. First, the study found that the professionals in the three sectors interpreted consumerism rather differently as they sought to negotiate and reconcile governmental discourse with established professional meanings and practices. For example, in health care, we found organization managers and professionals debating how far existing policies went—on patient participation or choice of service provider—

meaning that they were already "doing" consumerism, so little further change was required (Newman and Vidler 2006). This was not a straightforward matter of resistance to or rejection of government policy; the interview transcripts showed respondents engaged in quite subtle deliberations about the meaning of policy and of professional practice.

Second, the study showed how the users of welfare services tended to hold multiple subject positions: as citizens, as members of local communities, as members of the public, and sometimes as consumers. The significance of this finding is that it shows how discursive strategies or narrative structures do not necessarily produce their intended effects. Interviewees were shown to have multiple identities, interests, and beliefs, and to offer different (and sometimes irreconcilable) meanings when asked to interpret their worlds. Those whom policy seeks to address may translate it in unanticipated ways in order to make new claims or restore older meanings and practices that they see as being eroded.

A different approach to the study of meaning can be found in studies of policy as narrative. My example here is Needham's (2011) analysis of the emergence of "personalisation" as a policy narrative in the United Kingdom in the New Labour years (1997–2010). This narrative was used to legitimate reform in a wide range of social policy arenas, including health, social care, housing, education, and employment. Needham shows how it constructed the past in ways that condemned what had gone before, and went on to highlight personalization as the viable path to the resolution of the problems past forms of welfare provision had generated. However, she also notes that a focus on narrative alone tends to minimize the role of contexts and agents. Her interpretive study traces how different policy actors (including civil servants, activists, managers, frontline staff, and service users) gave meaning to narratives and to the reforms they heralded. In the process, Needham shows how actors "translate" (interpret and modify the meanings of) policy as it moves from one sector or profession to another. Context is important here, in that the emergence of personalization derives in part from the work of social movements. But its takeup within the professions and government was "due to its ability to cohere with the broader political climate in which individual rights are twinned with responsibilities in an unstable mix" (Needham 2011:85), as well as its potential to deliver cost savings. This created what Needham terms a "purposive ambivalence" (p. 86) that generated both the possibility of enlarged spaces of action for both frontline staff and service users and, at the same time, created difficulties and dilemmas.

Such studies point to the importance of actors who negotiate the border between would-be hegemonic discourses (choice, personalization) and alternative meanings rooted in social democratic, professional, and popular discourses (those that neoliberal political projects are seeking to residualize). The meanings of "choice," "personalization," and "coproduction" are not fixed; they can be mobilized as progressive forms of change that respond to social movement demands or radical professional interventions. And they can become tied to neoliberalizing projects of public service retrenchment coupled to individualizing models of citizenship. These different meanings are negotiated and enacted in multiple "spaces of power" in increasingly complex welfare systems.

SPACES OF POWER

The concept border work draws attention to the ongoing work of those working for change in the "spaces of power" where conflicting rationalities converge and are negotiated in increasingly complex welfare systems. Such spaces are not only those where professional meets client but also those in which professional change is negotiated, where policy networks converge, where partnership boards meet, where training schemes are designed and delivered, where nongovernmental organizations (NGOs) and think tanks commission and interpret research, where social movements engage with policy actors to put forward new claims, where community-based and volunteer organizations negotiate contracts with those commissioning services, where frontline staff interpret managerial rules, and many others. Such spaces are relational (they stretch beyond individual encounters) and political (they are where power is both exercised and challenged). Spaces of power are those in which conflicting meanings are negotiated and in which the colonization or appropriation of what might be viewed as progressive reform may be both enacted and resisted.

In *Working the Spaces of Power* (Newman 2012), I report on a study of how women over four generations had taken activist commitments into their working lives in community and volunteer organizations, local and national government, policy networks, research organizations, think tanks, and academia. The interviews show how the participants in the study worked across different organizations, sectors, nations, and institutions. For example, the study explored the work of women trying to work across the borders between governmental norms of community and more grassroots, activist conceptions of local action. It showed how women had attempted to influence policy, bringing feminist and other social movement perspectives to bear on social policy. It traced ways in which women had influenced the reshaping of organizational practice toward greater concern with issues of equality and diversity, more participative and person-centered leadership, and had brought socialist, feminist, and antiracist politics into particular spaces within the state. These were not easy places to be: borders were not only between sectors or institutions but also between different identifications and loyalties. Across the accounts, the notions of "we" and "them," of inside and outside, were rather slippery, especially where participants sought to render boundaries more permeable in order to extend the influence of social and political movements on dominant ruling relations. Despite their engagements with governmental power, they also sought to stay in touch with the places where, in the words of participants, "reality bites," to build bridges between policy actors and the grass roots, to link community-based actors and those in poverty to resource streams, and to enlarge opportunities for "voice."

Border work therefore has to be understood as political rather than sectoral or geographical: the "inside," "outside," "edges," "middle," and so on referred to by participants were less concerned with defined places than with political possibilities. They were spaces of agency, of power, but also spaces of ambiguity, discomfort, and emotional work. There is a long tradition of highlighting the "emotional labor" at stake in the delivery of human services (Hochschild 1983; Henderson 2001; Hoggett 2000). Border work offers a rather more expansive concept than that of emotional labor. It relies on cognitive, sensory, and bodily capacities, network skills, and the capacity to accumulate relational experience and learning and to translate it in new contexts. It is a set of capacities that are required not only in professional–client relationships but in all forms of policy, managerial, and organizational work, and in the work of user and advocacy groups. However, like emotional labor, it tends to remain unrecognized, marginal, and often highly gendered.

It became evident during this research that border work could produce profound discomfort as different identifications—as insiders and outsiders, as both different from and as part of the dominant order—were lived and performed. Being "inside-outside"—of the nation, the organization, the polity, activist networks, the academy—clearly brought feelings of both inclusion and exclusion. The transcripts suggest multiple and partial positionings of the self: as at the same time an activist and a paid worker, as an insider and an outsider, as a stranger and a professional, as an individual making her own decisions and compromises and as part of collective entities. Participant accounts also referenced *affective* dimensions of border work: being "shocked" and finding it "difficult," taking risks and finding things "bizarre" or "weird," being proud and "fulfilled," not being able to "bear" one sector and feeling "stifled" by another, of being viewed (and perhaps viewing the self) as compromised because of decisions made. For example, one woman who had spent years attempting to foster local social action spoke about her anger when UK prime minister David Cameron began to speak about the need for a "Big Society" and how this was part of a set of policies designed to use projects such as hers to replace state support and funding. Yet she had to speak the language of "Big Society" in order to bid for funding to continue the work of the organization she led—something about which she was profoundly ambivalent.

Paying attention to such representations of emotion and affect suggests some of the forms of "self work" at stake. Participants draw discourses and repertoires from different worlds, forming new configurations of what "work" means and how it is to be conducted. Indeed, it is this capacity to span different worlds and identities that generated the spaces of power with which I was concerned.

SPEAKING TO THE PRESENT: THE CONTEMPORARY DYNAMICS OF BORDER WORK

This analysis of this chapter points to the dangers of viewing contemporary shifts in normative discourse—for example, those promulgating coproduction and personalization—as practices that flatten difference, that transcend questions of difference and power. They are not about making everything equivalent by abolishing expertise. Rather, they are policy discourses and sets of practice that reorder the relational dynamics of human services far beyond the point of service delivery.

Therefore, they are the site of significant lines of tension and forms of ambivalence, especially under conditions of austerity. In the United Kingdom, the ideals of coproduction, for example, have been somewhat tempered by the effects of severe cuts to state services, the withdrawal of funding to many volunteer and community organizations, and the increasing impoverishment of those reliant on state benefits. It has become increasingly difficult for those working in cash-strapped public services to find, let alone tap into, the "hidden resources" of families and communities in order to "empower" them to participate in the production of positive social outcomes. There is an argument that austerity and cuts make the idea of coproduction more attractive both for policymakers (pursuing projects of slimming down the state) and for organizational managers (seeking to do "more with less" as the cuts bite). It also opens up space for other agents—civil society actors, social entrepreneurs, and NGOs—to pursue radical forms of innovation. However, organizational downsizing and welfare retrenchment reduce the capacity of state agents to support their side of the "co" of coproduction. Under conditions of austerity, coproduction may herald not a new partnership between state and civil society, between organizations and users, but instead a politics of abandonment and abjection.

Austerity and cuts are also having a malign impact on "border workers" in public human services. Many have lost their jobs or seen their jobs move to private sector providers, with the consequential worsening of conditions and new demands for "flexibility"—zero hour contracts, short-term contracts, and so on. Those that remain are presented with new challenges to their legitimacy and a circumscribed sphere of decision-making power. Some have stepped away from the performance pressures of service organizations and become part of the growing social economy of nonprofit or social enterprise organizations struggling to find a place in a shrinking market for state-funded services.

However, border workers are not just the passive recipients of such shifts. Whether paid or unpaid, whether part of the formal or informal economy, they are active agents in the shaping of potential new social and political settlements, "performing new worlds" within the constraints of the present (Newman 2013). Some are shaping new projects that fit with a culture of austerity governance—encouraging citizens and service users to become more independent, to rely less on the state. Others are engaged in new forms of political activism that disrupt the established norms of a discredited political and economic system. Those working with vulnerable and dispossessed peoples are trying to balance the protection of vulnerable clients and communities with the creation of new forms of mutual care or self-care. Those working in or for local neighborhoods are struggling to find new sources of resilience to meet the needs of citizens most affected by the cuts (Lowndes and McCaughie 2014). Policy entrepreneurs (in think tanks, political parties, trade unions, NGOs, campaign organizations, and other "spaces of power") are working toward new settlements based on environmental and economic sustainability, working the borders of the existing political system to influence long-term change. All are immersed in new forms of knowledge economy that tend to dissolve boundaries between work and nonwork, and all are having to make difficult judgments about the relationship between paid and unpaid work, between care for others and care for the self, as they manage the affective, as well as material, consequences of austerity.

• • •

The predominant focus in the "human service" literature is on the borders between professional and service user, and how inequalities of power and expertise might be overcome. This chapter has attempted to look beyond these individual relationships to the contradictory politics that shape the processes of welfare reform, and to the work of those managing the dilemmas and constraints that these politics produce. This has consequences for how questions of power and agency are imagined. Rather than a strong—and relatively fixed—set of boundaries between governmental power and sociopolitical agency, my focus in this chapter has been concerned with how such boundaries are remade or reshaped through everyday, reflexive forms of practice (see Garrow, Chapter 5, this volume). And rather than a simple (and individualized) conception of borders between the state and society, or between sectors and services, the chapter has been concerned with multiple borders: those between social movements and government policy, between activism and incorporation, between strategic centers and organizational peripheries, and perhaps between "tradition" and "innovation."

My focus on borders and border work has two important qualifications. First, it is context-specific. Different nations and political administrations draw the boundaries between state and citizen in very different ways, with some continuing to shape services around norms of public welfare while others privilege notions of responsibility and choice (Newman and Tonkens 2011). They also generate very different conditions in which border work takes place. For example, in the early twenty-first century, at least in Britain, work opportunities in the state-funded volunteer sector have been significantly reduced as a result of funding cuts; social entrepreneurship offers an important but less developed substitute. In Britain and elsewhere, working life has become more precarious, making it more difficult to challenge dominant orthodoxies. However, there is likely to be significant divergence between different municipal or regional regimes, each with their own political and historical characteristics, such as the account of regional differences in care policies and practice within Italy (De Leonardis 2011) or of differences between nations of the disunited United Kingdom (Mooney and Scott 2012). A recent analysis of "exemplary practitioners" working in urban neighborhoods in England, Denmark, and the Netherlands emphasizes the importance of situating their characteristics and the nature of their work in local contexts rather than homogenizing them as heroic agents (Agger et al. 2014). Rather than new grand narratives, we need to understand how multiple principles and strategies are combined and condensed in specific locations (institutions, relationships, policy sites).

This takes me to the second set of qualifications, on the mutability of borders. Borders are redrawn repeatedly as politicians, professionals, voluntary bodies, and civic associations engage with new contracting or coproduction arrangements, and redrawn by citizens as they negotiate new norms and responsibilities. Coproduction, participation, and other potentially transformative discourses have implications for the borders between service provider and recipient as the expertise of service users is recognized, their participation in decision making is enhanced, and as service design as well as delivery becomes more collaborative—or even delegated entirely. But they also change the relationships between institutions and workers. For example, those promoting new practices of coproduction have to negotiate the interface with institutional cultures unsympathetic to the erosion of traditional hierarchies of power and authority, as well as coping with ceding and changing—the basis of their own power. At the same time, they have to look outward to mine communities for "hidden resources" and attempt to build new networks and capacities as, for example, in Durose's work on how "civic entrepreneurs" work to create new forms of social capital (Durose 2011).

The mutability of borders is particularly significant in the context of current processes of welfare reform. Borders are shifting not only as a result of organizational (re)design but also as a result of wider processes of state retrenchment. This implies changing relationships with "communities" whom organizations attempt to "activate," either to become part of the new market economy of welfare services or to provide for their own needs. The old emphasis on working across departmental and service boundaries in order to deliver "joined up" services is being destabilized as the boundaries become unsettled and institutions unmade. At stake are not just the borders between professional and client but those between strategic centers and "frontline" staff or between social and civic agents attempting to create new forms of capacity and resilience.

The intensification of new reform initiatives designed to destabilize old welfare systems is creating high levels of institutional churn. This produces new insecurities and uncertainties but also generates a proliferation of new borders and forms of border work. Work itself is being transformed not only through new forms of contracts and an intensification of the labor process but also new forms of knowledge work that dissolve the boundaries between work and nonwork, bringing work into the spaces of intimate life (Gregg 2011). Border work has always been the source of high levels of personal flexibility and freedom, but it is now the site of new forms of exploitation and oppression.

But none of these changes can be represented as a smooth shift from "old" to "new" patterns of power and authority. Instead, border work concerns the labor of working between different, and often incompatible, working principles and rationales. My particular concern in this chapter has been to understand border work as political labor: the labor of those with activist commitments as they negotiate forms of welfare reform that seek to draw on and rework the meaning of their political claims. Today, many continue to struggle for change, using openings in the process of political and organizational reform to pursue "other" projects and to create alternative possibilities. But they do so in the context of fragmented and insecure labor processes and in a climate dominated by political dismay and disaffection. Borders are not an easy place to be.

REFERENCES

Agger, A., L. de Graaf, C. Durose, O. Escobar, S. Jeffares, and M. van Hulst. 2014. "Five Ways to Make a Difference; Practitioners and Their Engagement in Urban Neighbourhoods." Paper presented at the 9th International Interpretive Policy Analysis Conference, Wageningen, the Netherlands.

Bang, H., and E. Sørensen. 1999. "The Everyday Maker: A New Challenge to Democratic Governance." *Administrative Theory and Practice* 21(3): 325–341.

Barnes, M., and R. Bowl. 2011. *Taking Over the Asylum: Empowerment and Mental Health*. Basingstoke: Palgrave.

Barnes, M., and D. Prior, eds. 2009. *Subversive Citizens: Power Agency and Resistance in Public Services*. Bristol: Policy.

Beresford, P. 2012. "Ignored or Just Forgotten?" *Journal of Integrated Care* 20(4): 202–214.

Cahn, E. 2000. *No More Throwaway People: The Coproduction Imperative*. Washington, DC: Essential.

Clarke, J., D. Bainton, N. Lendvai, and P. Stubbs. 2015. *Making Policy Move: Towards a Politics of Translation and Assemblage*. Bristol: Policy.

Clarke, J., J. Newman, N. Smith, E. Vidler, and L. Westmarland. 2007. *Creating Citizen-Consumers: Changing Publics and Changing Public Services*. London: Sage.

Cruikshank, B. 1990. *The Will to Empower*. Ithaca, NY: Cornell University Press.

De Leonardis, O. 2011. "Dividing or Combining Citizens: The Politics of Active Citizenship in Italy." In *Participation, Responsibility and Choice: Summoning the Active Citizen in Western Europe*, edited by J. Newman and E. Tonkens, 127–146. Amsterdam: Amsterdam University Press.

Durose, C. 2011. "Revisiting Lipsky: Front-Line Work in UK Local Governance." *Political Studies* 59(4): 978–995.

Fraser, N. 2009. "Feminism, Capitalism and the Cunning of History." *New Left Review* 56:97–117.

Gregg, M. 2011. *Works Intimacy*. Cambridge: Polity.

Henderson, A. 2001. "Emotional Labour and Nursing: An Underrepresented Aspect of Caring Work." *Nursing Enquiry* 8(2): 130–138.

Hochschild, A. 1983. *The Managed Heart*. Berkeley: University of California Press.

Hoggett, P. 2000. *Emotional Life and the Politics of Welfare*. Basingstoke: Macmillan.

Jensen, J. 1999. "Lost in Translation: The Social Investment Perspective and Gender Equality." *Social Politics* 16(4): 446–483.

Lendvai, N., and P. Stubbs. 2007. "Policy as Translation: Situating Transnational Social Policies." In *Policy Reconsidered: Meanings, Politics and Practice*, edited by S. Hodgson and Z. Irving, 173–190. Bristol: Policy.

Lewis, D. 2008. "Using Life Histories in Social Policy Research: The Case of Third Sector/Public Sector Boundary Crossing." *Journal of Social Policy* 37(4): 559–578.

Lipsky, M. 1980. *Street-Level Bureaucracy: Dilemmas of the Individual in Public Services*. New York: Russell Sage Foundation.

Lister, R. 2003. *Citizenship: Feminist Perspectives*, second edition. Basingstoke: Palgrave Macmillan.

Lowndes, V., and K. McCaughie. 2014. "Weathering the Perfect Storm? Austerity and Institutional Resilience in Local Government." In *Rethinking Policy and Politics*, edited by S. Ayres, 95–115. Bristol: Policy.

Maynard-Moody, S., and M. Musheno. 2000. "State Agent or Citizen Agent: Two Narratives of Discretion." *Journal of Public Administration Research and Theory* 10(2): 329–358.

McRobbie, A. 2009. *The Aftermath of Feminism: Gender, Culture and Social Change*. London: Sage.

Milligan, C., and D. Conradson, eds. 2006. *Landscapes of Voluntarism*. Bristol: Policy.

Mooney, G., and G. Scott. 2012. *Social Justice and Social Policy in Scotland*. Bristol: Policy.

Needham, C. 2011. *Public Services: The Personalisation Narrative*. Bristol: Policy.

New Economics Foundation. 2008. *Coproduction; a Manifesto for Growing the Core Economy*. London: Nef.

Newman, J. 2012. *Working the Spaces of Power: Activism, Neoliberalism and Gendered Labour*. London: Bloomsbury.

Newman, J. 2013. "Performing New Worlds? Policy, Politics and Creative Labour in Hard Times." *Policy and Politics* 41(4): 515–532.

Newman, J., and E. Tonkens, eds. 2011. *Participation, Responsibility and Choice: Summoning the Active Citizen in Western Europe*. Amsterdam: Amsterdam University Press.

Newman, J., and E. Vidler. 2006. "Discriminating Customers, Responsible Patients, Empowered Users: Consumerism and the Modernisation of Health Care." *Journal of Social Policy* 35(2): 193–209.

Ostrom, E. 1996. "Crossing the Great Divide: Co-production, Synergy and Development." *World Development* 24(6): 1073–1087.

Rose, N. 1999. *Powers of Freedom: Reframing Political Thought*. Cambridge: Cambridge University Press.

Vabo, M. 2011. "Active Citizenship in Norwegian Elderly Care: From Activation to Consumer Activism." In *Participation, Responsibility and Choice: Summoning the Active Citizen in Western Europe*, edited by J. Newman and E. Tonkens, 87–106. Amsterdam: Amsterdam University Press.

van Hulst, M., L. de Graaf, and G. van den Brink. 2012. "The Work of Exemplary Practitioners in Neighbourhood Governance." *Critical Policy Studies* 6(4): 434–451.

Wills, J. 2012. "The Geography of Community and Political Organization in London Today." *Political Geography* 31(2): 114–126.

CONTRIBUTORS

TONE ALM ANDREASSEN is professor and head of research for the interdisciplinary program in Care, Health and Welfare at Oslo and Akershus University College of Applied Sciences in Norway. She received her doctorate in Political Science from the Department of Sociology and Human Geography at the University of Oslo. Service user involvement has been a research interest of hers for years, along with studies of processes of organizational change and those of policymaking and policy implementation at the level of civil society organizations.

MARIAN BARNES is emeritus professor of social policy at the University of Brighton, United Kingdom. She previously held a chair in social research at the University of Birmingham and also has worked at the universities of Leeds and Sheffield. She is well known for her research on user involvement and user movements, public participation, citizenship, and new forms of democratic practices. In the last few years, her work has focused on the ethics of care, and aging and well-being. Barnes's many publications include *Power, Participation, and Political Renewal*, with Janet Newman and Helen Sullivan; *Caring and Social Justice*; and *Care in Everyday Life*.

E. SUMMERSON CARR is associate professor in the School of Social Service Administration at the University of Chicago, where she is also an affiliate of the Department of Anthropology, the Center for Gender Studies, and the Department of Comparative Human Development. She is the author of *Scripting Addiction: The Politics of Therapeutic Talk and American Sobriety* and several articles based on extensive ethnographic work in social service settings. She currently is co-editing a book on the anthropology of scale and is writing a monograph—tentatively titled *Motivating Apprentices: Science, Spirit, and the Institution of American Expertise*—based on her recent research on motivational interviewing.

RACHAEL COLLINS is currently pursuing her medical degree at Norwich medical school, having previously completed her BS in natural sciences at Durham

University, United Kingdom. She hopes to specialize in psychiatry and is currently conducting research into the views and experiences of psychiatrists on service user–led recovery.

ERIK ERIKSSON is a PhD candidate at the School of Social Work at Lund University, Sweden. His PhD studies concern the relationship between the service user movement and the welfare state. Through ethnographically inspired fieldwork, he examines how service user involvement is constructed within local human service organizations. From this study, Eriksson has published an article titled "To Tell the Right Story" in the *Journal of Comparative Social Work*.

CRISTI FLOOD is a graduate student in McMaster University's Department of Health, Aging, and Society and is a student member of the Gilbrea Centre for Studies on Aging and the Critical Health Research Network, Canada. Flood has an interdisciplinary background in critical gerontology, medical sociology, and cultural studies. Her current graduate work draws on interdisciplinary and transdisciplinary approaches to examine discourses and representations of Canada's physician-assisted suicide debate.

GERALDINE FOLEY is assistant professor in the Discipline of Occupational Therapy, School of Medicine, Trinity College Dublin, Ireland. She has worked as a clinical specialist occupational therapist in the Irish public health care system. Foley's research has focused on health care experiences among people with amyotrophic lateral sclerosis (ALS), and her work has identified key psychosocial processes that underpin how people with ALS engage with health care services. She has published widely on health care experiences among people with ALS. She has peer reviewed for a number of academic journals and is a regular reviewer for *Qualitative Health Research* and for *Amyotrophic Lateral Sclerosis and Frontotemporal Degeneration*. Foley holds a BS OT, MS OT, and PhD from Trinity College Dublin.

EVE E. GARROW is a researcher and policy analyst for the American Civil Liberties Union (ACLU) of Southern California, where she studies the design and implementation of policies that target vulnerable populations, including persons who are homeless. Before joining the ACLU, Garrow was on the social work faculty at the University of Michigan, where she engaged in research focusing on disparate access to social benefits and human service programs based on factors such as race and disability. The underlying concerns that have driven her research are the consequences of policy design and implementation for service recipients and the development of policies that can more effectively advance human rights.

IAN GREENER is professor and deputy pro-vice chancellor at Durham University, United Kingdom. He has written monographs on a range of topics, including the history of health services in the United Kingdom and public management after the 2008–2009 financial crisis, as well as articles and thought pieces on health care, health policy, and research methods. Greener is particularly interested in issues of human agency and their relationship with health and well-being, and he is the general editor of the international journal *Social Policy and Administration*.

AMANDA GRENIER is associate professor in the Department of Health, Aging and Society, Gilbrea Chair in Aging and Mental Health, and director of the Gilbrea Centre for the Study of Aging, McMaster University, Canada. Grenier is a social gerontologist interested in the intersections of theory, policy, organizational practice, and lived experience. Her research program has focused on the social constructions of frailty, home care, late life transitions, and older homelessness, and she has published a number of journal articles on these topics. Her recent books include *Transitions and the Life Course* and the co-edited collection *Ageing, Meaning and Social Structure*. She is currently experimenting with running a blog on critical gerontology (www.criticalgerontology.com).

JABER F. GUBRIUM is professor and chair of sociology at the University of Missouri. His long-standing program of research on the social organization of care in human service institutions has produced several ethnographies and related journal articles, including *Living and Dying at Murray Manor*; *Out of Control: Family Therapy and Domestic Disorder*; *Caretakers: Treating Emotionally Disturbed Children*; *Speaking of Life: Horizons of Meaning for Nursing Home Residents*; *Describing Care: Image and Practice in Rehabilitation*; and *Oldtimers and Alzheimer's: The Descriptive Organization of Senility*. The program is an offshoot of his conceptualization of a sociology of description. Gubrium also has written extensively on the logic of qualitative inquiry and has contributed to the development of an institution-based approach to narrative analysis. He is founding and current editor of the *Journal of Aging Studies*.

KATARINA JACOBSSON is associate professor at the School of Social Work, Lund University, Sweden. She has a general interest in qualitative methodology and the sociology of knowledge, and her current project deals with documentation practices among human service workers. Her previous publications dealing with the sociology of bribery include the article "Accounts of Honesty" in the journal *Deviant Behavior.* Jacobsson also has published on the use of categories by medical staff (the article "Categories by Heart" in the journal *Professions and Professionalism*). One of her recent articles on methodology is titled "Interviewees with an Agenda," co-authored with Malin Åkerström, and was published in *Qualitative Research.*

MARGARETHA JÄRVINEN is professor of sociology at the University of Copenhagen, Denmark. Her research areas are client and state welfare encounters, symbolic interaction, alcohol and drug problems, and social marginalization. Her recent publications include *Turning Troubles into Problems: Clientization in Human Services,* co-edited with Jaber F. Gubrium (Routledge); "Explanations and Expectations: Drug Narratives Among Young Drug Users in Treatment," co-authored with Signe Ravn, in the journal *Sociology of Health and Illness;* and "Out of Sync: Time Management in the Lives of Young Drug Users," co-authored with Signe Ravn, in the journal *Time and Society.*

SIGNE MIE JENSEN holds a Master of Social Sciences degree from the Department of Political Communication and Management at the Copenhagen Business School, Denmark. Applying Niklas Luhmann's systems theory, she has explored the increasing complexity at the front line of welfare management that followed reforms inspired by New Public Management. Her thesis, completed in 2012, is titled "Welfare Management Under Pressure." Jensen has published several articles on this topic, a chapter for a Danish anthology, and dissemination reports.

PIA KONTOS is senior scientist at Toronto Rehabilitation Institute–University Health Network, and associate professor in the Dalla Lana School of Public Health at the University of Toronto, Canada. Central to her program of research is the transformation of the culture of dementia care so it is more humanistic and quality enhancing for individuals living with dementia, their family members, and health care practitioners. She draws significantly on the arts for their emotive and expressive nature, specifically music, dance, and improvisational play, to enrich the lives of individuals living in long-term care settings. She also draws on research-based drama and film as novel approaches to educational initiatives to effect change at a personal and organizational level. She has published across multiple disciplines on selfhood, dementia, embodiment, and arts-based innovations to improve dementia care.

KAREN-LEE MILLER is a critical health sociologist who specializes in qualitative research methods. Her work focuses on issues affecting women's health and social care across the life span, including frameworks of care and caring, emotion work, and gendered violence. She holds a PhD from the Dalla Lana School of Public Health, University of Toronto, Canada, and is a senior research associate with the Toronto Rehabilitation Institute–University Health Network.

JANET NEWMAN is emeritus professor in the Faculty of Social Sciences, The Open University, United Kingdom. She brings feminist and cultural forms of analysis to questions of governance, politics, and power, and is particularly concerned with engaging with policy and practice. Recently, her interests have centered on the relationships between austerity, activism, and participation. Her most recent book is *Working the Spaces of Power: Activism, Neoliberalism and Gendered Labour.*

TARJA PÖSÖ is professor of social work at the School of Social Sciences and Humanities, University of Tampere, Finland. She has long-standing experience studying child welfare from different perspectives, with a keen interest in cross-cultural perspectives and exploring methods and ethics for child welfare research. Her current research focuses on children in care and on decision making in child welfare. Pösö's most recent book is *Child Welfare Systems and Migrant Children*, co-edited with Marit Skivenes, Ravinder Barn, and Katrin Križ. She also is the editor of *Nordic Social Work Research.*

TOM SHAKESPEARE is senior lecturer in medical sociology at the University of East Anglia Medical School, United Kingdom. His research interests lie in disability studies, mental health, and bioethics. His books include *Disability Rights and Wrongs*, *The Sexual Politics of Disability*, and *Genetic Politics*. He currently is researching relationships between disabled people and their personal assistants.

PER KOREN SOLVANG is professor of rehabilitation in the Department of Physiotherapy, Oslo and Akershus University College of Applied Sciences, Norway. He is a sociologist and has held a position as professor of sociology at the University of Bergen. Solvang has published studies on a wide variety of themes related to disability. These include disability art, transnational meeting places for deaf people, life course perspectives on living with disabilities, and controversies on the medicalization of dyslexia.

VIRPI TIMONEN is professor in the School of Social Work and Social Policy at Trinity College Dublin, Ireland. Her research focuses on intergenerational relationships and policy pertaining to older adults. Timonen has authored or co-authored five books, including a major introductory textbook titled *Ageing Societies: A Comparative Introduction*, and co-edited (with Sara Arber) the first book on grandparenting in global contexts, titled *Contemporary Grandparenting*. The journals in which she has published include *Social Science and Medicine*, *Ageing and Society*, *Family Relations*, *Qualitative Health Research*, *Journal of Aging Studies*, *Social Politics*, *Research on Aging*, *Health and Social Care in the Community*, *Journal of Family Issues*, *Journal of Social Policy*, *Qualitative Research*, and *European Journal of Ageing*. From 2014 to 2017, she will be serving as the president of the Research Committee on the Sociology of Ageing (RC11) of the International Sociological Association.

KASPAR VILLADSEN is associate professor in the Department of Management, Politics and Philosophy, Copenhagen Business School, Denmark. Villadsen has published extensively on the genealogy of social work and on issues of power and technology in welfare institutions. His current research deals with the concept of the state and state phobia in Michel Foucault's writing (forthcoming book with Mitchell Dean from Stanford University Press). He is the author of *Power and Welfare: Understanding Citizens' Encounters with State Welfare* (with Nanna Mik-Meyer). Villadsen's articles have appeared in journals such as *Economy and Society*, *Constellations*, *New Political Science*, *Organization*, and *Social Theory and Health*.

INDEX

GPSR Authorized Representative: Easy Access System Europe, Mustamäe tee 50, 10621 Tallinn, Estonia, gpsr.requests@easproject.com

www.ingramcontent.com/pod-product-compliance
Ingram Content Group UK Ltd.
Pitfield, Milton Keynes, MK11 3LW, UK
UKHW040651130626
471925UK00022B/71/J
* 9 7 8 0 2 3 1 1 7 1 5 2 6 *